Blac

Care

Blackwell's Primary Care Essentials Series

Second Edition

Other books in Blackwell's Primary Care Essentials Series:

Blackwell's Primary Care Essentials: Cardiology
John Sutherland

Blackwell's Primary Care Essentials: The Complete Guide, 4/e
Daniel K. Onion

Blackwell's Primary Care Essentials: Emergency Medicine
Steven Diaz

Blackwell's Primary Care Essentials: Gastrointestinal Disease and Liver Disease
David W. Hay

Blackwell's Primary Care Essentials: Geriatrics, 2/e
Karen Gershman and Dennis M. McCullough

Blackwell's Primary Care Essentials: Sports Medicine
Thomas M. Howard and Janus D. Butcher

Blackwell's Primary Care Essentials: Travel Medicine
Robert P. Smith and Stephen D. Sears

Blackwell's Primary Care Essentials: Urology
Pamela Ellsworth and Stephen N. Rous

Blackwell's Primary Care Essentials: Psychiatry, Second Edition
David P. Moore

Blackwell's Primary Care Essentials: Dermatology

Second Edition

By

Stanford I. Lamberg, MD

Associate Professor, Dermatology
Johns Hopkins Medical Institutions
Baltimore, Maryland

Series Editor

Daniel K. Onion, MD, MPH, FACP
Professor of Community and Family Medicine
Dartmouth Medical School
Director of Maine-Dartmouth Family Practice Residency Program
Augusta, Maine

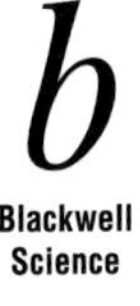

Blackwell
Science

Editorial Offices:
Commerce Place, 350 Main Street, Malden, Massachusetts 02148, USA
Osney Mead, Oxford OX2 0EL, England
25 John Street, London WC1N 2BS, England
23 Ainslie Place, Edinburgh EH3 6AJ, Scotland
54 University Street, Carlton, Victoria 3053, Australia

Other Editorial Offices:
Blackwell Wissenschafts-Verlag GmbH, Kurfürstendamm 57, 10707 Berlin, Germany
Blackwell Science KK, MG Kodenmacho Building, 7-10 Kodenmacho Nihombashi, Chuo-ku, Tokyo 104, Japan
Iowa State University Press, A Blackwell Science Company, 2121 S. State Avenue, Ames, Iowa 50014-8300, USA

Distributors:
The Americas
Blackwell Publishing
c/o AIDC
P.O. Box 20
50 Winter Sport Lane
Williston, VT 05495-0020
(Telephone orders: 800-216-2522; fax orders: 802-864-7626)

Australia
Blackwell Science Pty, Ltd.
54 University Street
Carlton, Victoria 3053
(Telephone orders: 03-9347-0300; fax orders: 03-9349-3016)

Outside The Americas and Australia
Blackwell Science, Ltd.
c/o Marston Book Services, Ltd.
P.O. Box 269
Abingdon
Oxon OX14 4YN
England
(Telephone orders: 44-01235-465500; fax orders: 44-01235-465555)

Acquisitions: Nancy Anastasi Duffy
Development: Julia Casson
Production: Elissa Gershowitz
Manufacturing: Lisa Flanagan
Marketing Manager: Kathleen Mulcahy
Cover design by Leslie Haimes
Text design and typesetting by Graphicraft Limited, Hong Kong
Printed and bound by Edwards Brothers, Inc.

Printed in the United States of America
02 03 04 05 5 4 3 2 1

Library of Congress Cataloging-in-Publication Data

Lamberg, Stanford I.
Blackwell's primary care essentials. Dermatology / Stanford I. Lamberg. — 2nd ed.
p. ; cm. — (Blackwell's primary care essentials series)
Rev. ed. of: The little black book of dermatology. c2000. Includes index.
ISBN 0-632-04629-5 (pbk.)
1. Dermatology—Handbooks, manuals, etc. 2. Skin—Diseases—Handbooks, manuals, etc.
[DNLM: 1. Skin Diseases—diagnosis—Handbooks. 2. Primary Health Care—Handbooks. 3. Skin Diseases— therapy—Handbooks. WR 39 L221b 2002]
I. Title: Primary care essentials. II. Title: Dermatology. III. Lamberg, Stanford I. Little black book of dermatology. IV. Title. V. Series.
RL74 .L55 2002
616.5—dc21

2001006469

Contents

How to Use This Book

This book aims to help primary health care providers—physicians, nurses, and physician assistants—who work in family medicine, internal medicine, pediatrics, and emergency medicine. The traditional dermatology textbook is organized by disease and often requires a diagnosis to locate the appropriate chapter. This book, however, is entirely problem-oriented. No dermatologic training is required. The book provides detailed information on treatments, prescribing information, and side effects of medications, but only brief discussions of pathophysiology and pharmacology.

Because patients complain of "hair loss," "itchy feet," or "groin irritation," not alopecia areata, lichen planus, or intertrigo, this book starts with the patient's presenting complaint and certain obvious signs and symptoms. It then leads the practitioner to the diagnosis, covering more than 300 disorders.

- Use the Contents graphic to find the appropriate chapter: a body site, a sign, or symptom.
- Use the graphic algorithm at the beginning of the chapter to lead you to a differential, usually listed in order of frequency of occurrence. A chapter's algorithm may refer you to sections in other chapters.
- Determine the most likely diagnosis in the differential by turning to the indicated section within the chapter and reading the clinical description of each disorder. After the clinical description, you will find information that may include cause, epidemiology, pathophysiology, signs and symptoms, course, complications, lab workup, and treatment.

Because disorders may present at several locations or with a variety of signs and symptoms, many are mentioned in more than one chapter. A description of psoriasis, for example, appears in 10 chapters: Axilla, Body, Diaper, Ear, Feet, Genital, Groin, Hand, Nail, and Scalp. Each emphasizes only the features pertinent to that chapter. To save space, the complete description of the disorder is presented in only one chapter; in the case of psoriasis, that is the Body chapter (**bold-faced** in the Index).

The book contains extensive cross-referencing. A numerical code will speed your finding each disorder. In 5.3.c., for example, the "5" refers to the chapter, the "3" to the section within the chapter, and the "c" to the disorder itself. You may notice that some letters are skipped. This will allow the later addition of disorders without renumbering the entire book. The sections are in sequence to ease scanning. Use the marginal tabbing to move about rapidly from chapter to chapter. You will find the most frequently cross-referenced chapters, DX and RX, near the back of the book. You may photocopy the Instruction sheets in the RX chapter for your patients.

The text notes when specialist referral is appropriate, most frequently to a dermatologist. This may seem self-serving since the author of this book is a dermatologist, but much time can be saved in a PCP office by treating those conditions that are easily and quickly treated and referring those that likely will prove time-consuming and frustrating. The book helps you recognize conditions that are potentially serious, more likely to be complicated, or generally unresponsive to usual therapy. Examples include patients with widespread blisters, children with hirsutism, and women with virilization.

I hope you will find the text both helpful and easy to use. I welcome your suggestions for additions to the next edition.

Stanford I. Lamberg, M.D.
Lamberg@mail.jhmi.edu

Abbreviations

$	costs from $ (least) to $$$$ (most)
1°	primary
2°	secondary
3°	tertiary
AAD	American Academy of Dermatology
abn	abnormalities
ACE	angiotensin-converting enzyme
AIDS	acquired immunodeficiency syndrome
ALT	alanine aminotransferase
AM	morning
ANA	antinuclear antibody
ANCA	antineutrophil cytoplasmic antibodies
ANUG	acute necrotizing ulcerative gingivitis
ASA	acetylsalicylic acid (aspirin)
ASO	anti–streptolysin-O titer
assoc	associated
AST	aspartate aminotransferase
asx	asymptomatic
AZT	zidovudine
BCE	basal cell epithelioma
bcp's	birth control pills
BFP	biologic false positive
bid	twice a day
BP	blood pressure
bx	biopsy
C'	complement
cap	caplet
CBC	complete blood count
CDC	Centers for Disease Control and Prevention
CF	cystic fibrosis
CLIA	Clinical Laboratory Improvement Amendments

cm	centimeter
CMV	cytomegalovirus
CNS	central nervous system
cr	cream
c + s	culture and sensitivity
CS	corticosteroid
CSF	cerebrospinal fluid
CT	computed tomography
CTCL	cutaneous T-cell lymphoma
CVA	cerebrovascular accident
d	day(s)
D&C	desiccation and curettage
dc('d)	discontinue(d)
ddx	differential diagnosis
DHEA-S	dehydroepiandrosterone sulfate
DIC	disseminated intravascular coagulation
DIF	direct immunofluorescence
DIP	distal interphalangeal
dL	deciliter
DLE	discoid lupus erythematosus
DM	diabetes mellitus
dsDNA	double-stranded DNA
DSM-IV	*Diagnostic and Statistical Manual of Mental Disorders*, 4th ed.
dx	diagnosis
EB	epidermolysis bullosa
eg	such as; for example
EKG	electrocardiogram
EMG	electromyography
ENA	extractable nuclear antigen
ENT	otolaryngologist
eos	eosinophils
esp	especially
ESR	erythrocyte sedimentation rate
FBS	fasting blood sugar
FDA	Food and Drug Administration
FEP	fibroepithelial polyp (skin tag)
fhx	family history
FTA	fluorescent treponemal antibody (test for syphilis)
FTA-ABS	fluorescent treponemal antibody antiabsorption test

5-FU	5-fluorouracil
f/u	follow-up
G-6-PD	glucose-6-phosphate dehydrogenase
GI	gastrointestinal
gm	gram
GTT	glucose tolerance testing
h	hour(s)
H.	*Histoplasma*
HC	hydrocortisone
hgb	hemoglobin
HPV	human papillomavirus
hrs	hours
hs	at bedtime
HSV	herpes simplex virus
HTLV II	human T-cell lymphotropic virus
hx	history
HZ	herpes zoster
I&D	incision and drainage
ie	that is
IFA	immunofluorescence assay
IL	intralesional
im	intramuscular
impt	important
inc	including
IUD	intrauterine device
iv	intravenous
KOH	potassium hydroxide
KS	Kaposi's sarcoma
L	liter
Lab	laboratory
LE	lupus erythematosus
LFTs	liver function tests
LGV	lymphogranuloma venereum
LN	lymph node
LN↑	lymph node enlargement
LN2	liquid nitrogen
LP	lumbar puncture
M.	*Microsporum* or *Mycobacterium*
MAO	monoamine oxidase
med	medication

μg	microgram
MI	myocardial infarction
min	minute(s)
mL	milliliter
mo	month
mos	months
MRI	magnetic resonance imaging
MTX	methotrexate
neg	negative
ng	nanogram
NSAID	nonsteroidal anti-inflammatory drug
ob-gyn	obstetrician-gynecologist
occas	occasional(ly)
oint	ointment
OR	operating room
OTC	over the counter (nonprescription)
P.	*Pneumocystis*
PABA	para-aminobenzoic acid
PAP	Papanicolaou (test)
pc	after meals
PCP	primary care provider
PCR	polymerase chain reaction
PCT	porphyria cutanea tarda
PFB	pseudofolliculitis barbae
PHN	postherpetic neuralgia
PM	evening
PMLE	polymorphous light eruption
po	by mouth
pos	positive
PPD	tuberculin skin test
pt(s)	patient(s)
PUVA	oral psoralen + long-wave ultraviolet light
Px	physical exam
q	every
qd	daily
qid	4 times a day
qod	every other day
RA	rheumatoid arthritis
rbc	red blood cell
RF	rheumatoid factor

RFTs	renal function tests
RMSF	Rocky Mountain spotted fever
RNP	ribonucleoprotein
r/o	rule out
ROH	alcohol
ROS	review of systems
RPR	rapid plasma reagin (test for syphilis)
Rx	prescription drug, where noted with name of drug
rx	treatment
rx'd	treated
rxn	reaction
S.	*Staphylococcus* or *Sporothrix*
sc	subcutaneous
SCC	squamous cell carcinoma
sec	second(s)
Si (or si)	sign(s)
SLE	systemic lupus erythematosus
soln	solution
SPF	sun protective factor
SRP	signal recognition particle
ssDNA	single-stranded DNA
SSKI	saturated solution of potassium iodide
SSSS	staphylococcal scalded-skin syndrome
STD	sexually transmitted disease
STS	serum test for syphilis
Sx (or sx)	symptom or symptomatic
T.	*Trichophyton* or *Treponema*
tab	tablet
tbc	tuberculosis
TCA	trichloroacetic acid
TCS	topical corticosteroid
TEN	toxic epidermal necrolysis
TIBC	total iron-binding capacity
tid	3 times a day
tRNA	transfer RNA
tsp	teaspoon
TSR	tangential shave removal
TSS	toxic shock syndrome
UC	ulcerative colitis
URI	upper respiratory infection

U.S.	United States
UV	ultraviolet
UVA	ultraviolet, long wave (320–400 nm; tanning)
UVB	ultraviolet, short wave (290–320 nm; burning)
VDRL	Venereal Disease Research Laboratory (test for syphilis)
w	with
wbc	white blood cell
wk	week
wks	weeks
WNL	within normal limits
w/o	without
w/u	work-up
yr	year
yrs	years
yo	years old
ZnOx	zinc oxide

Journal Abbreviations

Acta Derm Venereol	Acta Dermato-Venereologica
Adv IM	Advances in Internal Medicine
Am Fam Phys	American Family Physician
Am J Clin Path	American Journal of Clinical Pathology
Am J Contact Derm	American Journal of Contact Dermatology
Am J Dermatopath	American Journal of Dermatopathology
Am J Dis Child	American Journal of Diseases of Children
Am J Med	American Journal of Medicine
Am J Med Sci	American Journal of Medical Science
Am J Psych	American Journal of Psychiatry
Am J Surg	American Journal of Surgery
Am Rev Respir Dis	American Review of Respiratory Diseases
Ann Allergy	Annals of Allergy
Ann IM	Annals of Internal Medicine
Ann Plast Surg	Annals of Plastic Surgery
Ann Surg	Annals of Surgery
Arch Derm	Archives of Dermatology
Arch Dis Child	Archives of Diseases of Children
Arch IM	Archives of Internal Medicine
Arch Neurol	Archives of Neurology
Arch Surg	Archives of Surgery
Arthritis Rheum	Arthritis and Rheumatism
BMJ	British Medical Journal
Br J Derm	British Journal of Dermatology
Circ	Circulation
Clin Derm	Clinical Dermatology
Clin Endocrinol	Clinical Endocrinology
Clin Exp Derma	Clinical and Experimental Dermatology (England)
Clin Infect Dis	Clinics in Infectious Disease
Clin Oto	Clinical Otolaryngology

Comp Ther	Comprehensive Therapeutics
Contact Derm	Contact Dermatitis (Denmark)
Curr Opin Ob Gyn	Current Opinions in Obstetrics and Gynecology
Curr Opin Rheum	Current Opinions in Rheumatology
Curr Probl Cancer	Current Problems in Cancer
Dent Clin N Am	Dental Clinics of North America
Derm	Dermatology (Switzerland)
Derm Clin	Dermatology Clinics
Endo Metab Clin N Am	Endocrinology and Metabolism Clinics of North America
Fertil Steril	Fertility and Sterility
Gastroenterol	Gastroenterology
Inf Dis Clin NA	Infectious Disease Clinics of North America
Int Angiol	International Angiology
Int J Derm	International Journal of Dermatology
Int J Oral Max Surg	International Journal of Oral and Maxillofacial Surgery
Int Rev Immunol	International Review of Immunology
Jada	Journal of the American Dental Association
Jama	Journal of the American Medical Association
Jaad	Journal of the American Academy of Dermatology
J Gerontol	Journal of Gerontology
J Infect Dis	Journal of Infectious Disease
J Invest Derm	Journal of Investigative Dermatology
J Natl Cancer Inst	Journal of the National Cancer Institute
J Oral Max Surg	Journal of Oral and Maxillofacial Surgery
J Oral Path	Journal of Oral Pathology
J Oral Path Med	Journal of Oral Pathology and Medicine
J Peds	Journal of Pediatrics
J Rheum	Journal of Rheumatology
Mayo Clin Proc	Mayo Clinic Proceedings
Med	Medicine
Med Clin N Am	Medical Clinics of North America
Mmwr	CDC Morbidity and Mortality Weekly Report
Nejm	New England Journal of Medicine
Oral Surg Omop	Oral Surgery Oral Medicine Oral Pathology
Otol Clin N Am	Otolaryngologic Clinics of North America
Peds	Pediatrics

Ped Clin North Am	Pediatric Clinics of North America
Ped Derm	Pediatric Dermatology
Ped Rev	Pediatric Review
Prim Care	Primary Care
Rheum Dis Clin N Am	Rheumatic Disease Clinics of North America
Scand J Rheum	Scandinavian Journal of Rheumatology
Semin Arth Rheum	Seminars in Arthritis and Rheumatology
Semin Derm	Seminars in Dermatology
Transf	Transfusion

Notice

The indications and dosages of all drugs in this book have been recommended in the medical literature and conform to the practices of the general community. The medications described and treatment prescriptions suggested do not necessarily have specific approval by the Food and Drug Administration for use in the diseases and dosages for which they are recommended. The package insert for each drug should be consulted for use and dosage as approved by the FDA. Because standards for usage change, it is advisable to keep abreast of revised recommendations, particularly those concerning new drugs.

1 Axilla

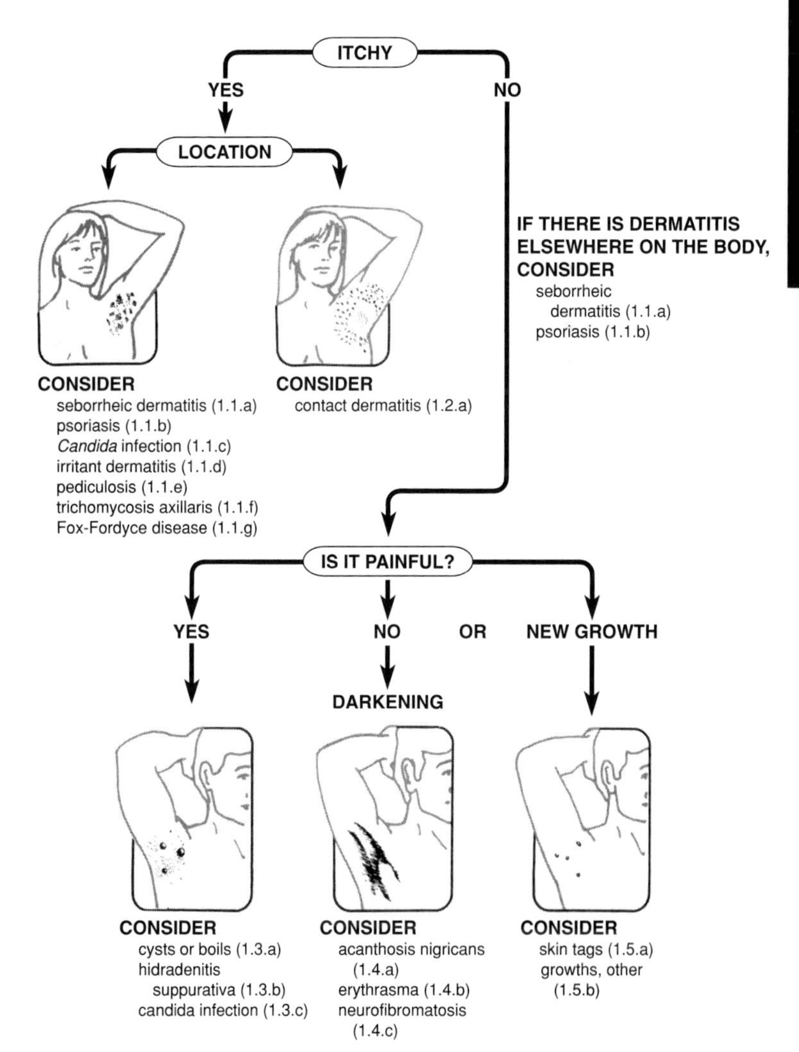
ITCHY
YES
NO
LOCATION
CONSIDER
seborrheic dermatitis (1.1.a)
psoriasis (1.1.b)
Candida infection (1.1.c)
irritant dermatitis (1.1.d)
pediculosis (1.1.e)
trichomycosis axillaris (1.1.f)
Fox-Fordyce disease (1.1.g)
CONSIDER
contact dermatitis (1.2.a)
IF THERE IS DERMATITIS ELSEWHERE ON THE BODY, CONSIDER
seborrheic dermatitis (1.1.a)
psoriasis (1.1.b)
IS IT PAINFUL?
YES
NO
OR
NEW GROWTH
DARKENING
CONSIDER
cysts or boils (1.3.a)
hidradenitis suppurativa (1.3.b)
candida infection (1.3.c)
CONSIDER
acanthosis nigricans (1.4.a)
erythrasma (1.4.b)
neurofibromatosis (1.4.c)
CONSIDER
skin tags (1.5.a)
growths, other (1.5.b)

ITCHY IN HAIRY AREAS

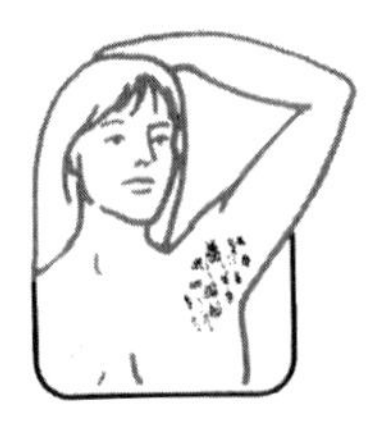

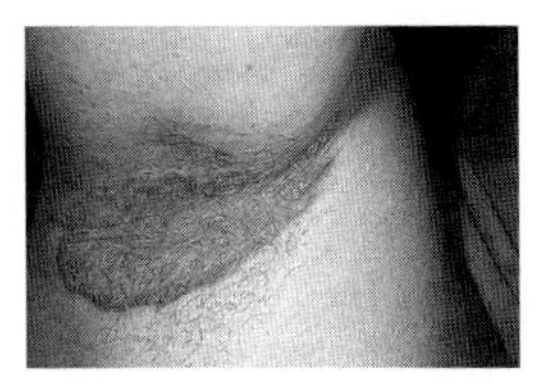

Psoriasis

1.1.A. SEBORRHEIC DERMATITIS

Summary: Usually diffuse but may be patchy; hairy areas most involved; yellowish greasy scale; mild redness and itching; similar scale and itching usually present at scalp, ear canals, retroauricular areas, eyebrows, nasolabial folds.

For additional details and rx, see FACE, 6.2.a., and SCALP, 24.3.b.

1.1.B. PSORIASIS

Summary: Because of moist location, silvery scale typical of psoriasis is replaced by red and glistening rash involving both hairy and nonhairy parts; irritating and itchy; look for typical psoriasis elsewhere, esp scalp, to confirm dx; some pts have concomitant seborrheic dermatitis; rx w low-potency TCS (class VI–VII), ie, 1%–2.5% HC cr, as more potent fluorinated TCSs may lead to atrophy and striae (see RX.5.).

For additional details and rx, see BODY, 3.1.d.

1.1.C. *CANDIDA* INFECTION

Summary: Moist, red, tender; edge often studded w tiny pustules; inframammary and groin regions in women and glans penis in men; pts often obese; may have DM; or on broad-spectrum antibiotics.

For additional details and rx, see GROIN RASH, 10.2.a.

AXILLA

1.1.D. IRRITANT DERMATITIS

Summary: *Irritant reactions*: involve both hairy and nonhairy parts; usually caused by antiperspirants; *allergic reactions*: involve nonhairy parts; usually caused by perfumes or preservatives in deodorants or formalin in permanent press clothing; both are itchy, pink to red, scaly, may become pigmented if chronic; look for rash elsewhere as seborrheic dermatitis or psoriasis may be present; rx as for contact dermatitis (see 1.2.a.); limit underarm deodorant to 2–3-cm area at peak of axillae where most of perspiration arises to prevent irritation on adjacent skin; use of roll-on instead of spray helps limit overapplication; use fragrance-free products.

1.1.E. PEDICULOSIS

Summary: Pinhead sized; brown; firmly adherent; flecks; examine w inverted microscope eyepiece; while 1° infestation is in pubic area, other areas often involved are axillae, nipples, eyelashes; consider scabies if anterior axillary fold but not hairy parts are involved.

For additional details and rx, see GROIN RASH, 10.5.a.

1.1.F. TRICHOMYCOSIS AXILLARIS

Cause: Bacterial infection from one of several *Corynebacterium* species (J Am Acad Derm 1988;18:778).

Epidem: Uncommon in U.S. but common worldwide.

Sx: Not itchy.

Si: Yellow, red, or black, barely visible, adherent granules coat hairs of the axilla and sometimes the pubis.

Crs: Persistent.

Lab: Pinhead-sized accretions attached along hair shaft visible under low-power microscope.

Rx: Shaving is fast and effective; washing w soap does not remove accretions; topical antibiotics only moderately helpful; refer suspected cases to dermatology.

1.1.G. FOX-FORDYCE DISEASE (APOCRINE MILIARIA)

Cause: Apocrine duct obstruction and hormonal factors (Jama 1973;223:924).

Epidem: Rare; nearly all cases are women between puberty and menopause.

Sx: Itchy, often severe.

Si: Uniform, skin colored, rice grain–sized papules; in areas high in apocrine glands: axillae, genital, areolae.

Crs: Persistent; flares w menstruation, emotional upset; often clears temporarily in latter part of pregnancy; may persist until menopause.

Lab: Dx: confirm w bx.

Rx: Estrogens (1.25–5 mg daily) or bcp's help some; TCS cr may help; topical antibiotics may help (Derm 1992;184:310); topical tretinoin may help; surgical excision may be required; generally followed by dermatologist.

ITCHY IN NONHAIRY AREAS

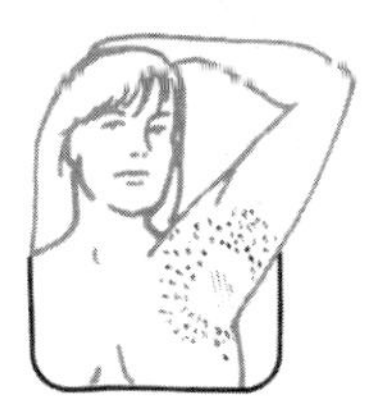

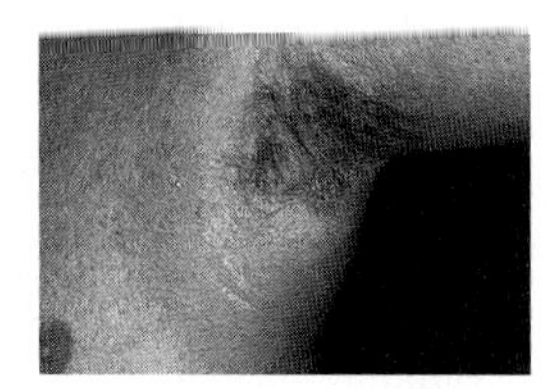

Contact dermatitis—*Rhus*

1.2.A. CONTACT DERMATITIS

Cause: Irritant or allergic (Contact Derm 1988;19:195).

- Irritant: usually from drying salts of antiperspirants.
- Allergic: preservatives, perfumes, elastics, formaldehyde in permanent press clothing, detergents released from clothing by perspiration and friction.

Sx: Itchy, burning.

Si: Red, scaly, rash; accentuated in axillary folds while relatively absent in hairy portion; pigmentation if chronic; *note*: rash in hairy areas usually is a 1° skin disorder, ie, psoriasis, seborrheic dermatitis.

Crs: Persistent; pts seldom get relief from changing brands as similar products contain similar ingredients.

Lab: Patch testing is not practical; individual components not available for testing.

Rx: TCS (class VI–VII); change antiperspirant/deodorant to fragrance-free product; limit underarm deodorant to 2–3-cm area at peak of axillae where most of perspiration arises to prevent irritation on adjacent skin; use of roll-on instead of spray helps limit overapplication; use fragrance-free products.

PAINFUL

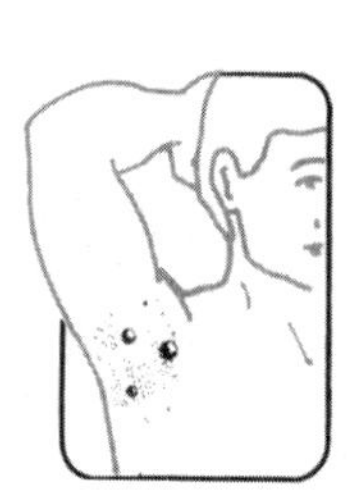

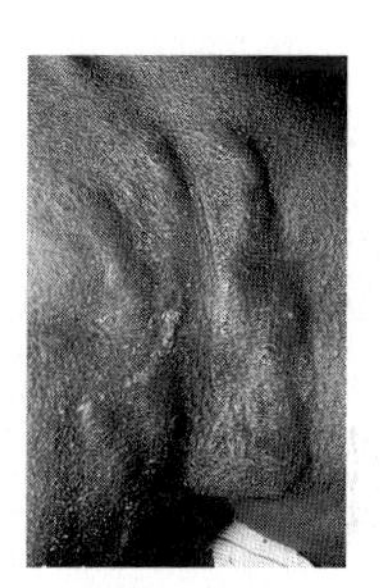

Hidradenitis suppurativa

1.3.A. CYSTS AND BOILS

Summary: *Isolated and sporadic*: rx by I&D; use systemic antibiotics only if pt has si of toxicity: fever, cellulitis, lymphangitis; *chronic and recurrent*: w scarring and fistulous tracts: consider hidradenitis suppurativa (see 1.3.b.).

1.3.B. HIDRADENITIS SUPPURATIVA

Cause: Apocrine gland obstruction w bacterial infection; obesity, acne, DM predisposes (J Am Acad Derm 1996;35:191; Arch Derm 1988;124:1043).

Sx: Painful abscesses.

Si: Recurring, draining abscesses; heals w scarring; areas involved: axillae, groin, mammary, buttocks; fever and systemic toxicity are infrequent; acne and cysts elsewhere often present (see SCALP, 24.4.b.).

Crs: Starts after puberty when apocrine glands develop; chronic, over many yrs; lesions heal by drainage or absorption over wks; fistulae, lymphedema, restriction of arm or leg movement from hypertrophic scars may develop; activity often wanes by late middle age.

Ddx: Other infections: tbc, actinomycosis, cat-scratch disease, granuloma inguinale.

Lab: CBC and differential and serum glucose level at least once; if you choose to I&D the abscess, obtain bacterial culture and antibiotic sensitivities.

Rx:

- Acute: I&D and systemic antibiotics, ie, erythromycin (250–500 mg qid) or dicloxacillin (500 mg bid) for 10–14 d; long-term antibiotic suppression is controversial; bid washing w hexachlorophene soap (PhisoHex) or a quaternary iodine scrub (Betadine or povidone) may help (Arch Derm 1988;124:1047).
- Chronic severe: excision of entire affected area and flap or skin grafting effects permanent cure (Ann Plast Surg 1988;20:82); isotretinoin po for several mos improves 50% of pts, esp if mild (J Am Acad Derm 1999;40:73); often are referred to dermatology and/or general or plastic surgeon.

1.3.C. *CANDIDA* INFECTION

Summary: Moist, red, tender; edge often studded w tiny pustules; inframammary and groin regions in women and glans penis in men; pts often obese, have DM, or on broad-spectrum antibiotics.

For additional details and rx, see GROIN RASH, 10.2.a.

NOT PAINFUL WITH DARKENING

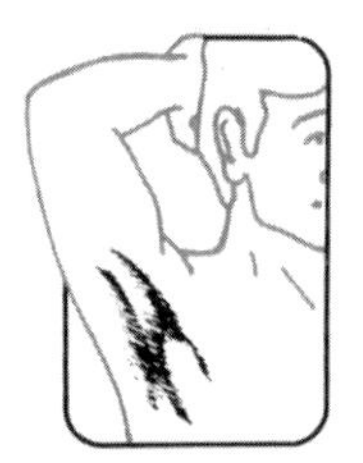

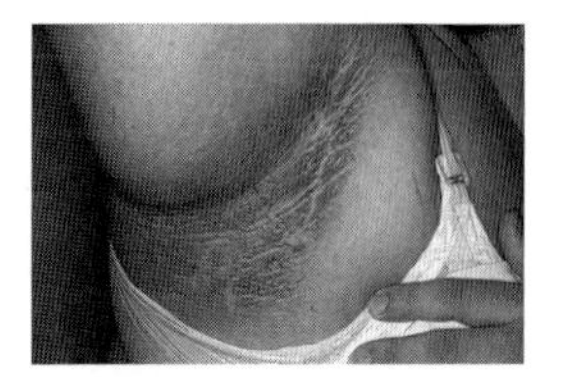

Acanthosis nigricans

1.4.A ACANTHOSIS NIGRICANS

Summary: Brown to black; velvety texture; most common in axillae, neck, groin; asx; most are obese adults w pigmentation for mos to yrs(benign); if thin pt >40 yo and recent onset: r/o underlying malignancy or endocrine disorder.

For additional details, see PIGMENT INCREASE, 22.2.b.

1.4.B. ERYTHRASMA

Summary: Brown scaly rash; asx; pt often obese; look for similar eruption in toe webs, groin, perianal regions; bacterial infection; confirm by coral-red fluorescence w Wood's light, if available; does not respond to antifungal meds.

For additional details and rx, see GROIN RASH, 10.3.a.

1.4.C. NEUROFIBROMATOSIS

Summary: Telltale freckles; not likely to be a 1° complaint.

For additional details, see GROWTHS, 11.9.b.

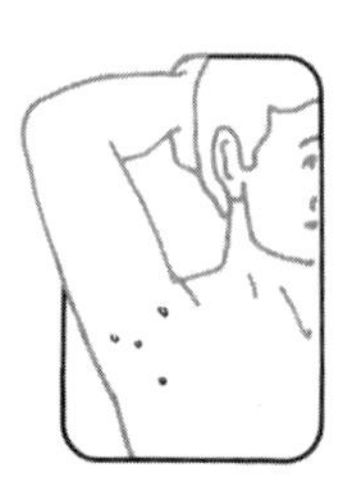

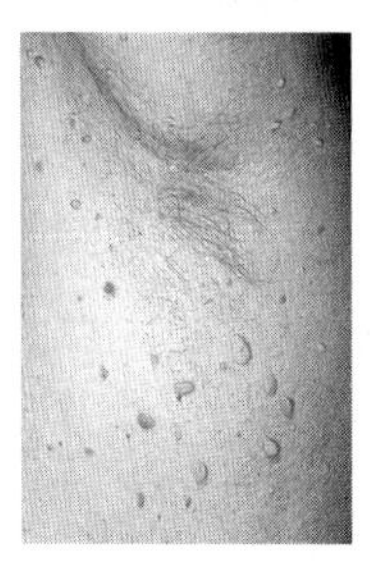

Skin tags (FEPs)

1.5.A. SKIN TAGS (FIBROEPITHELIAL POLYPS, FEPS)

Summary: Common, esp >30 yo; pinhead to BB sized; tan skin colored; sites: also at groin, neck, eyelids; rx w electrocautery w or w/o local anesthetic or prior EMLA cr.

For additional details and rx, see GROWTHS, 11.9.a.

1.5.B. GROWTHS, OTHER

Summary: **Nevi, seborrheic keratoses, fibromas** are common benign growths found in axilla (see GROWTHS, 11.); nuisance to pts; do not become malignant, even if frequently irritated or cut; easily removed.

2 Blisters

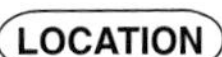

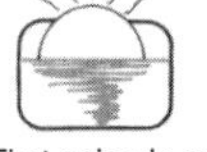

First episode or present for months (2.1)

Recurrent or present for months (2.2)

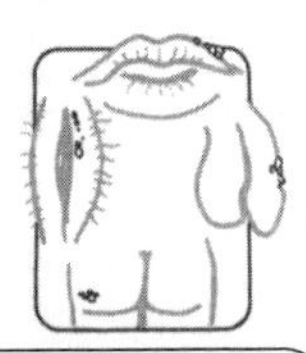

ORAL OR GENITAL, OR BOTH

CONSIDER (2.1)
- herpes simplex, primary (2.1.a)
- erythema multiforme (2.1.b)

CONSIDER (2.2)
- herpes simplex, recurrent (2.2.a)
- erythema multiforme (2.2.b)

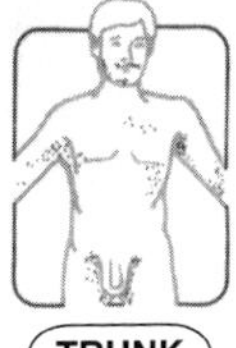

TRUNK

CONSIDER
- varicella (2.3.a)
- drug-induced eruption (2.3.b)
- erythema multiforme (2.3.c)
- zoster (2.3.d)
- toxic epidermal necrolysis (2.3.e)
- staphylococcal scalded skin syndrome (2.3.f)

CONSIDER
- erythema multiforme (2.4.a)
- dermatitis herpetiformis (2.4.b)
- epidermolysis bullosa (2.4.c)
- pemphigus (2.4.d)
- pemphigoid (2.4.d)

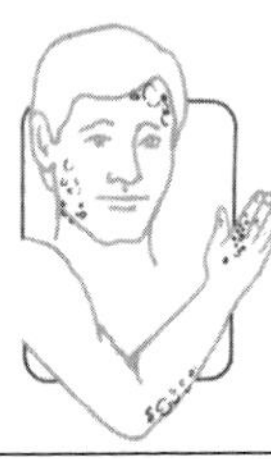

EXPOSED PARTS ONLY

CONSIDER
- contact dermatitis (2.5.a)
- impetigo (2.5.b)
- trauma (2.5.c)
  - light
  - burns
  - insect bites

CONSIDER
- contact dermatitis (2.6.a)
- porphyria (2.6.b)
- epidermolysis bullosa (2.6.c)

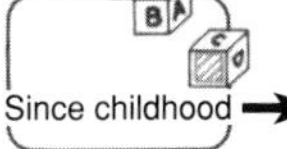

→ See neonatal blistering (2.7)

Acute blistering disorders generally are bacterial or viral, and both can be diagnosed by Gram's stain (see DX.1.) or cytology stain (see DX.2.) of the blister base; nonbacterial, nonviral acute blistering disorders encompass a wider diagnostic tree, and referral to dermatologist is appropriate; chronic blistering disorders are uncommon and generally serious; obtain dermatology consultation.

ORAL OR GENITAL, OR BOTH FIRST EPISODE OR PRESENT FOR DAYS OR RECURRENT

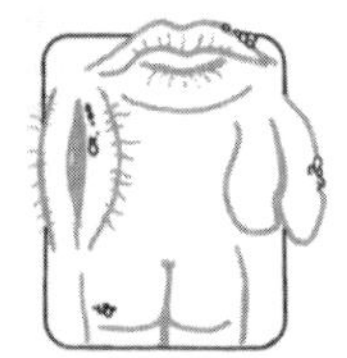

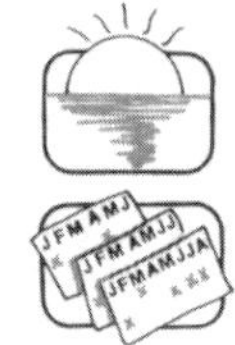

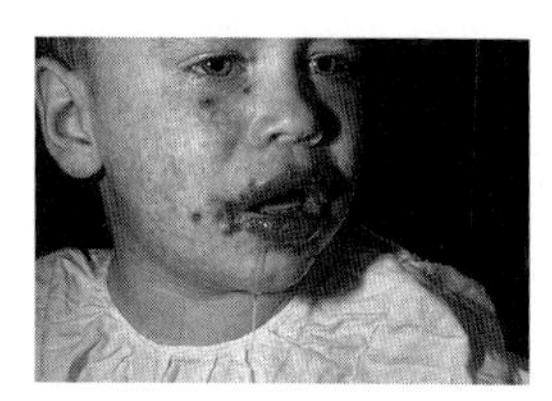

Herpes simplex

2.1.A. AND 2.2.A. HERPES SIMPLEX VIRUS (HSV)

Cause: Herpesvirus hominis; DNA virus; type 1—most oral-labial infections; type 2—most genital infections; 10% reversed (oral-genital contact).

Epidem: 90% of adults have antibodies against HSV; genital HSV affects 1/5 American adults; blisters and crusts contain viable virus; easily transmitted.

Pathophys: Virus is latent within regional nerve root ganglia after infection; periodic activation causes recurrent blisters.

Si:

Oral-labial:

- 1° infection: localized blisters about lips; fever; malaise; usually in childhood, often not remembered.
- Recurrence: prodrome of few hrs or days of localized burning and tingling; multiple small vesicles; 3–5 days; then crusting and clearing w/o scar.

Genital:
- 1° infection: localized blisters, fever, malaise, tender LN↑; resolve 1–3 wks; does not scar.
- Recurrence: like oral-labial.

Crs: Recurrence, esp if frequent, is most troublesome; may follow local trauma; high fever; acute illness; emotional stress; acute sun exposure; or spontaneous; frequency ↓ after 5 yrs regardless of rx (Ann IM 1999;131:14).

Compl: Esp susceptible: infants, atopic dermatitis, aged, immunosuppressed.

Lab: Viral culture is best and easiest; results back 3–5 days; false neg if lesion too old; Tzanck prep (Giemsa stain of vesicle contents) (see DX.2.): multinucleate giant cells and intranuclear inclusions specific for HSV or HZ; bx edge of ulcer (see DX.7.).

Rx: Antiviral drug review: 11 drugs are approved by FDA for rx of viral infections other than HIV infection (Review: BMJ 2000;321:619; also: Jaad 1999;41:511; Nejm 1999;340:1255; Mmwr 1998;47:RR-1:20; Arch Derm 1998;134:650).

1°: Acyclovir ($$) 400 mg tid for 7–10 d, or valacyclovir ($$)1 gm bid for 7–10 d, or famciclovir ($$) 500 mg tid for 7 d; none are approved in pregnancy; all reduce duration of viral shedding and lesion healing; none prevent virus latency or recurrences; analgesics; lukewarm saline compresses; ZnOx paste; special precautions in pregnancy: seek ob-gyn referral; special precautions if eye sx: seek ophthalmology referral.

Recurrent:
- Infrequent recurrences, every few mo or so: acyclovir 400 mg tid, or valacyclovir 500 mg bid, or famciclovir 125 mg bid for up to 5 d; start at onset of prodrome.
- Frequent recurrences, >5 episodes/yr: daily suppressive rx: acyclovir 400 mg bid, or valacyclovir 1 gm qd (500 mg qd if <10 recurrences/yr), or famciclovir 250 mg bid; daily rx ↓ recurrences >75%; *note*: suppressive rx does not eliminate asymptomatic viral shedding.
- Topical: penciclovir cr (Denavir 2 gm, Rx, $$) q2h while awake × 4 d may be tried (Jama 1997;277:1374); topical acyclovir does not shorten episodes.

Contact 1.877.699.HERO (toll-free) or www.cafeherpe.com for pt support information.

2.1.B. AND 2.2.B. ERYTHEMA MULTIFORME

Br J Derm 1993;128:542. Arch Derm 1993;129:92. Ped Rev 1990;1:217. Ped Clin North Am 1983;30:631.

Cause: 20% preceded by HSV infections (Br J Derm 1998;138:952); others assoc w drug allergy; bacterial, mycobacterial, or mycoplasma infections; internal malignancies; collagen/vascular disease; pregnancy; most cases are idiopathic.

Epidem: Idiopathic type most common in spring and fall.

Sx: May be tender, esp palmar, plantar, and mouth lesions; itching not as severe as w urticaria.

Si: Flat, dusky lesions; 1–3 cm; often resemble bull's-eyes or targets; persist longer than urticaria; sites: extensor sides of arms and legs or generalized; palmar and plantar areas: red, tender lesions; mucous membranes: erosions are frequent.

Crs: Often have prodrome of few d to 2 wk; resolution in 2–4 wk w or w/o rx; 1/4 have recurrences mos to yrs later.

Compl: Severe cases develop erosions, peeling, blistering; **Stevens-Johnson syndrome**: widespread lesions; mucous membrane erosions; fever.

Lab: Seek out and rx coexisting infections and underlying disease; dc medications if possible; HSV antibodies not useful; skin bx helpful to r/o vasculitis; other labs not helpful.

Rx: Eliminate precipitating causes, ie, consider HSV suppression w antiviral drugs to prevent episode of HSV that might trigger outbreak (Br J Derm 1995;132:267); TCSs have no effect; systemic CSs are controversial as toxic signs are reduced but may ↑ morbidity; severe cases need fluid support; consider referral to dermatologist to confirm dx.

TRUNK AND EXTREMITIES OR TRUNK ALONE FIRST EPISODE OR PRESENT FOR DAYS

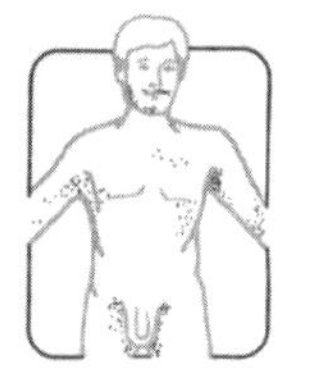

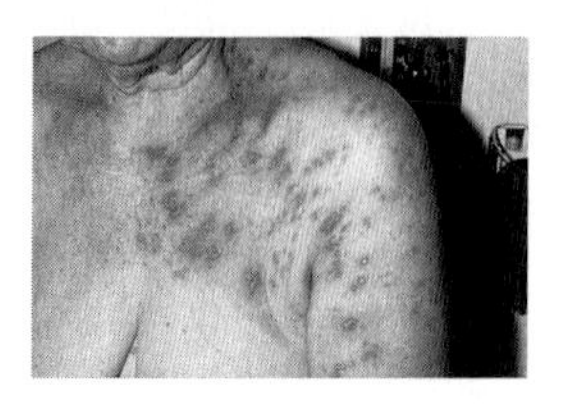

Zoster

J Infect Dis 1996;174:S306.

BLISTERS

2.3.A. VARICELLA (CHICKENPOX)

Cause: DNA herpesvirus group.

Epidem: Transmitted via respiratory tract or direct skin contact; during seasonal epidemics some children have only minimal or no rash w/o fever.

Sx: Itching, children > adults.

Si: Sick; febrile w scattered, not grouped, pea-sized blisters and pustules; central dell; initial lesion may be inflammatory, like pyoderma or abscess.

Crs: Rash appears 10–14 d after exposure following mild prodrome of fever and malaise for 1–3 d; starts centrally, on trunk and face; spreads quickly; forms crusts in 2–5 d while new blisters appear, generally peripherally; may leave small depressed scars on healing; fever persists while new blisters appear.

Compl: Fever after new lesions have stopped suggests 2° bacterial infection or complication: ataxia, neuritis, Reye's syndrome, myocarditis, vasculitis, inflammation of viscera; can be severe or fatal in immunosuppressed persons; more severe in adults than children; 1 bout of varicella confers lifelong immunity; varicella virus resides latently in nerve root ganglia and, if reactivated, reappears as HZ.

Lab: Usually not necessary; cytology smear or culture in unusual adult cases; chest x-ray for pulmonary sx in adult to r/o viral pneumonitis.

Rx: Acyclovir (800 mg po × 5/d for 1 wk) initiated within 24 h of rash onset shortened the clinical course (Ann IM 1992;117:358); antipyretics; antihistamines for itching; calamine lotion w or w/o 0.25% menthol; immunosuppressed persons: may develop severe, even fatal varicella infections, and may require consultation; vaccination is available (Inf Dis Clin NA 1996;10:631).

2.3.B. DRUG-INDUCED ERUPTION

Cause: Allergic, toxic, or idiosyncratic rxn to drug.

Sx: Usually itchy.

Si: Many forms, from a faint pink, evanescent, nonscaly rash, usually on the trunk, to blisters, itchy hives (see ITCH, 16.3.a.), pustules, erythema multiforme (see 2.1.b.) or purpura.

Crs: Usually improves or clears within 48 h after dc of offending drug; may last for days or wks, depending on rate of clearance of med.

Lab: None; penicillin skin testing may be used just prior to necessary rx w penicillin.

Rx: Elimination of suspected drugs; risk of serious systemic rxns if attempt to rx w antihistamines or systemic CS while continuing drug.

For additional details, med specifics, and rx, see BODY, 3.1.b.

2.3.C. ERYTHEMA MULTIFORME

Summary: Lesions usually first appear on extremities and mucosal surfaces, rather than trunk (see 2.1.b.).

2.3.D.(1). ZOSTER (HERPES ZOSTER, HZ, SHINGLES)

J Am Acad Derm 1999;41:1.

Cause: Reactivation of varicella virus, harbored in a latent state within nerve ganglia since 1° infection, usually in childhood.

Epidem: Varicella may be contracted from pt w HZ; HZ is not contracted from pt w varicella; reactivation often assoc w blunting of immune system, ie, old age, acute systemic illness, lymphoma-leukemia, immunosuppressive therapy, AIDS.

Sx: Pain, often lancinating.

Si: Group of small blisters, each w central dimple; sharp demarcation at midline, following distribution of a peripheral nerve.

Crs: Onset follows prodrome lasting 1–4 d w tingling, tenderness, itch restricted to nerve segment; vesicles (within 12–24 h); pustules (in 3–4 d); crusts (in 7–10 d); pain may last (see 2.3.d.(2)); most severe in immunocompromised and elderly pts (Nejm 1982;307:971).

Compl: PHN is most troublesome; pts w lesions about eye or nose may have corneal involvement and should be examined by an ophthalmologist.

Ddx: Before hallmark eruption, pain may resemble MI, peritonitis, sciatica, acute arthritis; HSV also may show a dermatome pattern.

Lab: Usually not necessary in typical dermatomal case; confirm in unusual case, ie, dissemination in immunosuppressed persons; viral culture is best and easiest; results back 3–5 d; false neg if lesion too old; Tzanck prep (Giemsa stain of vesicle contents): multinucleate giant cells and intranuclear inclusions specific for HSV or HZ; HZ is not a sufficient indicator of underlying malignancy to warrant special studies in otherwise normal persons.

Rx: Initiate antiviral medication within 72 h of first vesicle (do not rx w antivirals if blisters began >5 d ago); consider rx between 72 h and 5 d if lesions not crusted, pt >50 yo, immunocompromised, or has trigeminal zoster; dosage: acyclovir 800 mg 5x/d for 7 d, or valacyclovir 1 gm tid for 7 d, or famciclovir 500 mg tid for 7 d; early rx may ↓ PHN (Ann IM 1995;123:89); ↓ dose in pts w renal insufficiency; consider iv acyclovir for immunocompromised pts at risk for dissemination or foscarnet (J Infect Dis 1990;161:1078); narcotic analgesia usually needed for pain, esp in aged; nighttime sedation w diphenhydramine; cool saline compresses followed by a thick coat of ZnOx paste to ↓ sticking of blister fluids to clothing; adding systemic CS does not ↓ PHN (Ann IM 1996;125:376; Nejm 1994;330:896).

2.3.D.(2). POSTHERPETIC NEURALGIA (PHN)

Neim 2000;342:635; Nejm 1996;335:32.

Cause: Neuralgia after HZ; probably from late fibrosis and scarring of nerves.

Sx: Severe and persistent nerve root pain; often lancinating.

Si: Scars from previous bout of HZ often present.

Crs: Usually improves over wks to mos, but may continue for yrs in older persons (Comp Ther 1996;22:183).

Rx: Difficult; systemic CSs do not ↓ development of PHN; topical capsaicin (Zostrix, OTC) qid to noneroded skin (J Am Acad Derm 1989;21:265); 5% lidocaine patches (Lidoderm, $$$), up to 3 patches, each about the size of a postcard, applied for 12 h within each 24-h period (Pain 1999;80:533); topical EMLA cr (Rx, $$) (Pain 1989;39:301); nortriptyline 10 mg at dinner, increasing to 50–100 mg as tolerated (Pain 1992;48:29); carbamazepine, useful in tic douloureux, may be beneficial in dose of 100–200 mg bid, increasing wkly up to 800 mg qd; gabapentin (Neurontin, Rx) in dose of 300 mg and ↑ by 300 mg/d to maximum of 1800 mg/d (↓ w renal insufficiency) (Neurology 1996;46:1175); if severe and unresponsive, refer to neurosurgeon or anesthesiologist to consider injection of local anesthetic into nerve root for temporary relief, alcohol injection for permanent numbing, even surgical sectioning of nerve.

2.3.E. TOXIC EPIDERMAL NECROLYSIS (TEN)

Cause: Probably against antigen, most commonly drug; most frequent indicted drugs: barbiturates, butazones, hydantoins, sulfonamides; other cases assoc w burns, malignancy, viral infections, chemical toxins.

Epidem: Both sexes; all races; mostly adults.

Sx: Painful and burning blisters, like an extensive burn.

Si: Red, tender, burning rash first on face and extremities; eruption quickly becomes confluent; large, flaccid blisters develop; ruptured blisters leave large, denuded areas; skin easily sheared by sideway pressure (*Nikolsky sign*); mucous membranes: painful erosions and crusts; febrile.

Crs: Begins w fever, malaise, arthralgias; resolution is slow, over wks.

Compl: High mortality, up to 50%; may leave scarred eyes or mucous membranes; damage to lungs, GI tract, kidneys.

Lab: Skin bx may be diagnostic; lesions of TEN show necrosis of epidermis starting at lower layers; look for leukocytosis, ↑ liver enzymes, renal insufficiency, electrolyte imbalance.

Rx: Prompt referral to dermatologist or burn center; usually requires hospitalization often in burn unit if available; eliminate inciting cause; rx w systemic CSs is controversial and probably best avoided.

2.3.F. STAPHYLOCOCCAL SCALDED-SKIN SYNDROME (SSSS)

J Am Acad Derm 1998;39:383.

Cause: Exotoxin from phage group II, *Staphylococcus aureus* induces splitting of epidermis; ↓ renal function in very young and very old slows excretion of exotoxin and contributes to susceptibility.

Epidem: Bullous impetigo is localized form of SSSS; most are children <5 yo; may affect adults w renal failure or HIV infection.

Sx: Widespread skin tenderness.

Si: Widespread redness; large blisters w shedding of skin in sheets; mucosal surfaces *not* involved, unlike TEN or erythema multiforme.

Crs: Sudden onset; may start as purulent eruption of nose, eyes, throat; evolves in 1–2 d to widespread rash; course usually brief, <1 wk; mortality: 3% in children, 50% in adults.

Comp: SSSS develops in 1/2 of the cases of **Group A Streptoccal Necrotizing Fasciitis** "flesh-eating disease": rare, but highly destructive and potentially lethal; assoc w severe, unrelenting pain unresponsive to NSAIDs, fever, tachycardia, GI sx, myalgias, ↓ BP; confirm w blood culture, MRI; surgical debridement and clindamycin + penicillin may be effective (Infect Med 2001;18:198).

Lab: Seek source of infection, esp occult otitis or nasopharyngeal infection; skin bx shows cleft in upper layers of epidermis.

Rx: Distinguish SSSS from TEN as rx differs greatly (see 2.3.e.); penicillinase-resistant penicillin, ie, dicloxacillin (12.5–25 mg/kg/d) or methicillin sodium (50–150 mg/kg/d) in children; avoid systemic CSs; consider early dermatologic and infectious disease consultation.

TRUNK AND EXTREMITIES OR TRUNK ALONE RECURRENT OR PRESENT FOR MONTHS

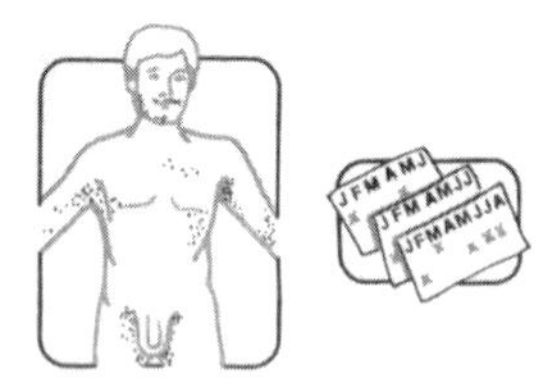

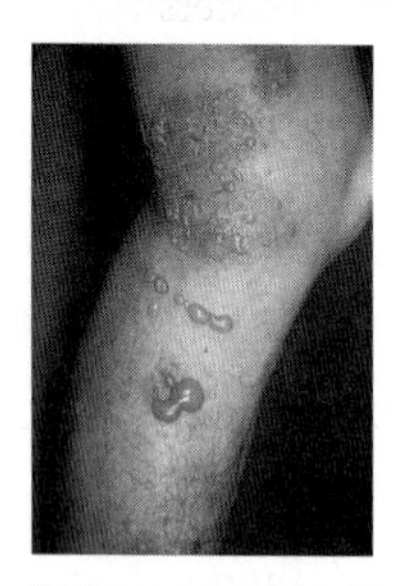

Bullous pemphigoid

2.4.A. ERYTHEMA MULTIFORME

Summary: Lesions usually first appear on extremities and mucosal surfaces, rather than trunk (see 2.1.b.).

2.4.B. DERMATITIS HERPETIFORMIS

Summary: Intensely itchy and burning; groups of pea-sized papules, small blisters, scratch marks; on forearms, elbows, knees, scalp, sacrum; may have irritable bowel w intermittent abdominal pain and diarrhea; chronic, persistent course.

For additional details and rx, see BODY, 3.1.m.

2.4.C. EPIDERMOLYSIS BULLOSA (EB)

Summary: Most appear on extremities, rather than trunk, because lesions are induced by trauma (see 2.6.c).

2.4.D. PEMPHIGUS AND PEMPHIGOID

Derm Clin 1993;11:429. Derm Clin 1990;8:689.

See color plate section.

Cause: Autoimmune disorders w antibodies against antigens of epidermal cells (pemphigus) or against dermal-epidermal junction (pemphigoid).

Epidem: Pemphigus usually age 40–50; pemphigoid usually age 60–70.

Sx: Painful blisters and erosions.

Si: Skin can be sheared by sideways pressure (*Nikolsky sign*).

- Pemphigus: blisters anywhere on body; rupture easily; often painful oral ulcers.
- Pemphigoid: blisters predilection for flexural areas (groin and axillae); tend to be tense and remain intact; less likely to have oral lesions.

Crs:

- Pemphigus: chronic; long rx but rx-induced remissions occur; prior to CSs pemphigus was fatal from malnutrition, infection, fluid loss.
- Pemphigoid: tends to be self-limited; responds to CSs; often remits; a few cases are chronic or relapsing (Derm Clin 1993;11:483; Derm Clin 1990;8:701).

Compl: 5-yr mortality from pemphigus is about 10%; mortality from pemphigoid is less.

Lab: Skin bx for routine and DIF and IFA of serum for antiepidermal antibodies.

Rx: Oral pulse MTX (J Am Acad Derm 1999;40:741) or systemic CS (sometimes >100 mg/d prednisone) (Derm Clin 1993;11:483) may be required; cyclophosphamide or azathioprine may be required for immunosuppressive and steroid-sparing effects; complications of high-dose CSs must be anticipated and often overshadow debility from disease; most cases are followed by a dermatologist.

Contact the National Pemphigus Foundation (POB 9606; Berkeley CA 94709-0606; 510.527.4970; www.pemphigus.org) for pt support information.

EXPOSED PARTS ONLY
FIRST EPISODE OR PRESENT FOR DAYS

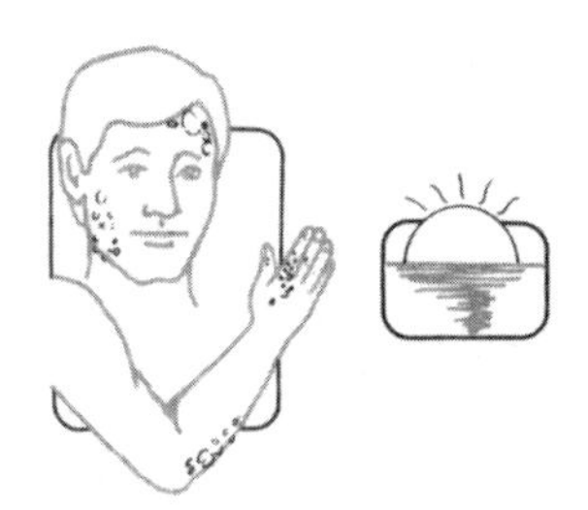

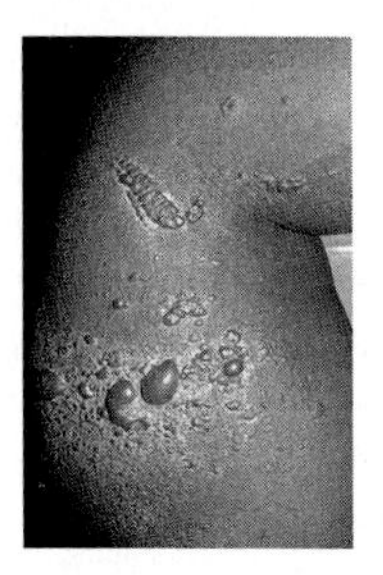

Contact dermatitis—*Rhus*

2.5.A. CONTACT DERMATITIS

Cause:

- Irritant contact: detergents, solvents.
- Allergic contact: plants, esp poison ivy (*Rhus*) most common; also nickel or chrome in jewelry, latex, acrylics.

Pathophys:

- Irritant contact: affect all persons; rxn soon after contact; first exposure; mild irritant may require repeated or prolonged exposure.

- Allergic contact: affect some persons; rxn delayed after contact; does not occur w 1st exposure.

Sx: Intensely itchy; may be edematous, painful.

Si: Exposed part of body (face, arms, legs); palms, soles, scalp, hairy part of axillae, mucous membranes are relatively resistant to contact dermatitis; eruption often has bizarrely shaped and angular lesions.

Crs: Poison ivy (*Rhus*) induced blisters may appear for up to 3 wk because of continued exposure to antigen via contaminated clothing, tools, sports equipment, fur of the family pet; blister fluid does not "spread" rash to other sites as content of blisters is only edema transudate.

Ddx: Irritant and allergic dermatitis often are identical in appearance; distinction depends on hx and rxn to patch testing.

Lab: Dermatologist or allergist may perform patch testing to identify an inciting antigen but most causes are discovered by hx.

For additional details and rx, see BODY, 3.1.a.

BLISTERS

2.5.B. IMPETIGO

Summary: Either blisters (usually a pathogenic strain of *S. aureus*) or honey-colored, stuck-on crusty patches (usually group A β-hemolytic streptococci); usually multiple but sometimes single; mildly irritating; most common location: face; most are in young children; may be regional LN↑; not febrile; abrupt onset w rapid spread; heals w/o scars; glomerulonephritis may follow streptococcal impetigo.

For additional details and rx, see FACE, 6.6.a.

2.5.C. TRAUMA

Summary: Cause of blisters induced by trauma generally are obvious; include **sunburn** (see LIGHT REACTIONS, 18.1.a.), **chemical**, **electrical**, or **heat burns, insect bites** (see LEG RASH, 17.2.a.); sunburns do not scar, unless infected; burns extend into the epidermis (1st degree) or into the dermis (2nd degree), heal w/o scars, unless infected; burns through the dermis (3rd degree) heal slowly w scars; 3rd-degree burns or burns covering more than just a few % of the body, other than sunburns, should be referred to plastic surgeon or hospital burn center.

EXPOSED PARTS ONLY
RECURRENT OR PRESENT FOR MONTHS

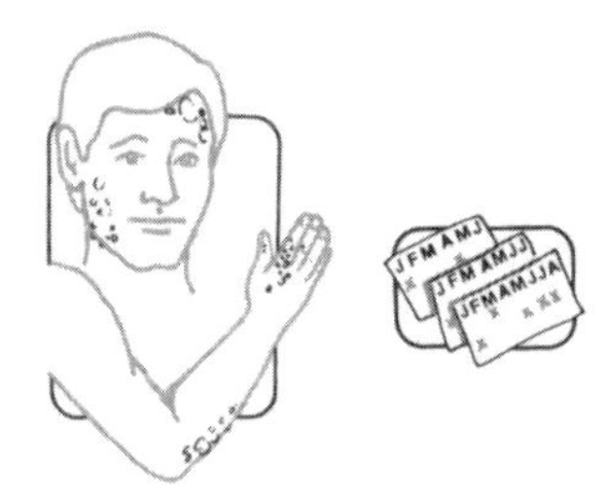

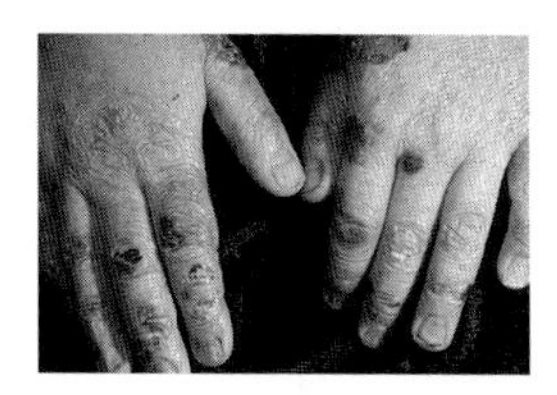

Epidermolysis bullosa

2.6.A. CONTACT DERMATITIS

Summary: Contact dermatitis recurs w re-exposure to irritant or allergen (see 2.5.a.).

2.6.B. PORPHYRIA

Summary: Only **porphyria cutanea tarda** (PCT) is assoc w blisters; appears on sun-exposed skin hrs or days after exposure; chronic; usually w thin scars from fragile skin that shears easily; hyperpigmentation of face and backs of hands; exposed skin is thickened w ↑ hair, eyebrows may meet each other or hair at temples may meet eyebrows, giving pts a "werewolf" facies; urine may be dark, like red wine, esp during flares; often assoc w DM or alcoholism.

For additional details and rx, see LIGHT REACTIONS, 18.1.c.

2.6.C. EPIDERMOLYSIS BULLOSA (EB)

See color plate section.

Cause: Group of genetic disorders of weakened cutaneous integrity; molecular biology for many has been clarified.

Epidem: Rare, affects about 25,000 persons in U.S.

Pathophys: Subtypes show different but distinctive ultramicroscopically visible epidermal and dermal splitting or loss of fine collagen-anchoring fibrils; generally, recessively inherited types have skin splitting at deepest levels and are more likely to heal w scarring and contractures.

Si: Blisters induced by mild trauma or appear spontaneously; ease of blistering and scarring depends on subtype.

Crs: Most serious forms appear at birth or soon after; mild forms may not be apparent until pt is exposed to trauma, ie, sports; rare "acquired" form appears during adulthood (Br J Derm 1995;133:19); however, some variation between pts w same genetic subtype so pts judge own tolerance to trauma.

Compl: Scars and milia at sites of repeated trauma more common in recessive dystrophic variants; severe forms: mouth, esophagus involved, adhesions cover digits, retarded height.

Lab: Refer to specialized centers to determine dx and subtype.

Rx: Nearly all pts w such blisters will already be cared for by a dermatologist and geneticist, as well as GI, orthopedics, and other specialties, usually at university medical centers.

Contact D.E.B.R.A.—Dystrophic Epidermolysis Bullosa Research Association (40 Rector Street, 14th Floor, New York, NY 10006; 212.513.4090; www.debra.org) for pt education materials.

SINCE CHILDHOOD

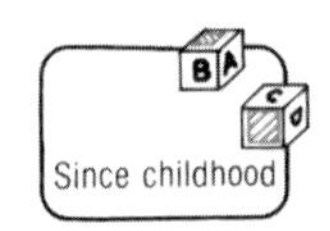

2.7. NEONATAL BLISTERING

Summary: Life-threatening disorder cared for by a pediatrician and/or a dermatologist; ddx includes bacterial infection, *Candida* infection, viral infection, ie, HSV, neonatal syphilis, EB, epidermolytic hyperkeratosis, lamellar ichthyosis.

3 Body

SCALY PATCHES

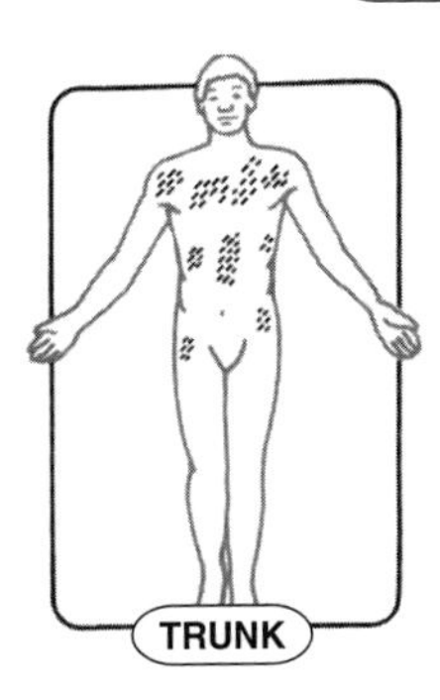

CONSIDER

COMMON

contact dermatitis (3.1.a)
drug reaction (3.1.b)
pityriasis rosea (3.1.c)
psoriasis (3.1.d)
scabies (3.1.e)
syphilis, secondary (3.1.f)
tinea corporis (3.1.g)
tinea versicolor (3.1.h)
Grover's disease (3.1.i)

UNCOMMON

dermatitis herpetiformis (3.1.m)
parapsoriasis (3.1.n)
pityriasis rubra pilaris (3.1.o)
mycosis fungoides (3.1.p)

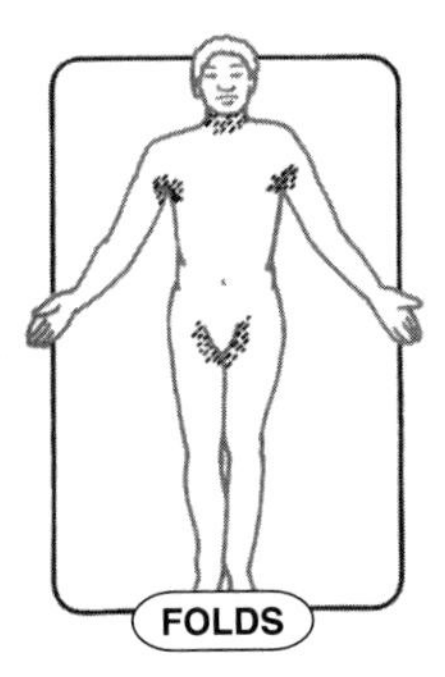

CONSIDER

atopic dermatitis (3.2.a)
contact dermatitis (3.2.b)
miliaria (3.2.c)
psoriasis (3.2.d)
seborrheic dermatitis (3.2.e)

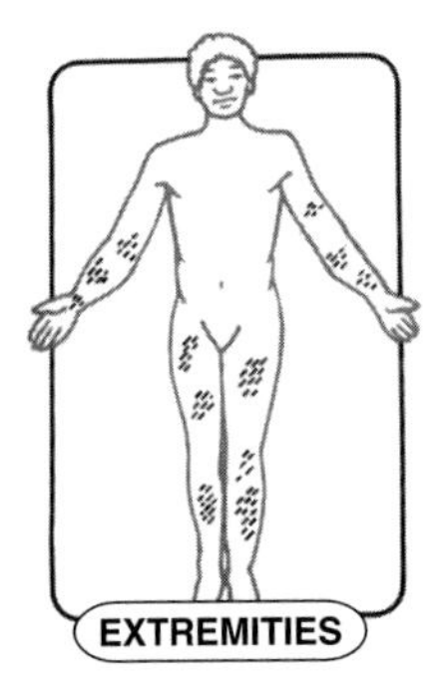

CONSIDER

COMMON

atopic dermatitis (3.3.a)
contact dermatitis (3.3.b)
nummular eczema (3.3.c)
psoriasis (3.3.d)
scabies (3.3.e)
syphilis, secondary (3.3.f)
tinea infection (3.3.g)
keratosis pilaris (3.3.h)

UNCOMMON

dermatitis herpetiformis (3.3.m)
lichen planus (3.3.n)
sarcoid (3.3.o)
xanthoma (3.3.p)
leprosy (3.3.q)

SCALY PATCHES ON TRUNK COMMON ERUPTIONS

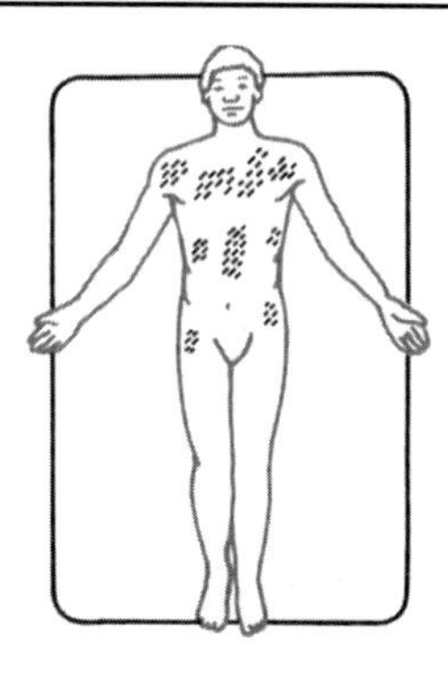

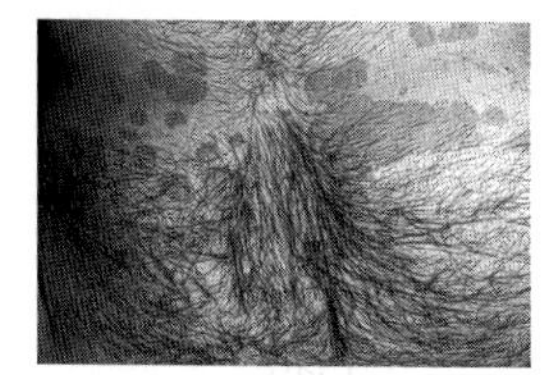

Tinea versicolor

See color plate section.

3.1.A. CONTACT DERMATITIS

Cause: Cutaneous rxn to an external agent, may be irritant or allergen; pattern often suggests dx: *face, neck, forearms, hands*—light induced or airborne allergen or irritant; *axillae*—deodorant or perfume; *earlobes*—nickel or chrome in jewelry; *ring finger*—nickel, chrome, detergent: *shoes*—leather or adhesives; *eyelids*—cosmetics, fingernail polish, dust, pollen.

- Irritant: affects everyone exposed; rxn soon after contact; mild irritants may require repeated or prolonged exposure.
- Allergic: prior sensitization required; rxn delayed for hrs to days; atopic background and occupations w frequent exposure (dentists, florists, printers) predispose.

Common Contactants

Plants: Poison ivy, oak, sumac most potent plant allergens; often severe w blisters, bizarre and linear, angular shaped from direct transfer; blister fluid does not "spread" rash; new lesions appear for days to wks from unintentional re-exposure to resin on clothing, tools, sports equipment, fur of family pet; resin takes up to 3 wk to evaporate.

Rx: Wash tools w soapy water; leave shoes outside; remove clothes for washing; shower immediately after exposure; hyposensitization not yet practical; *mild* cases: antihistamine po and TCS; *severe* cases w blisters that interfere w work or sleep: systemic CS (prednisone 40 mg for 4 d, then 30 mg for 1 wk, then 20 mg for 1 wk in a typical healthy adult) in addition to above.

Metals: Allergy usually chronic w scaling, pigmentation, itching; earlobe, neck, wrist, and under hooks, zippers, jewelry; dermatitis under a ring: metal allergy or trapped soap residue.

Rx: Change to higher gold content; plastic or hypoallergenic jewelry; clear tape on skin side of jewelry; TCS (class IV–V); patch testing is not practical in a PCP office, although a nickel covered w occlusive tape for 48 h may show red, scaly, itching rxn 1–3 d later.

Topical Meds: Subacute w redness, scaling, itch to acute w blisters; rxns to systemic meds are usually widespread on the trunk, not localized as w topical meds; common allergens: neomycin; anesthetics (benzocaine, tetracaine), preservatives (parabens, thimerosal (Merthiolate), benzyl alcohol, ethylenediamine); TCS masks underlying contact dermatitis.

Rx: Stop all topical meds, including moisturizers, scented soap, perfumes.

Cosmetics: Pink, scaly, pigmented, itchy; worse at site of application; eyelids often involved w allergy to *any* cosmetic, inc hair dye, fingernail polish, moisturizer, etc; cosmetic rxns are allergic, not irritant; pt typically attempts to deal w cosmetic rxns by substituting other products or by avoiding the product for a wk or so; she often fails to find a nonreacting product, because most products for the same use have similar ingredients.

Cause: Average woman uses 14 cosmetics simultaneously (American Academy of Dermatology); most common allergens:

- Fragrance (40% of rxns): look for products labeled “fragrance free” and not just “unscented”; unscented products, although not having an obvious smell, may still contain fragrance, used by manufacturer to cover odor of ingredients.
- Preservatives: quaternium-15, imidazole urea, parabens, methylisothiazolinone (Kathon CG).
- Nail cosmetics: look for polish that says *toluene and formaldehyde free*.

- Others: *Colophony*: mascaras, epilating waxes; hair dyes w *paraphenylenediamine*: pt should follow package instructions and test before using; *propylene glycol*: shampoos and hair gels.
  Rx: Substituting one makeup for another does not help as most cosmetics contain similar ingredients; stopping some makeup for a few days does not help as eruption may not clear w avoidance <1 wk; most women have a closet full of partially used cosmetics; try the following protocol:
- Wk 1: TCS (class IV–V) cr; pt lists all cosmetic products used and dc all those she can do w/o for 2 wk.
- Wk 2: stop TCS but maintain elimination program to determine if TCS is masking allergic rxn; if rxn recurs, pt must eliminate more cosmetics; if clear, proceed to wk 3.
- Wk 3: restart 1 new cosmetic each wk until rash reappears; if pt cannot identify culprit, refer to dermatologist who might perform patch testing.

Epidem: Irritant rxns more frequent than allergic rxns in both workplace and home.

Sx: Itching and painful cracking.

Si:

- Acute: blisters, edema, itch, even pain.
- Chronic: scaly, pigmented, thickened, lichenified; depths of skinfolds are protected from external contactant and remain clear; areas resistant to contact rxn are palms, soles, scalp, hairy part of axillae, mucous membranes.

Crs: Persists up to 2 wk after exposure ceases; see individual contactants above.

Lab: Patch testing is not practical in PCP office but most cases are diagnosed by hx; a dermatologist or allergist has access to testing materials.

Rx:

- Acute: saline compresses 20 min q 2–4 h; antihistamine; topical lotion (calamine w 0.25% menthol); TCS (class II–III) if mild; systemic CS if severe: prednisone 40 mg/d for 2–5 d until relief is attained, then tapered for 2–3 wk.
- Chronic: TCS (class IV–V); seek to establish cause.

3.1.B. DRUG REACTION

Cause: 10%–20% of hospitalized pts develop an adverse drug rxn, and of these, half were to drugs that were contraindicated or were unnecessary; eventually 40% of pts in general practice develop some type of drug rxn; incidence of adverse rxns ↑ w age (Breathnach SM, Drug reactions, in Fitzpatrick's dermatology in general medicine, McGraw-Hill, New York, 1999:3349).

Allergic, toxic, idiosyncratic, or photo rxn; *IgE-mediated allergic* rxns: urticaria, angioedema, anaphylaxis; *non-IgE-mediated allergic* rxns: flat, bumpy, petechial, blistering; allergic rxns are not dose related; *toxic*: dose related, any morphology but not urticaria; *idiosyncratic*: low incidence and not predictable; *photo-rxn*: requires light in combination w drug; *chemotherapeutic* drugs: given to cancer pts induce numerous and varied drug eruptions (J Am Acad Derm 1999;40:367); recognition and care generally provided by oncologists prescribing the agents.

- According to the Boston Collaborative Drug Surveillance Program (Jama 1986;256:3358), based on 15,438 consecutive inpts, drugs or agents assoc w highest frequency of skin rxn are:

Drug or Agent	Rxns per 1000 Recipients*
Amoxicillin	51
Trimethoprim/sulfamethoxazole	34
Ampicillin	33
Ipodate	28
Blood	22
Cephalosporins	21
Penicillin, semisynthetic	21
Erythromycin	20
Dihydralazine hydrochloride	19
Cyanocobalamin	18
Penicillin G	17
Quinidine	13
Hyoscine butylbromide	13
Cimetidine	13
Phenylbutazone	12
Phenazopyridine hydrochloride	9
Acetylcysteine	9
Allopurinol	8
Hydralazine hydrochloride	8
Carbocysteine	7
Bromhexine hydrochloride	6
Vincristine sulfate	6

Drug or Agent	Rxns per 1000 Recipients*
Isoniazid	6
Cyclophosphamide	5
Doxycycline	5
Gentamicin sulfate	5
Pentazocine hydrochloride	5
Barbiturates	4

*Allergic skin rxns >4 per 1000 recipients to drugs received by 100–1000 pts (combined Tables 1–3; Jama 1986;256:3358).

Si: Many appearances; most start on trunk, rather than extremities; most are itchy; may proceed to life-threatening eruption (Stevens-Johnson syndrome, TEN, serum sickness).

Crs: Usually improve or clear within 48 h after dc of offending drug, but may last for days to wks if drug is cleared slowly; sometimes rash clears while drug is continued but systemic toxicity progresses (eg, see below, Anticonvulsant hypersensitivity reaction).

Lab: Skin testing for penicillin allergy w fresh penicillin and a penicilloyl determinant preparation (Pre-pen, Kremers-Urban) is available, but should be used just prior to need and only when penicillin is essential; no practical lab tests for other drug allergies.

Rx: Eliminate suspected drug(s) or agent(s); risky to attempt suppression of rxn w antihistamines or systemic CS while continuing drug; both help relieve discomfort and speed resolution if offending agents have been dc'd.

Anticonvulsant hypersensitivity reaction: Phenytoin, carbamazepine, barbiturates; usually begins 1–3 wk after start of med; assoc w fever, liver and renal toxicity; may be fatal if drug not dc'd.

3.1.C. PITYRIASIS ROSEA

Cause: Unknown, but infectious etiology suspected as there are seasonal epidemics and only rare recurrences (Arch Derm 1999;135:1070).

Epidem: Usually young adult.

Sx: Often itchy, sometimes interfering w work and sleep; otherwise feel fine.

Si: Up to size of a quarter, pink-to-brown, round-to-oval, scaly patches; fernlike pattern starting on trunk; face involvement infrequent, except in blacks; palms and soles not involved; no LN↑.

Crs: Many start w a "herald patch," 2–6-cm, round, scaly plaque on trunk or proximal extremity 1–2 wk before rest of eruption; typical course is 6–8 wk w spread from trunk to extremities in 1st mo and clearing from trunk to extremities in the 2nd mo.

Ddx: 2° syphilis: palmar/plantar lesions and LN↑ (see 3.1.f.), drug eruption.

Lab: STS to r/o 2° syphilis; bx is nonspecific.

Rx: *Mild* sx: no rx needed; *moderate* itch: antihistamines at dinner or hs, TCS (class II–III), calamine lotion w menthol; *severe itch* that interferes w work and sleep: systemic CS (prednisone 40 mg/d for few d until comfortable, then taper over 3–4 wk); UVB phototherapy or tanning salon for 1–3 wk speeds relief.

3.1.D. PSORIASIS

Med Clin N Am 1998;82:1135.

Cause: Unknown; genetic factors exist as 1/3 have fhx and certain HLA loci are assoc; dietary factors not important; but smoking may be a factor in as many as 1 in 5 cases (Arch Derm 1999;135:1479); guttate may be assoc w streptococcal pharyngitis.

Epidem: About 2% affected.

Sx: Mild itching, irritation, embarrassment.

Si: *Plaque form*: red, slightly raised, distinct margin, loosely adherent, silvery scale; plaques most common on elbows, knees, scalp, but all areas may be involved; *guttate form*: many raindrop sized, scattered, rapid onset; *pustular form*; *exfoliative form*: *nails*: often affected w pinpoint pits, nail separation from nail bed, or gross dystrophy (see NAIL, 20.2.a.)(Derm 1996;193:300); *oral lesions*: rare; *arthritis*: 5%, polyarticular, predilection for DIP joints, most pts have extensive psoriasis, RF neg, ANA neg, often HLA-27 pos.

Crs: Chronic, persistent; onset usually in early adult life; childhood onset assoc w more extensive disease.

Lab: Histology is characteristic but not diagnostic; dx may require dermatologic confirmation in atypical cases; uric acid excretion but not gout is ↑; HLA typing is not practical; obtain throat culture in pts w suspected guttate psoriasis, but such pts usually are referred to a dermatologist.

Rx:

- *Plaques of limited extent*: TCS (class I–III) except in flexural areas, genitals, face where class IV–VII are safer; oint form is most effective, but cr is less sticky and greasy in intertriginous areas.
- *Unresponsive plaques on nonflexural areas*: TCS occluded w tape (Blenderm, 3M) or kitchen plastic wrap overnight; TCSs usually do not induce complete resolution and plaque returns to pre-rx appearance in days after discontinuance of rx; TCSs, esp class I, are expensive ($60/60 gm); systemic absorption from TCSs usually not significant, but has been assoc w growth retardation in children.
- *Alternatives for plaques*: calcipotriene (Dovonex, $$$) cr, oint, or soln, a vitamin D analog; bid or hs w clobetasol oint AM; do not exceed 100 gm/wk to avoid ↑calcium (J Am Acad Derm 1996;35:268; Derm 1997;37:S55); *note*: dc calcipotriene if pregnancy occurs (Clin Derm 1997;15:705); improved results were recently reported using a schedule of calcipotriene oint bid for a week followed by betamethasone dipropionate (TCS, class I) hs for a week, then rotating, instead of using them together (Jaad 2000;43:61); tazarotene (Tazorac, $$$) gel; hs, starting w 0.05% and increasing to 0.1% as tolerated; often used w clobetasol oint AM to boost effect and ↓ inflammation assoc w tazarotene; *note*: topical tazarotene may be teratogenic, female users need pregnancy tests and warnings about birth control; tar preparations and anthralin are messy and not often used except by dermatologists (J Am Acad Derm 1997;37:85).
- *Special consideration*: see AXILLA, 1.1.b; FEET, 7.1.d.; HANDS, 14.7.c.; NAILS, 20.2.a.; SCALP, 24.3.a.
- *Extensive, disabling types*: refer such pts to a dermatologist; rx options include UVB, psoralen, and long-wave ultraviolet light (PUVA, $$$), systemic acitretin (Soriatane, Roche, $$$), MTX ($$) (J Am Acad Derm 1998;38:478); cyclosporine; do not use systemic CS as pts rebound w worse psoriasis; rheumatologic consultation also may be needed.

Contact National Psoriasis Foundation (6600 SW 92nd Avenue, Suite 300, Portland, OR 97223-7195; 800.723.9166 or 503.244.7404; www.psoriasis.org) for pt support information.

3.1.E. SCABIES

Jaad 1999;41:661; Med Clin N Am 1998;82:1081. Inf Dis Clin NA 1994;8:533.

Cause: A mite, *Sarcoptes scabiei* var. *hominis*, transmitted only between humans; sensitization to mite must develop before itch; <10 mites in normal adult but large numbers in immunosuppressed pts (including AIDS).

Epidem: Conjugal partners almost invariably involved, but other family members may or may not be infested, depending on living conditions.

Sx: Pruritus, sometimes severe, w or w/o extensive rash; itch often worse at night; often involves finger webs, elbows, buttocks, genital area.

Si: Scaly lichenified patches, excoriated, pink, rice grain– to pea-sized papules, some w threadlike extension or burrow; pts may only have scratch marks; most common areas: genitalia, finger webs, elbows, areolae, umbilicus, lower abdomen, wrists, antecubital fossae, gluteal cleft.

Crs: Sensitization followed by pruritus may take wks after 1st exposure but only days w reinfestation.

Compl: Untreated scratching may lead to 2° infection and lichenification.

Lab: Finding mites or eggs under the microscope clinches the dx but this is difficult, esp in PCP office, as mites are few and most lesions are hidden by crusting and scratch marks; generally rx on clinical suspicion; consider obtaining STS, smear for gonococcus, or HIV test as pts w scabies are often in a high-risk group.

Rx: Only rx pt and contacts who are itching:

- Ivermectin po (Stromectol, 3 and 6 mg, Merck, Rx, $$) 200 μg/kg in 1 dose (Nejm 1995;333:26).
- Permethrin cr (5%) (Acticin cr or Elimite cr, Rx, $$): safest alternative; apply 30 gm hs from neck to toes and all crevices and shower off 8–12 h later, a single rx usually is sufficient.
- Lindane cr or lotion (1% γ benzene hexachloride) (Kwell, Rx, $): effective but potentially neurotoxic; do not bathe prior to application or apply to broken skin; do not use in pregnant or lactating women or children <2 yo; apply 30 gm hs from neck to toes and all crevices and shower off 8–12 h later, repeat in 1 wk; dispense only enough for 2 rxs as overuse is irritating.
- Sulfur (6% in petrolatum, $): safe but messy alternative for children and pregnant or lactating women; apply from chin down for 3 consecutive nights and remove by bathing each AM.

- Wash or dry clean bed linens, towels, and worn clothing; itching takes 1–3 wk to clear as allergic response fades.
- Relieve mild itching w TCS (class IV–V) and antihistamine; severe itching requires systemic CS (prednisone 20–40 mg/d tapered over 2–3 wk).

3.1.F. SYPHILIS, SECONDARY

Jaad 1999;41:511; Am Fam Phys 1999;59:2233; CDC, MMWR 1998; No. RR-1;47:31; Med Clin N Am 1998;82:1081.

Cause: *Treponema pallidum*, a spirochete.

Epidem: Incidence of syphilis has been declining since 1990 (Arch Derm 2000;136:565)

Sx: Constitutional si and sx are mild or absent.

See color plate section.

Si: Lesions are notoriously varied; most common is widespread, slightly scaly, tan or copper-colored, non-itchy patches, each dime to quarter in size; similar lesions on palms and soles; pt may still have healing genital ulcer, also moist, wart-like genital growths (*condylomata lata*), painless oral erosions, mucous patches, "moth-eaten" alopecia; LN↑is common, esp epitrochlear nodes found on the inner side of the arm within a few fingerbreadths above the elbow; except in infants, blisters are never seen in 2° syphilis.

Crs: 2° lesions appear within a few wks of the 1° although the eruption may be fleeting or in about 1/3 never appears; the rash of untreated 2° syphilis disappears in a few wks, sometimes reappearing and disappearing again; about 1/3 of pts w unrx syphilis develop late sequelae: cardiovascular, neurological, or gummatous; **gummas** of skin and mucosa are destructive, infiltrated and scarring, frequently extending to underlying bone.

Lab:

- **Non-specific antibodies** against lipoidal antigens: Venereal Disease Research Laboratory (VDRL) or Rapid Plasma Reagin (RPR) test; nearly always pos when 2°; rare false neg unless titer is extremely high (*prozone phenomenon*); inexpensive, sensitive and can be quantitated: if pos, repeat and obtain FTA: if pos, pt has or has had a treponemal disease

- **Specific antibodies**: Fluorescein Treponemal Antigen (FTA or FTA-ABS) test; always pos w 2° syphilis
- **Darkfield**: Rapid and reliable but now only rarely performed
- **Biologic false-positive** (BFP) rxn to VDRL/RPR is common; FTA almost always neg; BFP rxns of <6 mo: infections, esp. viral infections, vaccinations, malignancy, narcotic abuse, or even pregnancy; chronic BFP rxns of >6 mo: collagen vascular disease, leprosy (see FEVER, 8.3.a.)
- All pts w syphilis should be tested for HIV (J Infect Dis 1989;160:530)

For rx, see GENITAL, 9.2.a.

3.1.G. TINEA CORPORIS (RINGWORM)

Med Clin N Am 1998;82:1001.

Cause: Most are fungi of 2 types: *Trichophyton rubrum*, most common fungal saprophyte of man, or *Microsporum canis*, one of many fungi carried by animals.

Epidem: Fungi from animal sources induce severe rxns on humans, but are only itchy and scaly on animal host.

Sx: Itching and discomfort.
See color plate section.

Si: Scaly, inflammatory, fine pustules, oozing, crusting; differs from tinea infections in moist areas, ie, feet and groin, which are scaly, pigmented, and itchy, but less inflammatory; "ringworm" shape develops as infection spreads outward and the inner part clears.

Crs: Inflammatory tinea corporis may eventually clear spontaneously but may leave scar.

Ddx: **Pityrosporum folliculitis**: scattered follicular pustules on upper trunk; young adults, esp after sunny vacation; may be assoc w recent po antibiotics, esp w long-term acne rx; caused by *Pityrosporum ovale*; Rx: dc antibiotics; try ketoconazole shampoo 1st but may need ketoconazole or itraconazole po, responds slowly and may require 1–2 mo of med; **hot tub folliculitis**: follicular pustules; worse on skin covered by swimsuit; start 1–2 d

BODY

after exposure; multiple persons infected; assoc w improper care of hot tub allowing *Pseudomonas aeruginosa* to multiply; no rx available; clears in 1–2 wk.

Lab: Confirm dx w KOH (DX.3) exam or submit scale in dry sterile tube or taped between 2 microscope slides to mycology lab for KOH, culture, and identification.

Rx: Advise exam of family pets; topical rx alone generally insufficient but speeds clearing (see RX.10); systemic antifungal agent usually required (see RX.11)

3.1.H. TINEA VERSICOLOR

Fam Pract 1996;43:127. J Am Acad Derm 1994;31:S18

Cause: Yeast form of normal skin fungus, *Pityrosporum orbiculare (Malassezia furfur)*; change of color due to blockage of UV tanning and disruption of existing pigment by fungus.

Epidem: Common, esp in summer and humid environment; curiously, conjugal partner not often infected.

Sx: Sometimes mildly itchy.

Si: Scaly, flat patches; light to dark pink to tan; color varies from 1 pt to another but is uniform in individual pt; area usually above waist; face may be involved in blacks.

Crs: Worsens during hot, humid summers, recedes in winter; reappearance common.

Lab: Dx easily confirmed w KOH exam (see DX.3.): short fungal hyphae mixed w spores, a "spaghetti and meatballs" appearance; fungus not cultured by commercial labs.

Rx: Scaling and itch clears w rx but discoloration persists until sun exposure.

- Topical: ketoconazole 1%–2% shampoo (2% Nizoral shampoo, Rx, $$, or 1%, OTC) applied to dampened skin from neck to wrists to waist, left on for 5 min, then rinsed off in shower; 1 application cures 80% (J Am Acad Derm 1998;39:944); topical imidazole cr and ciclopirox cr bid × 2 wk are effective but are more expensive.
- Systemic: ketoconazole (Nizoral, 200 mg, $$) or itraconazole (Sporanox, 100 mg, $$), qd × 5 d and repeated for another 3 d 1 and 2 mos later (J Am Acad Derm 1996;34:287).

3.1.I GROVER'S DISEASE (TRANSIENT ACANTHOLYTIC DERMATOSIS)

Sx: Itchy

Si: Sparse eruption; limited to chest and back; consisting of pink to red, discrete, scattered papules, rice-grain or smaller, occasional tiny blisters which are so fragile that usually only excoriations are evident

Crs: Comes and goes, worse with changes of seasons

Compli: None

Cause: Unknown

Epidem: Nearly all cases are in middle-aged to elderly men

Lab: Bx may be diagnostic by confirming the presence of an acantholytic vesicle, but is usually not necessary

Rx: TCS offer moderate relief and may be used when symptomatic but will not fully clear the eruption.

SCALY PATCHES ON TRUNK UNCOMMON ERUPTIONS

The remaining disorders in this section (3.1.) are uncommon; generally are cared for by a dermatologist; only brief summaries are provided.

BODY

3.1.M. DERMATITIS HERPETIFORMIS

Derm Clin 1993;11:511.

Summary: Autoimmune disease; IgA present at dermal-epidermal junction; some w circulating serum IgA anti–basement membrane antibodies; certain HLA haplotypes are overrepresented, but familial cases are rare; intense itching and burning; itching is severe yet the rash may appear trivial; groups of pea-sized papules and occasional small blisters, along w scratch marks on forearms, elbows, knees, scalp, sacrum; gluten-sensitive enteropathy w atrophy of jejunal villi occurs in most cases, but only 10%–20% have GI sx; chronic, usually lifelong; intensity varies; assoc w thyroiditis, gastritis; skin bx is diagnostic; responds dramatically to dapsone or sulfapyridine; response helps confirm dx; pts w dermatitis herpetiformis are followed by a dermatologist; GI and dietitians may be involved if pt has GI sx or attempts gluten-free diet (J Am Acad Derm 1993;29:447).

Contact Gluten Intolerance Group of North America (15110 10th Avenue SW, Suite A, Seattle, WA 98166-1820; 206.246.6652; gig@accessone.com or www.medhlp.netusa.net/agsg/agsg168.htm) for pt education materials.

3.1.N.(1). PARAPSORIASIS, ACUTE (PITYRIASIS LICHENOIDES ET VARIOLIFORMIS ACUTA, PLEVA, MUCHA-HABERMANN DISEASE)

Summary: Acute onset w crops of papules and blisters; scattered, not grouped; slightly painful, not itchy; malaise and low-grade fever may precede eruption; most are young adults; hypopigmentation and scars may remain; episode may persist wks to mos, but course may continue off and on for yrs; cause is unknown; skin bx of acute lesion assists dx; r/o 2° syphilis; rx is difficult but tetracycline, systemic CS, cytotoxic agents have been used; refer pts to dermatology for confirmation of dx and rx.

3.1.N.(2). PARAPSORIASIS, CHRONIC

Summary: Asx, slightly scaly patches, 2 forms: *guttate*: small, dime sized, not assoc w systemic disease; *large plaque*: palm-sized or larger patches, slightly itchy, may be or eventuate into a lymphoma, inc mycosis fungoides or Hodgkin's disease; resembles psoriasis, but scale is finer and distribution differs; pathology may not be diagnostic; refer suspected cases to dermatology.

3.1.O. PITYRIASIS RUBRA PILARIS

Summary: Scaly, red, roughened from minute horny accretions in hair follicles; scalp is esp scaly; yellow-pink thickening of palms and soles; resembles seborrheic dermatitis and psoriasis; remits in 2–4 yr in 80%; may develop generalized erythroderma; cause unknown; rx includes retinoids, cytotoxic agents; systemic CS and PUVA not helpful; refer suspected cases to dermatology.

3.1.P. MYCOSIS FUNGOIDES

Summary: T-cell lymphoma usually starting as itchy thickened patches; may remain stable or progress to thickened plaques, tumors, and exfoliative erythroderma; appears to start in skin and progress to viscera; men > women; average age 55 yo.

For additional details, see GROWTHS, 11.14.b.

SCALY PATCHES ON BODY FOLDS

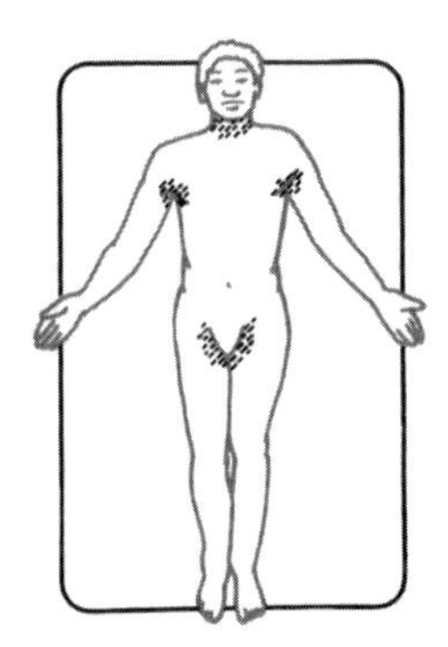

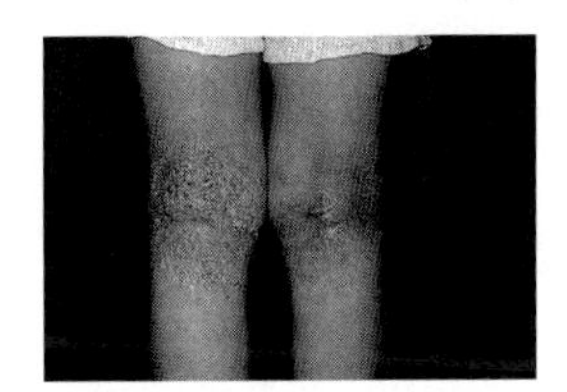

Atopic dermatitis

3.2.A. ATOPIC DERMATITIS

J Am Acad Derm 1999;41:72. Med Clin N Am 1998;82:1105. J Am Acad Derm 1995;33:1008.

Cause: Probably immunologic; elevated IgE levels in most, but not all; genetics play role as 90% have fhx of hay fever, wheezing, eczema; about half of offspring are affected to some degree.

Sx: Pruritus may be severe and interfere w sleep; triggered by sweating, irritants, ie, scratchy wool clothing, low winter humidity, overbathing.

Si: *Acute*: reddened, oozy, scaly; *chronic*: thickened, lichenified, pink where scratched; not toxic or febrile unless infected; children gain weight normally; redundant crease or fold below lower eyelids (Dennie-Morgan fold).

- Distribution: *<1 yo*: involves exposed skin, ie, face and extensor surfaces of arms and legs, diaper area is clear; *older child*: flexural areas, ie, antecubitals, popliteals, neck.

Crs: Not present at birth but may start as early as 2nd mo, most start by 5 yo; 2/3 clear by puberty but 2/3 recur after puberty w respiratory, skin, or both disorders; rash and itch tend to improve in summer but bacterial pyoderma is more common; adults w atopic dermatitis often clear by 40 yo.

Compl: Capsular cataracts from atopic dermatitis or complication of rx w CS; HSV infection may be severe (**eczema herpeticum**).

Ddx: Contact dermatitis, seborrheic dermatitis, rarely Letterer-Siwe disease.

Lab: IgE often ↑ but test not necessary.

Rx: Role of dietary factors is controversial; elimination diets may control some pts; skin testing and desensitization do not help; *acute exacerbations*: cooling baths, TCS cr; search for contacts or infections that induced flare; short courses of systemic CSs occasionally are necessary for severe flares but should not be used for long-term rx; adults: start w 30–40 mg prednisone or its equivalent in single AM dose and reduce dose by 5–10 mg/d w improvement and stop within 3–4 wk; *chronic*: TCS (class II–III) oint; use cr when weepy and crusty, use oint when dry, scaly, chronic; reduce frequency of bathing and use of soap by offering techniques suggested for rx of **xerosis** (see ITCH, 16.1.a. and RX.2); Tacrolimus oint (Protopic 0.03% for children, 0.1% for adults, 30 and 60 gm, $$$), an immunosuppressant used in organ transplant surgery, now available for topical use in moderate to severe atopic dermatitis, may supplant TCS in some cases (Arch Derm 2000;136:999). Application is bid; skin must be dry to ↓ the burning sensation felt by some pts; avoid sun/artificial tanning as Tacrolimus potentiates UV carcinogenicity in animals. *Pyoderma* w oozing and crusting: erythromycin (250 mg qid × 10 d for adults) or erythromycin suspension (30 mg/kg qid × 10 d for children) usually is adequate; bacterial cultures from skin reflect surface bacteria and are not useful; antihistamines are sedating and help, esp hs: use hydroxyzine 10 mg tid or diphenhydramine 50 mg tid, increasing dose 2–3-fold hs if needed; more expensive, nonsedating antihistamines are not effective (Arch Derm 1999;135:1522); UV phototherapy is an alternative rx for severe atopic dermatitis; topical tacrolimus; cases severe enough for systemic CSs usually are cared for by a dermatologist or allergist.

Contact National Eczema Association (1220 SW Morrison Street, Suite 433, Portland, OR 97205-2235; 800.818.7546 or 503.228.4430; www.eczema-assn.org) for pt education materials.

3.2.B. CONTACT DERMATITIS

Summary: Irritant or allergic rxns to deodorants, perfumes, topical meds are common in flexural regions due to occlusion and moisture; body folds are less involved w airborne contactants as they are partially protected from exposure.

For additional details, see 3.1.a.

3.2.C. MILIARIA (PRICKLY HEAT)

Cause: Eccrine sweat duct occlusion w rupture or leakage of sweat into surrounding tissue; type of miliaria depends on level of obstruction within the duct.

Epidem: Develops in persons working or exercising daily in hot, humid environment, or in pts wrapped w occlusive bandages, lying on or under plastic sheets, or pts w high fever.

Sx: Prickling and itchy.

Si: Depends on level of sweat duct obstruction: *miliaria rubra*: red, prickly eruption on occluded or rubbing skin surfaces; *miliaria crystallina*: myriad of pustular, pinhead-sized, clear fluid-containing vesicles, resembling water droplets.

Crs: Clears when person is cooled and ventilated.

Lab: None; lesions are sterile.

Rx: Cooling and ventilating skin quickly clears lesions; 8 h each d in an air-conditioned sleeping room prevents development of miliaria regardless of working conditions; propylene glycol in water (50%) tid may help clear sweat duct blockage.

3.2.D. PSORIASIS

Summary: Usually affects extensor surfaces but may be flexural in pts w psoriasis concomitant w another skin condition that tends to affect skinfolds, ie, seborrheic dermatitis, atopic dermatitis, *Candida* infection; because of moist location, silvery scale typical of psoriasis is replaced by red, glistening rash involving both hairy and nonhairy parts; irritating and itchy; look for typical psoriasis elsewhere; groin psoriasis is cause of considerable discomfort and embarrassment; rx w low-potency TCS (class VI–VII), ie, 1%–2.5% HC cr, as more potent fluorinated TCS may lead to atrophy and striae (see RX.5.).

For additional details and rx, see 3.1.d.; AXILLA, 1.1.b.; GROIN RASH 10.4.c.

3.2.E. SEBORRHEIC DERMATITIS

Summary: Usually diffuse but may be patchy; hairy areas most involved; yellowish greasy scale; mild redness and itching; similar scale and itching usually present at scalp, ear canals, retroauricular areas, eyebrows, nasolabial folds; look for si of psoriasis elsewhere; consider *Candida* infection if pustules are present; rx: TCS cr (class VI–VII); avoid stronger TCS, which may cause atrophy and striae in flexural areas.

For additional details and rx, see FACE, 6.2.a., and SCALP, 24.3.b.

SCALY PATCHES ON EXTREMITIES COMMON ERUPTIONS

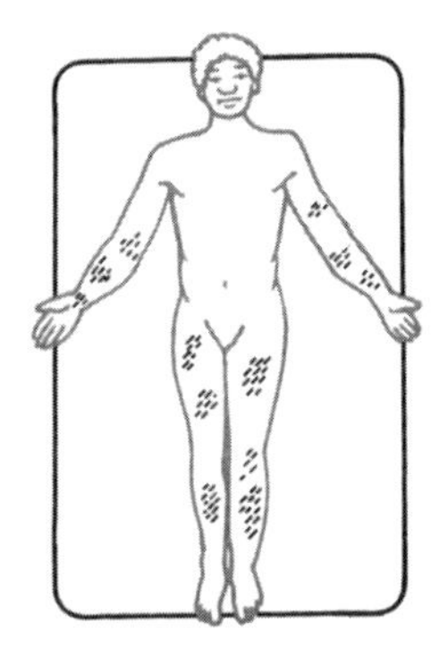

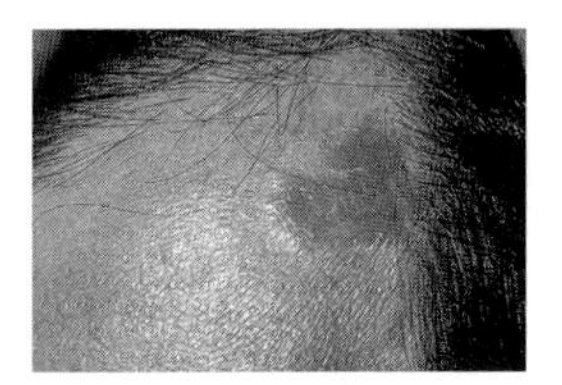

Sarcoid

BODY

3.3.A. ATOPIC DERMATITIS

Summary: Itchy; thickened; chronic; antecubital and/or popliteal areas in adult or child >1–2 yo.

For additional details and rx, see 3.2.a.

3.3.B. CONTACT DERMATITIS

Summary: Extremities often involved depending on source of irritant or antigen; causes include occupational contacts, shoes, jewelry, poison ivy.

For additional details and rx, see 3.1.a.

3.3.C. NUMMULAR ECZEMA

Cause: None proved.

Epidem: Late middle-aged men or young adult women.

Sx: Mild irritation and itching.

Si: Coin-shaped (nummular) patches; <20 or so; mostly on arms and legs; start w minute blisters and pustules that spread to become scaly and thickened.

Crs: Develops over a few wk; persist for >2 yr in about 1/2, often w remissions and recurrences.

Lab: Skin bx is nonspecific.

Rx: The PCP is justified to try a TCS oint bid–tid, even a highly potent TCS (class I), but if dermatitis is extensive, persistent, or does not remain clear after such a trial, refer to dermatology.

3.3.D. PSORIASIS

Summary: Chronic, sharply demarcated, scaly, thickened plaques on extremities, esp elbows, knees, hands, nails; may be widespread (see 3.1.d.).

3.3.E. SCABIES

Summary: Itchy, eczematous areas on extremities, esp elbows and finger webs; look for additional lesions in groin, waist, anterior axillary areas.

For additional details and rx, see 3.1.e.

3.3.F. SYPHILIS, SECONDARY

Summary: Many patterns; most common: widespread, slightly scaly, tan, copper-colored, nonitchy patches, lesions on palms and/or soles; recent or healing genital ulcer; moist, wartlike genital growths (condylomata lata); painless oral erosions and mucous patches; "moth-eaten" scalp hair loss; mild or absent constitutional si and sx; LN↑, esp epitrochlear nodes; no blisters except in newborn; 2° lesions appear few wk after 1°; rash disappears.

For additional details, see 3.1.f.

3.3.G. TINEA INFECTION

Summary: Acute, inflamed annular patches w fine pustules, oozing, crusting, itching; chronic tinea infections on feet and groin are less inflammatory, less scaly, less itchy; source usually is family dog, cat, horse; dx: confirm w KOH exam (DX.3) or culture by sending scale scraped w blade into sterile red-topped tube to clinical lab.

For additional details and rx, see 3.1.g.

3.3.H. KERATOSIS PILARIS

Summary: Mildly irritating; discrete; pinhead sized; hard or horny, raised plugs, some pink; feels like sandpaper; most located on extensor surfaces of upper arms, thighs, but may be generalized; most appear by age 10 yo; lesions are chronic but improve w age, most improve during summer; autosomal dominant

For additional details and rx, see ITCH, 16.1.b.

SCALY PATCHES ON EXTREMITIES UNCOMMON ERUPTIONS

3.3.M. DERMATITIS HERPETIFORMIS

Summary: Groups of pea-sized papules w an occasional blister on elbows, forearms, knees but also on sacrum and scalp; intensely itchy; rare.

For additional details and rx, see 3.1.m.

3.3.N. LICHEN PLANUS

Cause: Probably an immune disorder; T lymphocytes predominate and IgM and C3 bind to basement membrane; histologically similar to graft-vs-host rxn; some cases are assoc w meds, esp antimalarials, benoxaprofen, benzodiazepines, captopril, chlorpropamide, gold, quinidine, thiazides; ↑ assoc w hepatitis C (J Am Acad Derm 1999;41:787).

Sx: Itch, often severe.

Si: Pink to purple, flat-topped papules about size of a lentil; individual or tightly grouped coalescing into plaques; most involved: wrists, lower legs, ankles; some papules form into lines where there is a cut or scratch (*Koebner's phenomenon*); hypertrophic form: thickened, persistently itchy patches, less common, mostly in blacks; nails may be involved w loss, thinning, or scarring (see NAIL, 20.6.c.); buccal mucosa may have lacy, white patches (see MOUTH, 19.1.i.).

Crs: *Acute onset*: over days to wks; tends to remit after wks to mos; *slow onset*: over mos, tends to persist, sometimes for yrs; overall 2/3 clear within a yr but 20% of those recur.

Compl: No systemic manifestations.

Lab: Skin bx is diagnostic.

Rx: Itching is difficult to control; TCS (class I–III) cr or oint or less potent TCS w plastic wrap occlusion; antihistamines for sedation hs; occasionally systemic CS but rx may be prolonged; UV light or even PUVA is useful if widespread and is safer than long-term systemic CSs; pts w lichen planus generally are treated by a dermatologist.

3.3.O. SARCOID

Jaad 2001;44:725; Med 1999;78:65. Arch Derm 1997;133:882. Callen JP, Sarcoidosis, in Dermatological signs of internal disease, WB Saunders, Philadelphia, 1995.

See color plate section.

Cause: Unknown, presumably immunologic; activated T cells; vitamin D sensitivity.

Epidem: 25% of pts w sarcoid have skin involvement; blacks 10 × >> whites; women >> men; ↑ incidence: southern U.S., northern Europe, Australia.

Sx: Asx or slightly itchy; fatigue; weight loss; fever if systemic.

Si: Variable; most lesions are pink to yellow; firm papules or plaques; pinhead to pea sized or larger; may develop within preexisting scars; sometimes severe and may distort facial features; may be deep; may ulcerate; may lead to local hair loss; 10% of U.S. cases manifest as infiltrated, painful nodules over shins (**erythema nodosum**) (see LEG RASH, 17.3.a.); most common visceral changes: LN↑ hilar and peripheral; pulmonary nodules; uveitis; parotid enlargement; neurologic and cardiac involvement; infiltrates of kidney, spleen, and liver; bone cysts; various endocrinopathies.

Crs: Chronic but fluctuations are common; 60% resolve spontaneously and another 10–20% clear w systemic CS rx (Postgrad Med J 1996:72:196); acute sarcoidosis tends to resolve spontaneously; chronic forms vary from mild to disabling, depending on extent and nature of organ infiltration; pts w erythema nodosum tend to have early resolution of other manifestations of sarcoidosis.

Compl: May be confined to skin but most pts w skin involvement have internal involvement as well, esp lungs, kidneys, calcium control, neurologic, pituitary, joints.

Ddx: Presentation is notoriously varied; sarcoidosis is in ddx of many disorders.

Lab: Clinical dx is by exclusion, but confirmation requires histologic proof of characteristic noncaseating granulomas; minor salivary gland bx often pos; r/o foreign body granulomas induced by silica, talc, quartz, beryllium, zirconium by polarizing microscopy; r/o bacterial and fungal granulomas by culture and stains; consider: chest x-ray, pulmonary function tests, LFTs, RFTs, serum and urine calcium levels, EKG, eye examination, PPD; previously pos PPD may become neg because of anergy that often accompanies sarcoidosis.

Rx: Cutaneous sarcoid slowly responds to TCS, esp w plastic wrap or tape occlusion; large deforming nodules or plaques may require IL triamcinolone acetonide (Kenalog, 10 mg/mL diluted to 3–5 mg/mL) repeated monthly; systemic rx indicated if pulmonary, renal, cardiac, endocrine, or ocular involvement is symptomatic or progressive, if hypercalcemia is present, or if granulomas impinge on vital structures (Nejm 1986;315:727); systemic CSs are mainstay of systemic rx (Am Rev Respir Dis 1993;147:1598); other systemic agents sometimes effective include antimalarials for skin lesions (hydroxychloroquine 200 mg bid–qd), while monitoring eyes for retinal damage, and immunosuppressive agents, ie, MTX (Arch IM 1995;155:846); azathioprine; chlorambucil; a nonrandomized, open study showed efficacy of minocycline and doxycycline, 100 mg bid, in 12 cases of cutaneous sarcoid (Arch Derm 2001;137:69); care of pt requires multiple specialty consultations, esp dermatology, ophthalmology, pulmonary medicine.

3.3.P. XANTHOMA

Summary: Numerous variations; plasma lipid and lipoprotein abn are not specific to clinical appearance; however, certain clinical patterns exist: cutaneous *xanthomas* are yellow elevated lesions, except for deep *tendon* or *tuberous xanthomas* where skin is normal in color; **xanthelasma**: most common; about eyelids; 40% have abn serum lipids (see FACE, 6.9.i.); **eruptive xanthomas**: appear abruptly; over days to wks; elbows, knees, back, buttocks; yellow orange; size of split pea; itchy; nearly always assoc w serum lipid abn; may be assoc w uncontrolled DM, hypertriglyceridemia (types I, III, IV, V), or familial lipoprotein lipase deficiency; **palmar and planar xanthomas**: palms or body creases; assoc w type III hyperlipidemia, obstructive liver disease, or paraproteinemia; **tendon xanthomas**: deep within tendons or subcutaneous tissue; often assoc w ↑ cholesterol and ↑ low-density or β-lipoproteins; **tuberous xanthomas**: yellow to red, large firm nodules; extensor surfaces, assoc w ↑ cholesterol (type II) or triglycerides (Greer KE, Lipids, in Dermatological signs of internal disease, WB Saunders, Philadelphia, 1995).

3.3.Q. LEPROSY (HANSEN'S DISEASE)

Summary: Rare in U.S. (150 cases/yr); most cases are immigrants from Central and South America or tropical countries; 2 million affected worldwide, esp India, Brazil, Bangladesh, Indonesia; chronic granulomatous infection; caused by *Mycobacterium leprae*; clinical spectrum:

- *Early/indeterminate*: subtle; cutaneous; hypopigmented or hyperpigmented macules or plaques; patch may be anesthetic or paresthetic.

- *Tuberculoid*: early: may be hypopigmented hypoesthetic patch; later: anesthetic plaque w depressed center; single or few lesions; palpable peripheral nerves; assoc w neuritic pain, muscle atrophy, contractures, neurogenic ulcers.
- *Lepromatous*: extensive cutaneous involvement; variable lesions from macules to plaques; skin diffusely infiltrated and thickened; loss of lateral portions of eyebrows; late: lion-like facies; enlarged earlobes; nasal obstruction; hoarseness; septal perforation and nasal collapse; keratitis; LN↑; testicular scarring and sterility.

Dx and Rx: Not likely to be seen by PCPs; most often suspected because of an affected family member; dx: skin bx is most direct; dx and rx require a multidisciplinary approach.

4 Diaper Rash

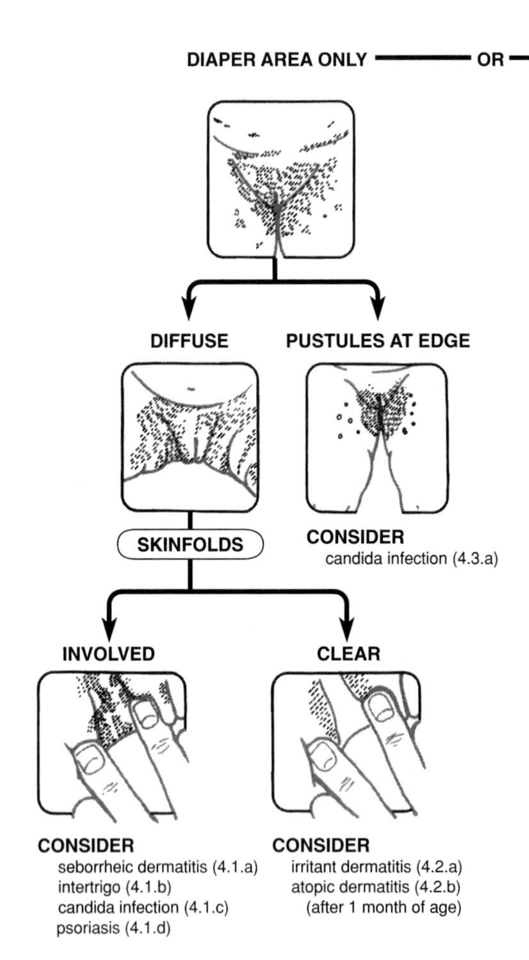

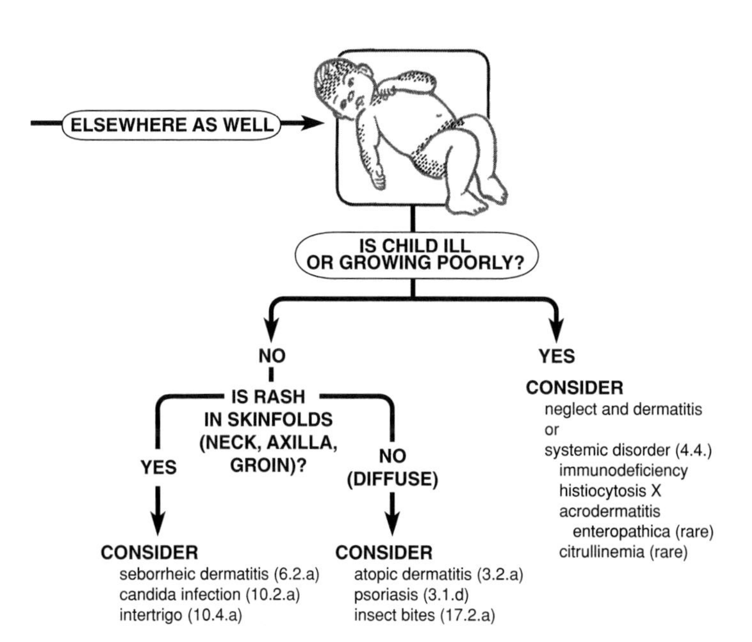

Note: If rash is present for longer than 3 weeks and does not respond to treatment, refer the patient to a pediatrician or dermatologist.

An occasional bout of diaper rash is common, and its presence usually has no significance. Persistent or erosive dermatitis in diaper area may indicate only that diaper has not been changed often enough, or it may be a sign of a systemic disorder, particularly if child also appears ill or is growing poorly.

DIAPER AREA ONLY, DIFFUSE RASH, SKINFOLDS INVOLVED

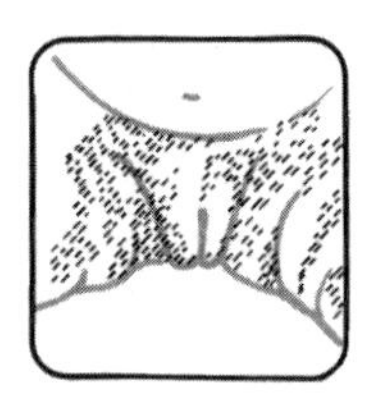

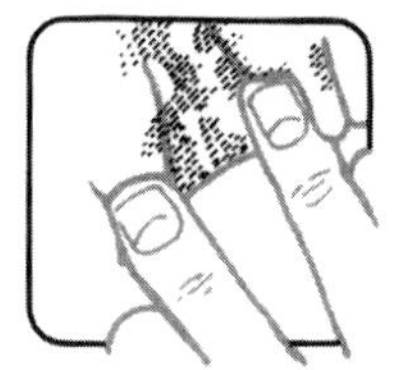

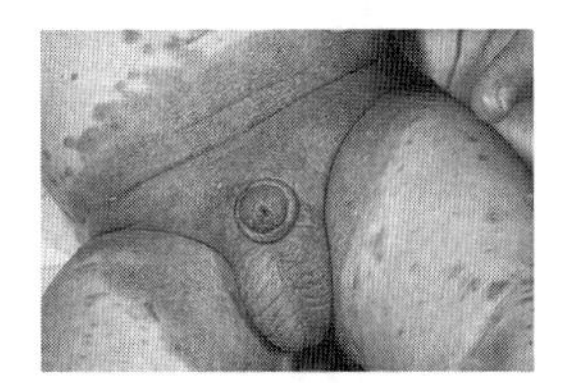

Seborrheic dermatitis

4.1.A. SEBORRHEIC DERMATITIS

Ddx: Pustules: consider *Candida* infection; petechiae plus rash: consider Letterer-Siwe form of histiocytosis X; severe and not responding to rx: consider psoriasis.

Si: Red, moist or glistening rash w yellowish greasy scale.

Crs: Infancy to age 1; occurs again at puberty.

Compl: Look for rash on scalp, face, neck, and axillae.

Rx: 1% HC cr or TCS (class VI–VII) sparingly w each diaper change; if not clearing, see Ddx.

4.1.B. INTERTRIGO

Cause: Heat, moisture, friction between rubbing skin surfaces; overdressing, tight-fitting plastic-covered diapers, hot moist weather; often a superimposed mixed bacterial or yeast infection.

Epidem: Mostly in summer or in hot, moist environment.

Si: Shiny, red, macerated, moist, uncomfortable; worse in folds where skin rubs skin; involved area sharply separated from normal skin.

Crs: Acute onset.

Lab: Neg KOH and Wood's light exam.

Rx: Reduce maceration and friction w temporary use of less occlusive diapers, ie, cloth diapers without a plastic cover; adsorbent dusting powder, ie, talc or miconazole nitrate (Zeasorb), and temporary use of a protective paste, ie, ZnOx paste or oint, or Desitin to keep urine and feces away from skin; apply oint thickly, like icing a cake, and reapply w each diaper change and hs; remove previously applied residue w mineral oil or "baby" oil on a cotton ball; if inflammation is severe, add 1% HC cr w each diaper change, before applying protective paste.

4.1.C. *CANDIDA* INFECTION

Summary: Moist, red, tender; edge often studded w tiny pustules; baby may have been on broad-spectrum antibiotics.

For additional details and rx, see 4.3.a. and GROIN RASH, 10.2.a.

4.1.D. PSORIASIS

Summary: Because of moist location, silvery scale typical of psoriasis is replaced by a red and glistening rash; asx or irritating and itchy; look for typical psoriasis elsewhere, esp scalp, to confirm dx but may be confined to diaper area, rx w low-potency TCS (class VI–VII), ie, 1%–2.5% HC cr, as more potent fluorinated TCSs may lead to atrophy and striae (see RX.5).

For additional details and rx, see BODY, 3.1.d.

DIAPER AREA ONLY, DIFFUSE RASH, SKINFOLDS CLEAR

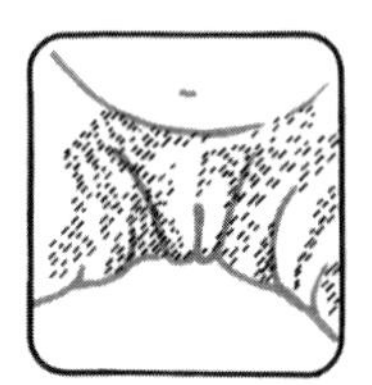

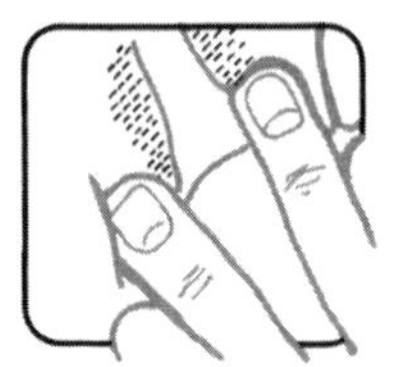

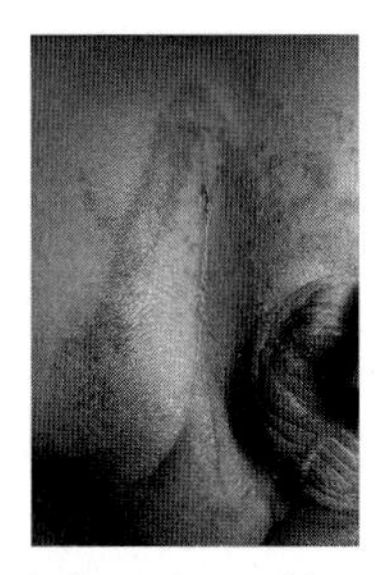

Irritant dermatitis

4.2.A. IRRITANT DERMATITIS

Cause: Irritants in urine and stool; occlusion by plastic-covered disposable diapers or by plastic covers over cloth diapers compounds heat, moisture, and irritation; soap and laundry detergent are not causes.

Sx: Uncomfortable.

Si: Shiny, red, moist; lower abdomen, perineum, buttocks, upper thighs; deeper portions of skinfolds are protected from irritation and are clear.

Compl: 2° infection w *Candida* is common (see 4.3.a.).

Rx: Same as for intertrigo (see 4.1.b.).

4.2.B. ATOPIC DERMATITIS

Sx: Itching except in diaper area.

Si: Redness, oozing, and scaly thickened skin widespread, esp on face, neck, and extensor surfaces of extremities, but diaper area is clear; child is irritable and sleeps poorly.

Crs: Not before 1–2 mo; only 1/3 of infants w atopic dermatitis persist w disorder during childhood.

Ddx: Dermatitis restricted to diaper area is not atopic dermatitis.

Rx: Cleanse diaper area w baby oil or mineral oil or a mild soap, ie, Basis; apply 1%–2.5% HC cr after each diaper change and cover cream w thick layer of ZnOx paste or oint to help retain TCS and minimize irritation from urine and feces.

For additional details and rx, see Body, 3.2.a.

DIAPER AREA ONLY, WITH PUSTULES

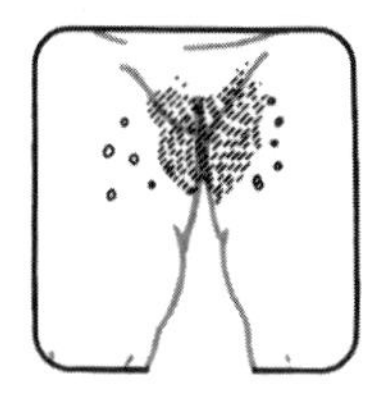

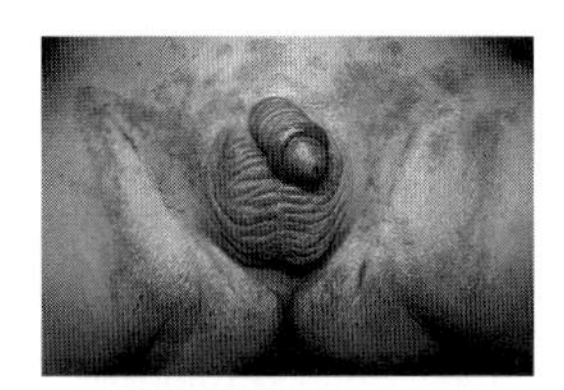

***Candida* infection**

4.3.A. *CANDIDA* INFECTION

Cause: Yeast, *Candida albicans*; warm, moist environment; common after systemic broad-spectrum antibiotics.

Si: Moist, beefy red; indistinct edge often studded w tiny pustules; look for thrush in mouth.

Crs: Acute, over a few days.

Lab: Generally rx on clinical suspicion; KOH prep (DX.3) from a macerated area or intact pustule shows short hyphae and spores in clumps and chains; culture is not useful as contamination is common.

Rx: Apply topical anticandidal agent (clotrimazole, econazole, miconazole, nystatin) (see RX.10.) w each diaper change; cover cr w ZnOx paste or oint thickly, like cake frosting, to adsorb serous oozing and protect skin from urine and feces (see RX.4.); if accompanying inflammation is severe, add 0.025% triamcinolone cr w antifungal agent for first few d; if oral candidal infection is present or diaper rash recurs, give nystatin oral suspension (100,000 units/mL, Rx 15 mL, $), using 1 mL qid for 3 d.

DIAPER AREA AND ELSEWHERE, CHILD NOT ILL

See algorithm.

DIAPER AREA AND ELSEWHERE, CHILD ILL/GROWING POORLY

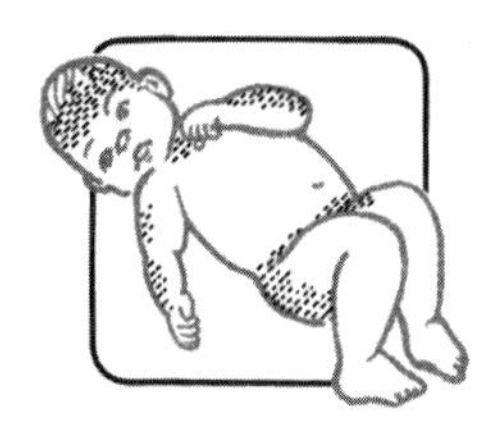

4.4. SYSTEMIC ILLNESS

None of the disorders described in this chapter are themselves causes of chronic illness or poor growth, although frequency of candidal infection is higher in sick children. Systemic disorders in which diaper dermatitis is associated w chronic illness or poor growth are rare. Systemic signs generally are so significant that need for pediatric or dermatologic consultation is evident. In general, consider referring to a dermatologist or pediatrician any infant w diaper dermatitis present for >3 wk and not responding to rx. Serious disorders associated w diaper dermatitis include immunodeficiency syndromes, histiocytosis X, acrodermatitis enteropathica (a zinc transport and deficiency syndrome), and citrullinemia.

5 Ear

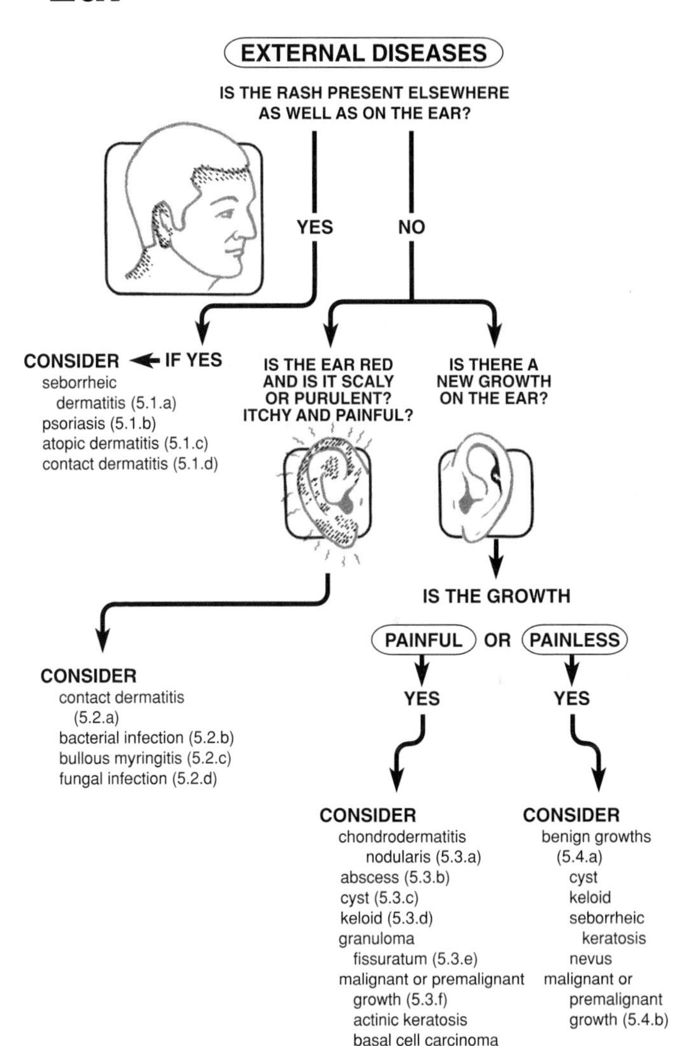

EXTERNAL DISEASES
IS THE RASH PRESENT ELSEWHERE AS WELL AS ON THE EAR?
YES
NO
CONSIDER
IF YES
seborrheic dermatitis (5.1.a)
psoriasis (5.1.b)
atopic dermatitis (5.1.c)
contact dermatitis (5.1.d)
IS THE EAR RED AND IS IT SCALY OR PURULENT? ITCHY AND PAINFUL?
IS THERE A NEW GROWTH ON THE EAR?
CONSIDER
contact dermatitis (5.2.a)
bacterial infection (5.2.b)
bullous myringitis (5.2.c)
fungal infection (5.2.d)
IS THE GROWTH
PAINFUL
OR
PAINLESS
YES
YES
CONSIDER
chondrodermatitis nodularis (5.3.a)
abscess (5.3.b)
cyst (5.3.c)
keloid (5.3.d)
granuloma fissuratum (5.3.e)
malignant or premalignant growth (5.3.f)
actinic keratosis
basal cell carcinoma
squamous cell carcinoma
melanoma
CONSIDER
benign growths (5.4.a)
cyst
keloid
seborrheic keratosis
nevus
malignant or premalignant growth (5.4.b)

Written in collaboration with Warren Rothman, MD, Assistant Professor of Otolaryngology, Head and Neck Surgery, The Johns Hopkins Medical Institutions, Baltimore, Maryland.

This chapter is limited to conditions of the external part of ear and ear canal up to the ear drum

Clin Oto 1997;22:497. Otol Clin N Am 1996;29:761. Otol Clin N Am 1996;29:783.

EAR RASH, RASH ELSEWHERE AS WELL

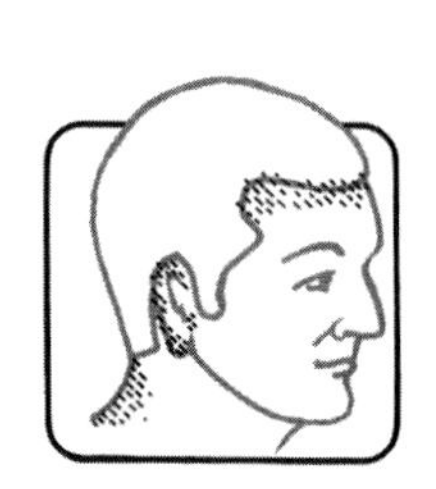

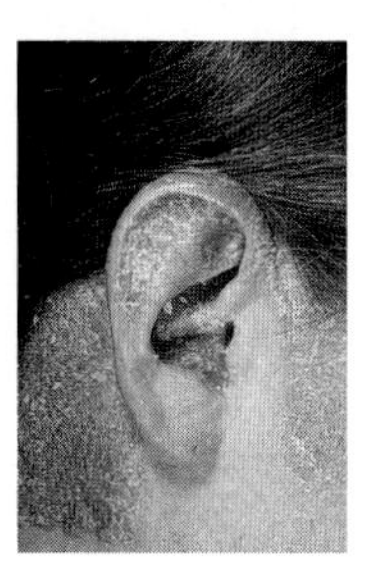

Psoriasis

5.1.A. SEBORRHEIC DERMATITIS

Summary: Usually diffuse but may be patchy; yellowish greasy scale; mild redness and itching; similar scale and itching often present on external auditory canal and postauricular areas; scalp, eyebrows, nasolabial fold.

For additional details and rx, see FACE, 6.2.a., and SCALP, 24.3.b.

5.1.B. PSORIASIS

Summary: Pink w coarse, silvery, nongreasy scale; external ear, canal; scaling may lead to partial closure; look for psoriasis elsewhere: scalp, elbows, knees, sacrum, nails; more resistant to rx than seborrheic dermatitis; TCS (class IV–V) lotion or soln, ie, fluocinolone soln (20 mL, 60 mL, $) bid; if resistant add calcipotriene soln (Dovonex, 60 mL, $$$) hs w TCS AM; refer persistent cases to dermatology or ENT.

For additional details and rx, see BODY, 3.1.d.

5.1.C. ATOPIC DERMATITIS

Summary: Behind ear, rather than canal or pinna; scaly, oozy, itchy; look for typical atopic dermatitis elsewhere; rx: TCS (class IV–V) cr or oint.

For additional details and rx, see BODY, 3.2.d.

5.1.D. CONTACT DERMATITIS

Summary: Confined to ears or present elsewhere as well; *acute*: red, scaly to weeping, crusty, edematous; *chronic*: scaly, pigmented, thickened (see 5.2.a.).

EAR

EAR RASH, NO RASH ELSEWHERE
RED AND SCALY/PURULENT, ITCHY/PAINFUL

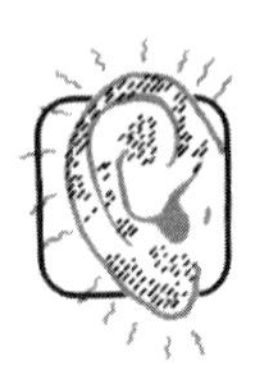

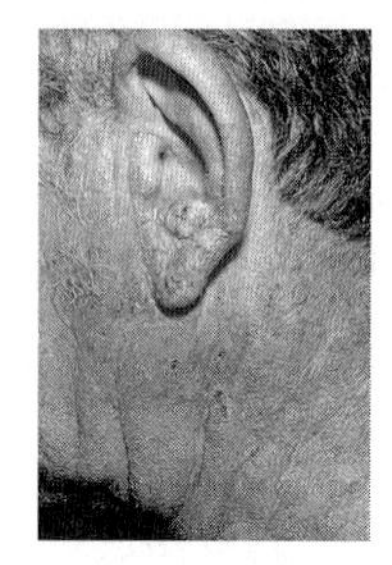

Contact dermatitis

5.2.A. CONTACT DERMATITIS

Oto Clin N Am 1998;31:157.

Cause: Irritant or allergen; use location as clue to cause:

- *Ear canal*: hearing aid mold or otic med, esp neomycin, or preservative, ie, paraben; rxns may be masked by TCS component in med.
- *Pinna*: poison ivy, ragweed, hair dyes, hair sprays, elastic headbands, hat.
- *Over or behind ear* (granuloma fissuratum, see 5.3.e.): eyeglass frames.
- *Lobes*: nickel, chromium, plastics in earrings; also look for dermatitis on wrists (watch and bracelets), fingers (rings), back (bra hooks), thighs (garter clips).

Sx: Itch.

Si: *Acute*: red and scaly to weeping, crusty, edematous; *chronic*: scaly, pigmented, thickened.

Lab: None necessary; allergy patch tests are available.

Rx: TCS (class IV–V) lotion or soln; eliminate suspected irritants or allergens.

For additional details and rx, see BODY, 3.1.a.

5.2.B. BACTERIAL INFECTION (SWIMMER'S EAR)

Cause: Most common: *Pseudomonas aeruginosa, Staphylococcus aureus.*

Epidem: Hot moist environment, often w ear-picking habit; may be severe w immunosuppression, DM (Inf Dis Clin NA 1995;9:195).

Sx: Itchy initially, then painful.

Si: *Gram-neg bacteria*: edema, purulent secretion, greenish w foul musty smell; *gram-pos bacteria*: localized abscess, yellowish crusting or ulceration w painful LN↑; hearing loss from edema or debris.

Crs: Acute, over days.

Compl: Look for perforated eardrum before using topical meds; if perforated, refer to ENT; also, refer if infection does not respond, recurs, or if hearing loss persists; *malignant form*: immunosuppressed pts; may invade bone, brain.

Lab: Obtain a culture for bacteria and fungi if resistant to rx or refer to ENT.

Rx:

- Red, scaly pinna only: compress w warm Domeboro's otic soln tid (60 mL) followed by 4 drops of an antibiotic soln (polymyxin B (Aerosporin), Cortisporin, or gentamicin sulfate (Garamycin), 10 mL); expect resolution in 5–7 d.
- Abscess: refer to ENT or I&D w culture for bacteria and fungi, followed by systemic antibiotic, ie, dicloxacillin (250 mg qid × 10 d) or cefuroxime (250 mg bid × 10 d).
- Canal swollen shut: refer to ENT for insertion of wick; no swimming until infection has subsided and pus and erythema have cleared.

5.2.C. BULLOUS MYRINGITIS

Clin Oto 1997;22:497.

Cause: Unknown; may be viral, *Mycoplasma pneumoniae*, other bacteria; all present w same clinical pattern.

Sx: Pain.

Si: Bloody discharge; hemorrhagic vesicles in tympanic membrane, external canal.

Crs: Lasts about 7 d, regardless of therapy.

Lab: Not necessary.

Rx: Auralgan, 4 drops tid (10 mL, $); pain medication, ie, codeine; myringotomy is contraindicated; advise early referral to ENT.

5.2.D. FUNGAL INFECTIONS

Oto Clin N Am 993;26:995.

Cause: Most common: *Aspergillus niger*; also: *Candida albicans*; assoc w moisture and chronic trauma.

Sx: Itch.

Si: *A. niger*: thick scaling of concha skin w desquamating skin in ear canal w gray membrane and black spots (spores); *C. albicans*: creamy white discharge.

Crs: Chronic, unless treated.

Rx: Irrigate to remove all necrotic debris and mycelium w lukewarm water; clotrimazole (Lotrimin) drops and systemic itraconazole (Sporanox) may be helpful; avoid antibiotic and HC ear drops; if not cleared in 1 wk, refer to ENT.

NEW GROWTH, PAINFUL

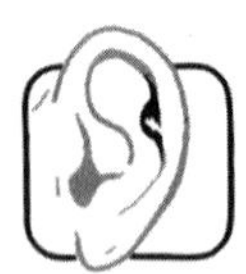

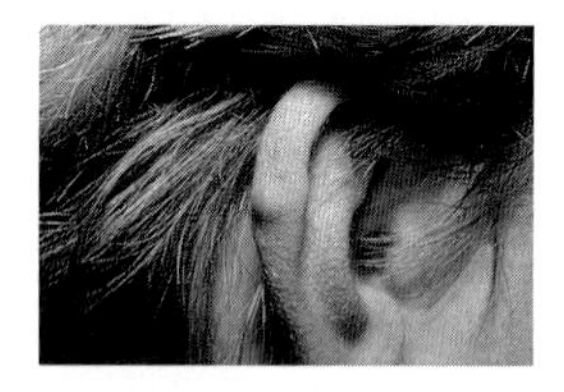

Chondrodermatitis nodularis

5.3.A. CHONDRODERMATITIS NODULARIS

Cause: Spontaneous or follows chronic trauma.

Epidem: Usually >40 yo.

Sx: Pain may interfere w sleeping or use of telephone.

Si: Solitary, painful, localized nodule often w erosion or hard crust on rim.

Crs: Chronic.

Rx: TCS cr class II or III w occlusion or a tape w steroid incorporated in adhesive (Cordran tape, 60 or 200 cm, Rx, $$), applied for 36 h and removed for 12 h to prevent maceration; for unresponsive cases, inject about 0.2 mL triamcinolone acetonide (Kenalog, 10 mg/mL) diluted to 5 mg/mL w saline; if 2 monthly injections do not produce relief, excision often gives permanent cure.

5.3.B. ABSCESS

Summary: Intensely painful; develops quickly (see 5.2.b.).

5.3.C. CYST

Summary: Usually behind ear or in earlobe.

For additional details and rx, see GROWTHS, 11.3.a.

5.3.D. KELOID

Cause: Nearly always follows trauma, most commonly ear piercing.

Epidem: Any race; blacks >> whites.

Sx: Painless to tender.

Si: Firm, fleshy, lump within or protruding from earlobe at site of ear piercing.

Crs: Grows for few mo, then persists.
Rx: If painful, often responds to IL injections w 10 mg/mL triamcinolone acetonide (use 1 mL Luer-lock tuberculin syringe and enough material to bulge out the keloid, repeat monthly for 3 mo); may require referral for surgical removal but recurrence is high; discourage attempts to repierce a treated ear.

5.3.E. GRANULOMA FISSURATUM

Cause: Chronic irritation or allergic rxn to eyeglass frames.
Sx: Discomfort.
Si: Fleshy lesion, in groove behind 1 or both ears.
Crs: Chronic and persistent.
Rx: Optician can modify frames or change to lighter plastic lenses; if concerned about skin cancer: bx or refer to dermatology or ENT.

5.3.F. MALIGNANT OR PREMALIGNANT GROWTHS

Summary: Often painless, but painful if eroded or infected; mostly men >50 yo w light complexions; upper outer rim of ear (most sun-exposed area); scaly, crusty, slowly growing; also look for actinic damage on face and hands (see 5.4.b.).

NEW GROWTH, PAINLESS

5.4.A. BENIGN GROWTHS

Ddx: Cyst, keloid, seborrheic keratosis, nevus, wart.

5.4.B. MALIGNANT OR PREMALIGNANT GROWTHS

Cause: Excessive occupational and/or recreational sun exposure.

Epidem: Mostly men >50 yo w light complexions.

Sx: Painful or painless.

Si: Upper outer rim of ear (most sun-exposed area); scaly, crusty, slowly growing; also actinic damage on face and hands.

- Actinic keratosis: low-grade premalignancy.
- BCE or SCC: thickened or dome-shaped lesion w central delling, necrosis, or crusting.
- Malignant melanoma: usually deeply pigmented.

Rx: Generally refer for bx and surgery.

6 Face

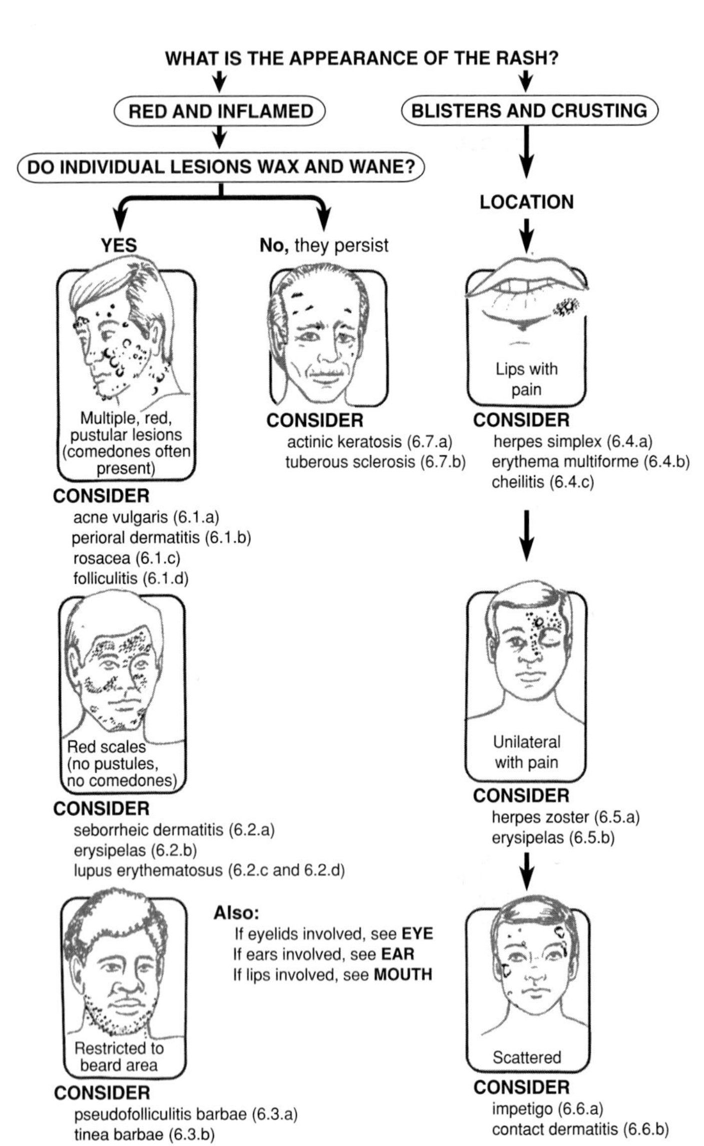

WHAT IS THE APPEARANCE OF THE RASH?
RED AND INFLAMED
BLISTERS AND CRUSTING
DO INDIVIDUAL LESIONS WAX AND WANE?
LOCATION
YES
No, they persist
Multiple, red, pustular lesions (comedones often present)
CONSIDER
acne vulgaris (6.1.a)
perioral dermatitis (6.1.b)
rosacea (6.1.c)
folliculitis (6.1.d)
Red scales (no pustules, no comedones)
CONSIDER
seborrheic dermatitis (6.2.a)
erysipelas (6.2.b)
lupus erythematosus (6.2.c and 6.2.d)
Restricted to beard area
CONSIDER
pseudofolliculitis barbae (6.3.a)
tinea barbae (6.3.b)
CONSIDER
actinic keratosis (6.7.a)
tuberous sclerosis (6.7.b)
Also:
If eyelids involved, see EYE
If ears involved, see EAR
If lips involved, see MOUTH
Lips with pain
CONSIDER
herpes simplex (6.4.a)
erythema multiforme (6.4.b)
cheilitis (6.4.c)
Unilateral with pain
CONSIDER
herpes zoster (6.5.a)
erysipelas (6.5.b)
Scattered
CONSIDER
impetigo (6.6.a)
contact dermatitis (6.6.b)

PRESENT SINCE CHILDHOOD OR PRESENT FOR YEARS AND UNCHANGED

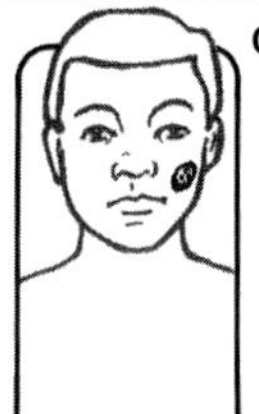

CONSIDER

- freckles or lentigines (6.8.a)
- melanocytic nevus (6.8.b)
- hemangioma (6.8.c)
- hereditary hemorrhagic telangiectasia (6.8.d)
- tuberous sclerosis (6.8.e)
- fibroma (6.8.f)
- seborrheic keratosis (6.8.g)
- dermatosis papulosa nigra (6.8.h)
- sweat gland tumor (6.8.i)
- cyst, dermoid (6.8.j)

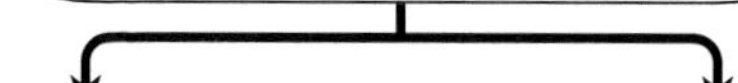

MULTIPLE

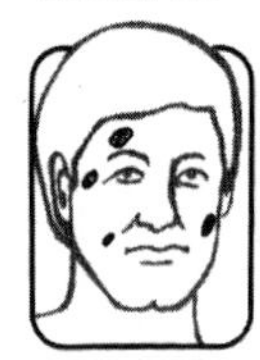

CONSIDER

- actinic keratosis (6.9.a)
- cyst (6.9.b)
- milia (6.9.c)
- molluscum contagiosum (6.9.d)
- nevus (6.9.e)
- sarcoid (6.9.f)
- seborrheic keratosis (6.9.g)
- wart, flat and filiform (6.9.h)
- xanthelasma (6.9.i)
- sebaceous hyperplasia (6.9.j)

SINGLE

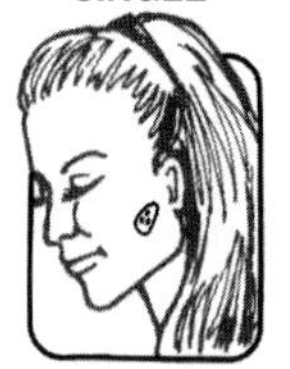

CONSIDER

- wart, filiform (6.10.a)
- fibroma (6.10.b)
- melanocytic nevus (6.10.c)
- seborrheic keratosis (6.10.d)
- pyogenic granuloma (6.10.e)
- skin cancer (6.10.f)
  - Bowen's disease (6.10.f.1)
  - basal cell carcinoma (6.10.f.2)
  - squamous cell carcinoma (6.10.f.3)
  - melanoma (6.10.f.4)

RASH, RED AND INFLAMED, LESIONS WAX AND WANE, PUSTULES

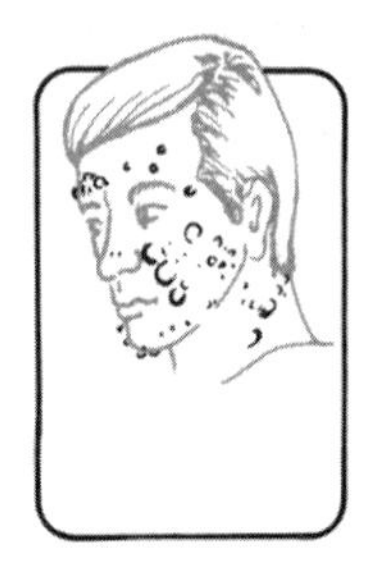

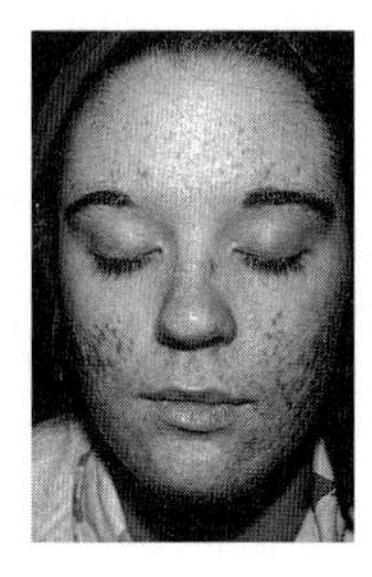

Acne

6.1.A. ACNE VULGARIS

Med Clin N Am 1998;82:1145. J Am Acad Derm 1994;31:826. Ped Derm 1991;8:332.

Cause: Disorder of sebaceous glands, initiated by androgens, usually at puberty, but also premenopausal; bacteria and their toxins also play a role, esp *Staphylococcus epidermidis* and an anaerobic diphtheroid, *Corynebacterium acnes*; systemic meds: CSs, androgenic steroids, phenytoin, iodide-containing decongestants, lithium, most low-dose bcp's do not cause acne to worsen; external causes: irritants, ie, creosote, tar, and industrial cutting oils can produce an acneiform eruption on exposed areas of face, arms, thighs (**chloracne**); acne at forehead and cheeks near the hairline, esp in blacks, may be caused or maintained by use of hair pomades (**pomade acne**); acne on the face in 20–40-yo women may be continuing by use of moisturizers, cold cr, heavy foundations, or use of waterless cleansing preparations, rather than soap and water (**acne cosmetica**).

Epidem: Nearly all adolescents have some degree of acne; boys = girls but often worse in boys.

Sx: Painful if lesions are deep; embarrassment.

Si: Areas involved are those where sebaceous glands are largest and most dense: face, chest, back; *comedone*: earliest visible sign of acne vulgaris; this blockage of sebaceous gland ducts produces engorgement that leads to raised, red *papules*; if gland walls leak or rupture, inflammation in surrounding tissue leads to *pustules*; some pts develop intensely inflammatory *nodules* or *cysts* deep in the dermis or in subcutaneous tissue (conglobate or **cystic acne**); such nodular and cystic lesions may evolve into depressed scars or epidermal inclusion cysts (see GROWTHS, 11.3.a.); cystic acne on the face is often accompanied by cysts elsewhere, particularly on the trunk and scalp, as well as by apocrine gland infections in the axillae and groin (see AXILLA, 1.3.b.).

Crs: Starts in early adolescence; may persist into adulthood or develop for first time in adults, esp premenopausal women.

Lab: Unnecessary except to r/o androgen excess in young woman w hirsutism (see HAIR INCREASE, 13.), high BP, irregular or absent periods; bacterial culture is rarely needed except if gram-neg folliculitis is suspected in a pt on long-standing broad-spectrum antibiotics.

Rx: OTC benzoyl peroxide is moderately effective for mild acne; for pt who comes to physician because acne is not responding to home rx, follow the plans outlined below. Goals of rx are to reduce number of lesions and to prevent scarring, physically and psychologically; complete clearing is not achievable in teenagers in midst of puberty.

General Measures: Firstly, discuss directly with the teenager that acne is not their fault, that it is not caused by poor hygiene or faulty diet but by normal hormonal changes. Secondly, since half of teenagers believe that acne is "curable" (Jaad 2001;44:439), help them understand that you cannot "switch off" acne but that you will do everything possible to control infection and scarring. Thirdly, tell them that any results from rx take at least 2 months to see. Instruct pt to wash face bid or tid gently w fingertips, rather than scrubbing or using an abrasive pad or machine, since such actions may rupture lesions within the skin, brand of soap is not important as soap removes only surface oils; suggest frequent hair washing, even daily washing does not harm hair; for women: advise selection of cosmetics labeled both "water based and oil free" while encouraging avoidance of all foundations, cold cr, and moisturizers; blusher and eye shadow do not seem to cause difficulties.

Mild Comedonal Acne: Comedones w few reddened papules but no pustules or cysts:

- Benzoyl peroxide, a desquamating and antibacterial agent (Benoxyl; Desquam-X or -E 5%–10% cr; Pan-Oxyl lotion; Persadox lotion, cr; Triaz gel; Xerac BP gel; all $); generally start w 5% concentration and tell pt to apply hs w a fingertip to entire face, not just lesions; some dryness during the d should become evident after 2 wk; overuse leads to erythema and uncomfortable peeling, not necessary for improvement; ↑ or ↓ % (2.5%–10%) as tolerated; older women may find benzoyl peroxide preparations too drying.
- Women: stop or curtail use of foundation cosmetics, cleansing cr, moisturizers; encourage soap and water washing w a mild nondetergent soap, ie, Dove, Ivory, or Purpose.

Mild Acne That Does Not Improve with Benzoyl Peroxide by 2 Mo or Acne Treated with Benzoyl Peroxide without Benefit before Pt Comes to Office:

- Topical retinoid (Avita cr, gel; Retin-A cr, gel, soln; Retin-A Micro; Differin gel, soln Tazorac cr, gel 0.05%, 0.1%, all $$$); retinoids interfere w follicular duct keratinization; all can be irritating so start qod hs and ↑ to qd as tolerated; applied to entire face, not just lesions; initial temporary flares may occur; expect some dryness but redness and peeling are not necessary for rx to be effective; advise blacks that excessive dryness and irritation may lead to temporary darkening of skin; advise pt to stop topical retinoids before concentrated sun exposure, ie, before a vacation at the beach; may be used in combination w below.
- Topical antibiotic: clindamycin (Cleocin T gel, lotion, soln); erythromycin (generic or A/T/S, Erygel, Emgel, Theramycin gel, soln); Benzamycin (erythromycin and benzoyl peroxide) (all $$); pt applies to entire face qd–bid; sodium sulfacetamide and sulfur (Sulfacet-R lotion w or w/o a tinted base).

Inflammatory Papular and Pustular Acne: Papules and pustules w comedones but no deep nodules or cysts.

- Use topical rx as outlined above and add a systemic antibiotic: tetracycline is the standard (about 1/4 of tetracycline prescribed in U.S. is used for rx of acne); *women*: no more than 250 mg qd or bid as higher doses may induce vaginal yeast infection, esp in women taking bcp's (interactions between antibiotic and bcp's are unproved); *men*: 1 gm/d and up to 3 gm/d if acne is severe and unresponsive to lower doses; tetracycline is best absorbed on an empty stomach, but pts who experience nausea may need to take med w food; once improved, slowly decrease dose as tolerated; drug has proved safe when taken for long periods, although resistance does develop.

- If tetracycline proves ineffective after 2 mo, alternative antibiotics include: erythromycin, minocycline, cephalexin, and ampicillin.

WARNINGS: Cycline antibiotics are incorporated into developing bones and teeth and stain and weaken them; as this does not happen until the 3rd mo of pregnancy, women may be placed on antibiotics but should be warned to stop them if they suspect they may be pregnant; cyclines also are phototoxic and cause ↑ risk of burning on sun exposure; an infrequent complication of broad-spectrum antibiotics is gram-neg folliculitis; watch for sudden worsening of acne and appearance of superficial and/or deep pustules, often worse about the nose; culture and appropriate antibiotics usually resolve this complication; minocycline has been assoc w serum sickness–like rxns and lupus-like syndrome in young acne pts (Arch IM 1999;159:493; Arch Derm 1996;132:934).

Nodular and Cystic Acne: Initial rx is systemic antibiotics as outlined above; for pts who are unresponsive or who are developing scars consider systemic isotretinoin (Accutane, 10/20/40 mg, $$$$); usual dose: 0.5–2 mg/kg for 4–6 mo; clears or greatly improves nearly all cases but 30% have mild recurrence needing topical or systemic rx again and 20% require re-rx w isotretinoin, esp teenage pts (Arch Derm 1998;134:376); side effects are universal: cheilitis, xerosis, dry eyes, nose bleeds, and less commonly, decreased night vision, reversible corneal opacities, inflammatory bowel disease, musculoskeletal sx, hair thinning, headache, depression (Jama 1998:279:1057) and suicidal thoughts; Labs: watch for ↑ lipids, LFTs, and ↓ RBCs and WBCs, but alterations that lead to discontinuation of the drug are infrequent (Br J Derm 1993;129:704).

WARNINGS:

- Additional warnings about depression and suicidal thoughts were added to the consent form by Roche and the FDA in 2001. Physicians prescribing Accutane must use these forms, available from Roche Medical Services at 1.800.526.6367; this issue remains controversial as large studies find no evidence for an association (Arch Derm 2000;136:1231).

- Isotretinoin is teratogenic; women of childbearing age must be on adequate birth control and monitored following guidelines of the FDA and Roche Pharmaceuticals (800.526.6367); suggested blood tests: pregnancy tests in women, blood lipids, liver enzymes; most side effects reverse shortly after rx stops, but may persist.

Additional Measures: Often used by dermatologists; include: expression of comedones; I&D or IL CS injection of cysts; superficial freezing w LN2; surgical, laser, or collagen injection of scars; estrogen-dominant anovulatory agents (ie, Ortho Tri-Cyclen) give some benefit. Refer pts w resistant or severe acne to a dermatologist.

6.1.B. PERIORAL DERMATITIS

Cause: Unclear but TCSs have been blamed.

Epidem: Almost always women 20–35 yo.

Sx: Mild discomfort if inflamed papules are present.

Si: Papular and mild pustular acneiform eruption, usually restricted to lower part of face, esp about lips and chin; area adjacent to lips often remains clear; some cases overlap w mild rosacea.

Crs: Chronic unless rx'd.

Ddx: Acne, rosacea.

Rx: Doxycycline 100 mg qd for 6 wk then tapered over another 6 wk, in combination w topical antibiotics (see 6.1.a.).

6.1.C. ROSACEA

Arch Derm 1998;134:679.

Cause: Not proved but may be infection w or sensitivity to *Pityrosporum ovale*; association w *Helicobacter pylori* infection not proved (Arch Derm 1999;135:659); most pts have a light complexion and blush easily, blushing further stimulated by alcoholic drinks and hot beverages (J Invest Derm 1981;76:15).

Epidem: Women > men; severity: men > women; age: most >35 yo.
Sx: Mild discomfort from inflammatory papules.
Si: Red papules and pustules w/o comedones; intermittent flushing is common; worse about central part of face; telangiectasia and persistent redness eventually appear; ocular or eyelid irritation is present in 1/4.
Crs: Progressive w flares assoc w ingesting hot, spicy foods or beverages, or alcoholic drinks; recurrences are common and long-term rx or repeated courses of several mo of med often are required; erythema and telangiectasia do not respond.
Compl: Chronic inflammation about nose may lead to a permanent, bulbous, tomato-like enlargement (**rhinophyma**).
Rx: Topical metronidazole (Metrocream, gel, lotion; Noritate cr, Rx, $$) hs–bid may be sufficient; response is slow, over 4–12 wk; if more severe, or unresponsive to topicals, or if eyes are involved, add tetracycline (250 mg) or doxycycline (100 mg) qd–bid (Arch Derm 1997;133:89); again, control is slow requiring 1–2 mo of rx; dose of oral med may then be reduced or dc'd depending on control; TCS (class VI–VII) may be needed to reduce irritation, but avoid more potent fluorinated TCSs which may lead to more telangiectasias; rx of *H. pylori* not helpful (Arch Derm 1999;135:659); consider referral to dermatologist if dx is uncertain or if rosacea is severe or resistant to rx.

6.1.D. FOLLICULITIS

Summary: Minute pustules centered at hair follicles; most of no significance as lesions usually heal quickly w/o scarring; consider gram-neg folliculitis in pts on broad-spectrum antibiotics (see 6.1.a.); and pseudofolliculitis barbae (see 6.3.a.).

RASH, RED AND INFLAMED, LESIONS WAX AND WANE, SCALY/NO PUSTULES

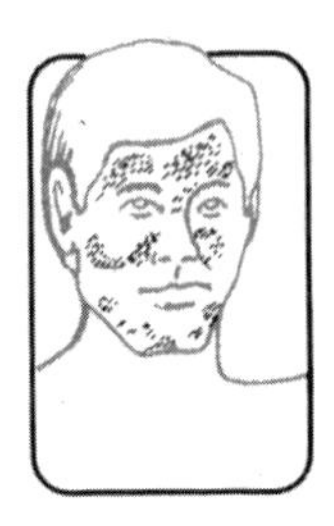

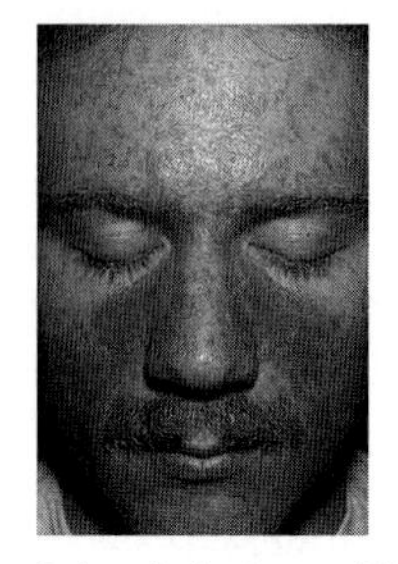

Seborrheic dermatitis

See color plate section.

6.2.A. SEBORRHEIC DERMATITIS

Cause: Unknown, but probably an infection or sensitivity to *P. ovale*; distribution of the disorder is same as distribution of large sebaceous glands: scalp, face, ears, eyebrows, chest, axillae, groin.

Epidem: Both sexes are affected; frequently seen in pts w neurologic disorder, esp Parkinson's disease, or after CVA, acute MI, or other acute medical illness.

Si: Erythema and yellow greasy scale, worse on middle of face, esp the nose, nasolabial folds, eyebrows, and other regions of large sebaceous glands.

Crs: May appear in infants up to 6 mo old; after that it does not appear until puberty; can persist or 1st appear in old age; most cases periodically clear and worsen; if unresponsive to rx and risk factors are present, consider seborrheic dermatitis as an early sign of HIV infection (see HIV, 15.).

Lab: None are useful or necessary.

Rx: Control usually can be achieved w a combination of topical ketoconazole cr or shampoo (Nizoral, $$) and TCS (class VI–VII); "cure" is not possible, but most pts respond adequately and can be maintained w minimal rx; avoid more potent fluorinated TCSs, which may induce persistent erythema and telangiectasia; for scalp involvement, see SCALP, 24.3.b.

6.2.B. ERYSIPELAS

Nejm 1996;334:240.

Cause: Usually *Streptococcus pyogenes*, but a few cases are caused by *S. aureus*.

Epidem: May follow skin wound; promoted by any systemic debility, ie, DM or malnutrition.

Sx: Pain.

Si: Rapidly spreading, single, warm, red, plaque w a sharp, indurated, advancing border often starting on the cheek or about the nose, but can appear anywhere; skin may look puckered, like an orange peel; regional LN↑; pt is toxic w chills and fever.

Crs: Sudden onset; pt becomes febrile and toxic within day; desquamation follows.

Compl: Infection may spread to viscera.

Lab: Culture any visible wound; consider blood cultures if pt is toxic; organisms sometimes may be recovered by injecting about 0.25 mL sterile saline into the advancing edge of the lesion and withdrawing fluid for culture; ASO titers do not ↑ after streptococcal skin infections; consider late glomerulonephritis, esp w epidemic streptococcal infection.

Rx: Do not wait for pos bacterial culture before starting rx; *infections w/o toxicity*: penicillin V (500 mg qid) or erythromycin (250–500 mg qid) orally; *infections and toxicity*: iv or im penicillin G (0.6–2 million units q 6 h × 10 d); if *S. aureus* is recovered, select an antibiotic according to sensitivities of the organism.

6.2.C. LUPUS ERYTHEMATOSUS, DISCOID (DLE)

Arch Derm 1994;130:1308. J Am Acad Derm 1993;28:477.

Cause: Local tissue autoantibodies; systemic antibodies are less common but 20% are ANA pos, generally at low titer, and 20% have antibody to ssDNA.

Epidem: Women >> men.

Sx: Minimal.

Si: Demarcated, pink to red, slightly scaly, round (*discoid*) plaques that often develop areas of atrophy on portions of the surface, esp the center, which becomes shiny, depressed, depigmented, hairless; telangiectasias on and about the plaques; worse on light-exposed parts, ie, face, scalp, and ear; hallmark lesions appear in the external ear canal.

Crs: Chronic; often worsens w sun exposure; leaves depigmented, depressed, disfiguring scars; conversion from DLE to SLE is uncommon, occurring in <5%.

Lab: Skin bx w DIF is diagnostic of DLE or SLE; obtain ANA as screen for SLE; neg ANA is strong but not absolute evidence against SLE; if ANA titer pos: obtain more specific tests, esp anti-dsDNA (native dsDNA) and anti-ENAs, which detects RNP and Sm; anti-dsDNA and anti-Sm are highly specific for SLE; anti-RNP is present in 100% of pts w *mixed connective tissue disease*; low (<1:40) titer is assoc w absence of SLE; C′ is normal in uncomplicated DLE; obtain RFTs and LFTs to establish baseline.

Rx: Treat to prevent or minimize disfigurement; restrict sunlight exposure w clothing and sunscreens (see RX.16.); TCSs usually are adequate, but some pts benefit from antimalarials (hydroxychloroquine 200 mg qd–bid); pts w DLE who smoke are less responsive to antimalarial rx (Jaad 2000;42:983); eye exams q 6–12 mo if on antimalarials; pts w DLE usually are followed by a dermatologist.

6.2.D. LUPUS ERYTHEMATOSUS, SYSTEMIC

Summary: Malar rash is characteristic of SLE but is nearly always accompanied by systemic si and sx of the disorder (see FEVER, 8.3.a.).

RASH, RED AND INFLAMED, LESIONS WAX AND WANE, BEARD AREA ONLY

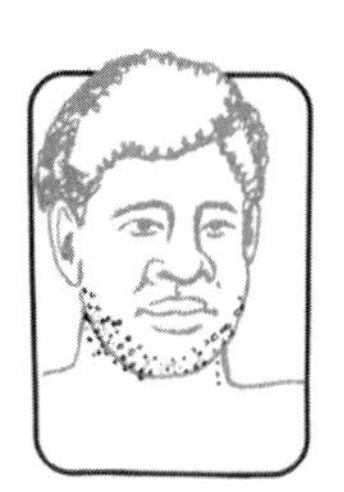

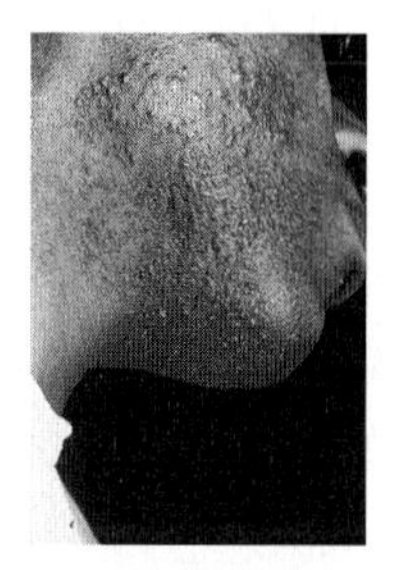

Pseudofolliculitis barbae

FACE

6.3.A. PSEUDOFOLLICULITIS BARBAE (PFB)

Cause: In-curving beard hairs, sharpened by shaving, push into skin adjacent to the hair follicle, hence the term "pseudo" folliculitis; ingrown hairs produce an inflammatory, foreign body rxn.

Epidem: Mostly black men but present in some whites and women.

Sx: Chronic irritation.

Si: Red to hyperpigmented papules and acne-like pustules neatly restricted to beard area.

Crs: Chronic and troublesome w continued shaving.

Lab: None.

Rx: "Cured" by growing a beard; partially controlled by changes in shaving method: use shaving techniques that do not give an overly close shave, do not stretch skin while shaving to prevent cutting beard below the surface, try an adjustable electric razor set at its least close shave position or a PFB razor (American Safety Razor Co., Staunton, VA), which does not allow close shaving, or a chemical depilatory to soften and remove beard hairs, including penetrating hair; additional relief w TCS (class VI–VII) cr after shaving or w topical antibiotics as used for acne vulgaris (see 6.1.a.).

6.3.B. TINEA BARBAE

Summary: Fungal infections of beard area are uncommon, but should be considered in any inflammatory and pustular dermatitis of beard area, esp in immunosuppressed pts and insulin-dependent DM; may be acquired from household pets or livestock.

For additional details and rx, see BODY, 3.1.g.

BLISTERS/CRUSTING INVOLVING LIPS (WITH PAIN)

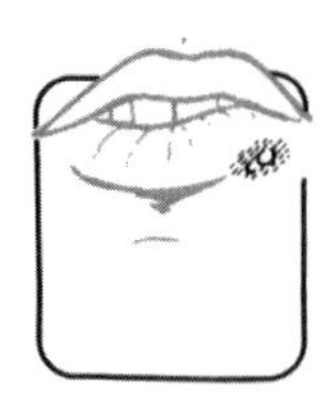

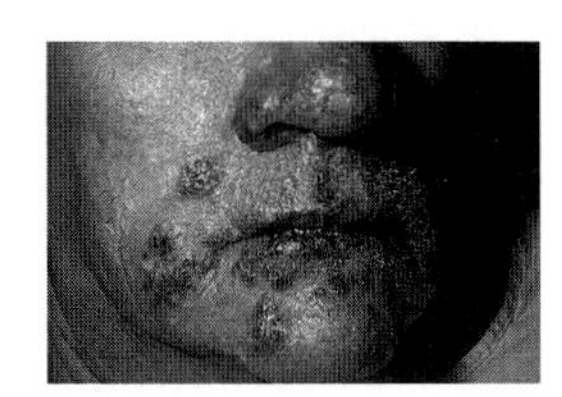

Herpes simplex

6.4.A. HERPES SIMPLEX

Summary: Groups of pinhead-sized blisters on lip, usually at vermilion border; hx of recurrence at same or nearly same site; may be assoc w malaise; LN↑.

For additional details and rx, see BLISTERS, 2.1.a.

6.4.B. ERYTHEMA MULTIFORME

Summary: Painful mucous membrane erosions, involving lip as well as any site within mouth; look for target-like skin lesions; ask about previous episodes.

For additional details and rx, see BLISTERS, 2.1.b.

6.4.C. CHEILITIS

Summary: Chapped cracked lips may be caused by repeated moistening and drying or may be induced by irritation or allergy from lipstick, toothpaste, or mouthwash.

For additional details and rx, see MOUTH, 19.8.f.

FACE

BLISTERS/CRUSTING, UNILATERAL (WITH PAIN)

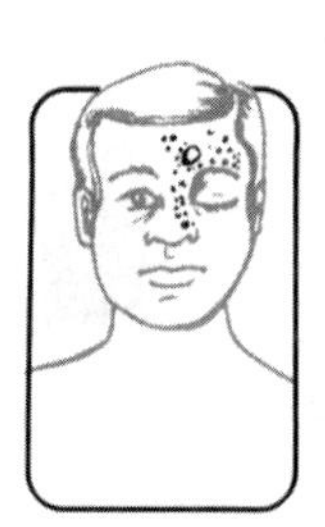

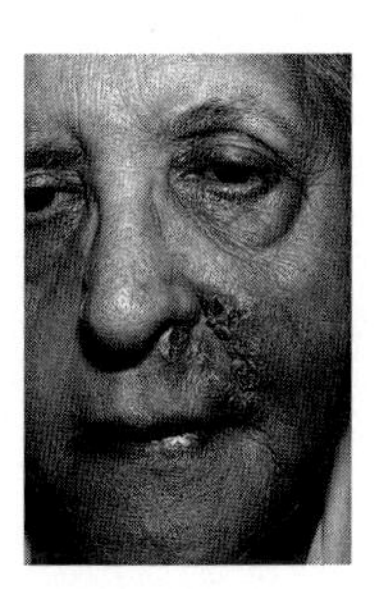

Zoster

6.5.A. ZOSTER (SHINGLES)

Summary: Prodrome of tingling, tenderness, or itch restricted to a nerve segment and lasting 1–4 d; grouped small blisters, each w a central dell; sharply demarcated at midline, following distribution of peripheral nerve; blisters on tip of nose indicate involvement of anterior ethmoidal branch of the nasociliary nerve, a sign that cornea is involved; **Ramsey-Hunt syndrome**: unilateral facial paralysis w auditory sx, herpes infection of geniculate ganglia.

If area about eye or tip of nose is involved or there are eye sx, refer to ophthalmology.

For additional details and rx, see BLISTERS, 2.3.d.

6.5.B. ERYSIPELAS

Summary: Rapidly spreading bacterial infection; warm, red, tender plaque; pt is febrile and toxic; for details and rx, see 6.2.b.

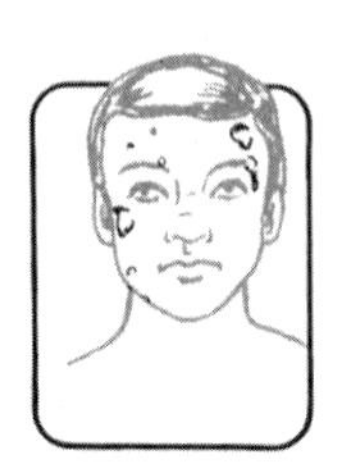

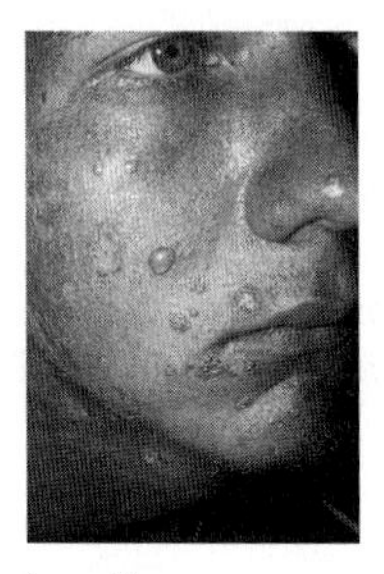

Impetigo

6.6.A. IMPETIGO

Ped Derm 1994;11:293.

Cause: Bacterial; *crusty* form: usually group A β-hemolytic streptococci; *blistering* form: *S. aureus* or *S. pyogenes.*

Epidem: Spreads from upper respiratory tract of carriers; also look for inciting cause, ie, pediculosis capitis or an infected playmate; highly contagious; school or daycare center should be informed.

Sx: From mildly irritating to painful.

Si: Either honey-colored crusts or blisters; most common on face; most cases are young children; may be regional LN↑; usually afebrile.

Crs: Abrupt onset w rapid spreading of new lesions; persists until rx'd; heals w/o scarring.

Compl: Glomerulonephritis may follow infection w epidemic streptococcal species; rheumatic fever does not follow streptococcal skin infections.

Lab:. Bacterial cultures generally not needed but may be done in epidemic outbreaks to identify presence of nephritogenic strains.

Rx: *Mild and few lesions*: topical rx usually suffices: soap and water cleansing tid followed by topical mupirocin (Bactroban, Rx, $$); *widespread lesions or epidemic*: systemic rx: penicillin or erythromycin is generally adequate, for streptococci; *staphylococci*: semisynthetic penicillin (dicloxacillin or cephalexin 12.5 mg/kg/d for children or 250 mg qid for adults × 10 d); identify and rx carriers; intranasal mupirocin bid × 5 d for pt and potential carriers (Clin Infect Dis 1993;17:466).

6.6.B. CONTACT DERMATITIS

See color plate section.

Cause: Common because of the wide variety of allergens to which the face is exposed: cosmetics, inc moisturizers, perfumes; shaving preparations, airborne materials, substances carried by hands to face, ie, nail polish; according to the AAD, the average woman applies 14 products to her body daily; changing to another brand of makeup may not be sufficient as similar cosmetic products, regardless of manufacturer, have same or similar ingredients; most pts also have underlying atopic or seborrheic dermatitis and many have become "addicted" to TCSs (J Am Acad Derm 1999;41:435).

Epidem: Women >> men.

Sx: Itching.

Si: Red, scaly, usually worse on eyelids; distribution may reveal source: lips: dermatitis from toothpaste, lipstick, candy; earlobes or neck: nickel or chrome.

Crs: Persistent until cause is identified and eliminated, often difficult.

Rx: Provide sx relief and find cause with following protocol: wk 1: TCS (class VI–VII) and eliminate as many cosmetic materials as tolerated; wk 2: if clear, dc TCS and maintain cosmetic elimination to determine if culprit has been excluded; wk 3: if still clear, restart 1 item each wk, but if not clear, eliminate additional cosmetic items until pt remains clear w/o need to use TCS; this program is difficult for some women who "need" their cosmetics; dx and rx are often best conducted by a dermatologist or allergist; successful rx will result in total cessation of all TCS.

For additional details and rx, see BODY, 3.1.a.

RASH, RED AND INFLAMED, LESIONS PERSIST

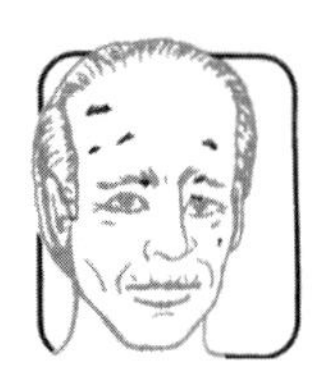

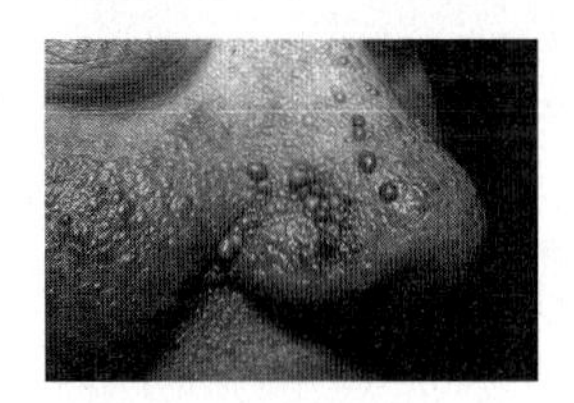

Adenoma sebaceum

6.7.A. ACTINIC KERATOSIS

Summary: Discrete; persistent; scaly, pink to red; esp in light-complexioned persons >40 yo; hx of excessive sun exposure; considered premalignant but few become SCC.

For additional details and rx, see GROWTHS, 11.11.a.

6.7.B. TUBEROUS SCLEROSIS (EPILOIA)

Summary: Multiple, pinhead to pea sized, red to skin colored and soft or firm; not pustular or painful; central part of face; confused w acne vulgaris, since, like acne, they appear and ↑ in number at puberty; assoc w mental retardation and/or seizures.

For additional details, see PIGMENT DECREASE, 21.3.b.

GROWTHS, YEARS OR SINCE CHILDHOOD

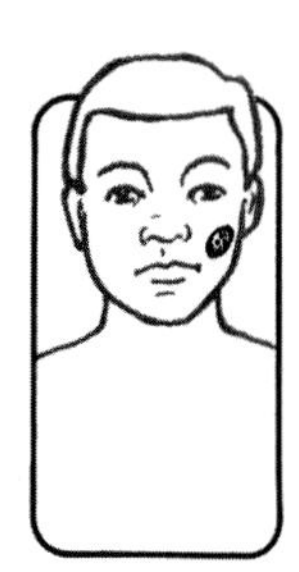

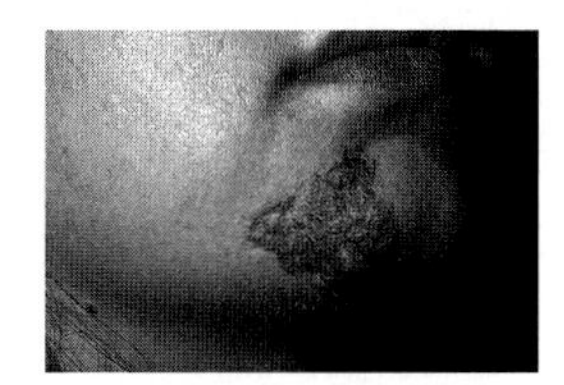

Hemangioma, capillary

6.8.A. FRECKLE/LENTIGO

Summary: *Freckle*: common; 1–3 mm; multiple; brown; flat; genetically determined on face; presence on trunk and arms indicates past intense sun exposure; not premalignant; rx not necessary or practical; *lentigo*: smaller and darker than freckle; fewer in number; not confined to sun-exposed areas; bx occasionally warranted to r/o melanoma.

For additional details and rx, see GROWTHS, 11.7.a.

6.8.B. NEVUS, MELANOCYTIC (MOLE—JUNCTIONAL, COMPOUND, AND INTRADERMAL)

Summary: Round; tan to dark brown; sharply outlined, present since young adulthood; average white adult has 20; prophylactic removal of all nevi is neither possible nor necessary; excise or bx a nevus that has changed, bled, or is irregular or black.

For additional details and rx, see GROWTHS, 11.1.a.

6.8.C. HEMANGIOMA, CAPILLARY AND CAVERNOUS

Summary: Blue to red vascular lesions that are present from birth or shortly afterward; some assoc w neurologic complications; lesions that appear in adulthood usually follow trauma.

For additional details and rx, see GROWTHS, 11.2.a.

6.8.D. HEREDITARY HEMORRHAGIC TELANGIECTASIA (OSLER-WEBER-RENDU SYNDROME)

Summary: Deep red to purple mats of blood vessels; flat to raised; pinhead to BB in size; single to grouped; located on lips, tongue, hands, nasal mucosa, upper trunk; bleed easily after minor trauma; assoc w glaucoma and arteriovenous shunts.

For additional details, see GROWTHS, 11.8.b.

6.8.E. TUBEROUS SCLEROSIS

Summary: Multiple, pinhead to pea sized, red to skin colored and soft or firm; not pustular or painful; central part of face; confused w acne vulgaris, since, like acne, they appear and ↑ in number at puberty; assoc w mental retardation and/or seizures.

For additional details, see PIGMENT DECREASE, 21.3.b.

6.8.F. FIBROMA

Summary: Fleshy, skin-colored, normal-appearing, noneroded surface; almost certainly benign; ddx: nevus, neurofibroma, FEP.

6.8.G. SEBORRHEIC KERATOSIS

Summary: Common benign growths, tan to dark brown, slightly roughened, waxy, crumbly; feels "stuck on" surface; usually fhx of similar lesions; most >40 yo.

For additional details and rx, see GROWTHS, 11.10.b.

6.8.H. DERMATOSIS PAPULOSA NIGRA

Summary: Dark papules; esp common in blacks; pos fhx of similar lesions; start in teens; resemble freckles but are raised; benign; persistent.

For additional details and rx, see GROWTHS, 11.7.e.

6.8.I. SWEAT GLAND TUMORS

Summary: Solid, cystic, or fluid filled; flesh colored; if fluid filled (**hidrocystoma**) may enlarge in hot environment; most are multiple; single tumor may resemble BCE; bx often needed to confirm dx.

6.8.J. CYST, DERMOID

Cause: Developmental sequestrations of surface epidermis.

Epidem: Most common orbital tumors of childhood but may not become evident until adulthood.

Si: Firm, rubbery, pea to marble sized, sc mass along upper lateral side of orbital rim but may develop in any quadrant about eye.

Rx: Confirmation of dx and surgical rx is performed by dermatologic, ophthalmologic, or plastic surgeons.

GROWTHS, RECENT, MULTIPLE

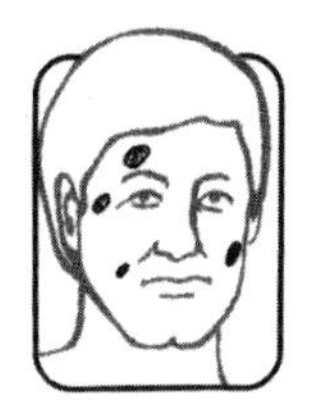

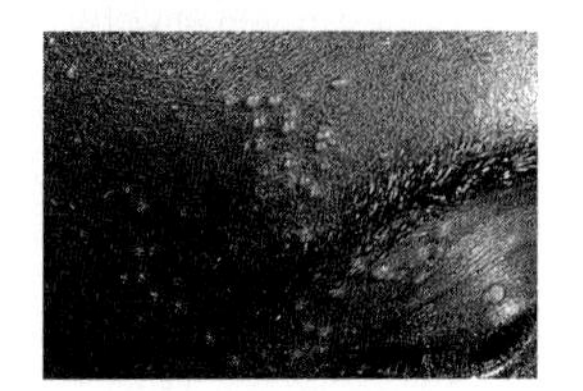

Molluscum contagiosum

6.9.A. ACTINIC KERATOSIS

Summary: Discrete; persistent; scaly, pink to red; esp in light-complexioned persons >40 yo; hx of excessive sun exposure; considered premalignant but few become SCC.

For additional details and rx, see GROWTHS, 11.11.a.

6.9.B. CYST, EPIDERMAL INCLUSION

Summary: Movable; firm to soft; dome shaped; pea to cherry tomato in size; single to multiple; surface is normal in color; may be a central, horny punctum; asx, unless ruptured; not premalignant; pts w multiple cysts often have or had severe acne vulgaris; main complaint is unsightly appearance esp when on face; removal, generally for cosmetic purposes, unless interfering w vision, usually is performed by dermatologic or plastic surgeon.

For additional details and rx, see GROWTHS, 11.3.a.

6.9.C. MILIUM (MILIA)

Cause: Small epidermal keratin inclusion cysts; develop spontaneously or follow use of occlusive cosmetics or face creams; may follow abrasive trauma, resolution of blisters of HZ, porphyria, epidermolysis bullosa, or pemphigus.

Epidem: Women > men.

Si: Pinhead- to rice grain–sized papule; yellow to white; firm to hard; most common on face, esp cheeks, forehead, and around eyes.
Crs: Persistent.
Rx: Easily removed by nicking w lancet and expressing contents, but may refill.

6.9.D. MOLLUSCUM CONTAGIOSUM

Summary: Pale to pink, shiny, elevated bump or papule w light-colored dimple in center; common on face in children; large numbers on face w HIV infection; look for lesions about genitals and lower abdomen in adults; asx unless traumatized; DNA poxvirus; transmission is by close person-to-person contact.
For additional details and rx, see GENITAL 9.7.b.

6.9.E. NEVUS, MELANOCYTIC

Summary: Round; tan to dark brown; sharply outlined, present since young adulthood; average white adult has 20; prophylactic removal of all nevi is neither possible nor necessary; excise or bx a nevus that has changed, bled, or is irregular or black.
For additional details and rx, see GROWTHS, 11.1.a.

6.9.F. SARCOID

Summary: Mimics other eruptions; most are pink to yellow; firm papules or plaques; pinhead to pea sized or larger; usually nape, face, extensor surfaces; minimal itching; may develop within preexisting scars; sometimes severe and may distort facial features; may be deep; may ulcerate; may lead to local hair loss; blacks >> whites.
For additional details and rx, see BODY, 3.3.o.

6.9.G. SEBORRHEIC KERATOSIS

Summary: Common benign growths, tan to dark brown, slightly roughened, waxy, crumbly; feels "stuck on" surface; usually fhx of similar lesions; most >40 yo.

For additional details and rx, see GROWTHS, 11.10.b.

6.9.H. WART, FILIFORM AND FLAT

Summary: *Filiform warts*: common on face, esp about eyes and mouth; usually have rough, broccoli-like surface, and project from the skin on hard stalks; single or few in number; for additional details and rx, see HANDS, 14.1.a.; *flat warts*: look like droplets of dried, skin-colored, rubber cement; multiple, smooth, round, slightly raised; common on face, neck, legs; asx.

For additional details and rx, see LEG RASH, 17.6.b.

6.9.I. XANTHELASMA

Cause: 50% have mildly ↑ low density (pre-β) lipoproteins; 25% have ↑ cholesterol.

Epidem: Middle aged or older; men = women; more common with familial hypercholesterolemia (esp type II), cardiovascular disease, DM.

Pathophys: Origin of lipid, plasma or local, is unclear.

Sx: None.

Si: Soft; yellow to orange; bilateral; well demarcated; flat plaques on or near eyelids; look at knees, elbows, tendons, palms for xanthomas.

Crs: Progress slowly, over many mos to yrs; does not disappear.

Lab: Obtain lipid screen.

Rx: Control hyperlipidemia, if present, by dietary or pharmacologic means; xanthelasma can be removed by surgical or chemical rx, but they return in mos to yrs; the following instructions are provided for the adventurous PCP, but most cases are rx'd by a dermatologist or plastic surgeon: apply 85% TCA *carefully* to plaques w wooden applicator (*WARNING*: a drop of TCA on cornea will produce immediate damage; protect eyes by covering them w dry gauze sponge and by not passing applicator over eyes); lesions become white and pt feels burning; after 30–60 sec, apply moistened gauze to halt the rxn.

6.9.J. SEBACEOUS HYPERPLASIA

Cause: Excessive UV light and sebaceous gland hyperactivity.
Sx: None.
Si: Yellow; pinhead sized; smooth papules; central dell; mostly in light-complexioned whites w hx of acne or oily skin.
Crs: Slowly ↑ in numbers.
Ddx: Resembles small BCEs and molluscum contagiosum.
Lab: Bx usually not necessary.
Rx: None needed; may improve appearance by touching w electrocautery, best done after partial numbing w EMLA, applied q 15 min for 2 h before procedure.

GROWTHS, RECENT, SINGLE

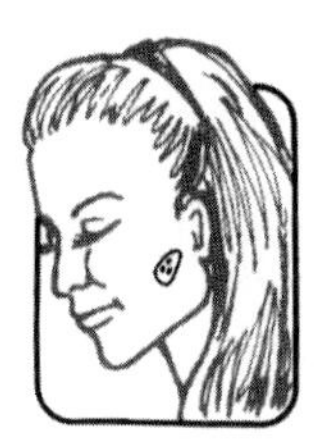

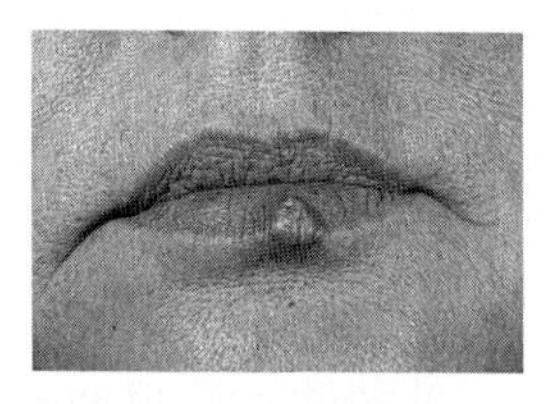

Squamous cell carcinoma

6.10.A. WART, FILIFORM

Summary: Common on face, esp about eyes and mouth; usually have rough, broccoli-like surface, and project from the skin on hard stalks; single or few in number.

For additional details and rx, see HANDS, 14.1.a.

6.10.B. FIBROMA

Summary: Fleshy, skin-colored, normal-appearing, noneroded surface; almost certainly benign; ddx: nevus, neurofibroma, FEP.

6.10.C. NEVUS, MELANOCYTIC

Summary: Round; tan to dark brown; sharply outlined, present since young adulthood; average white adult has 20; prophylactic removal of all nevi is neither possible nor necessary; excise or bx a nevus that has changed, bled, or that is irregular or black.

For additional details and rx, see GROWTHS, 11.1.a.

6.10.D. SEBORRHEIC KERATOSES

Summary: Common benign growths, tan to dark brown, slightly roughened, waxy, crumbly; feels "stuck on" surface; usually fhx of similar lesions; most >40 yo.

For additional details and rx, see GROWTHS, 11.10.b.

6.10.E. PYOGENIC GRANULOMA

Summary: Single, bright red, raspberry-like growth; pea or bean sized; often friable and bleeds easily when traumatized; most are on exposed parts, esp face, arms, legs, hands, fingers; any age group.

For additional details and rx, see GROWTHS, 11.5.a.

6.10.F. SKIN CANCER

6.10.F.(1). BOWEN'S DISEASE (SQUAMOUS CELL CARCINOMA IN SITU)

Summary: Single, thickened, sharply defined, dull red, scaly plaque; resembles psoriasis (see BODY, 3.1.d.) but usually only single; Bowen's disease is a persistent, slowly growing neoplasia w potential to become invasive SCC; confirm dx by skin bx (see DX.7.).

For additional details and rx, see GROWTHS, 11.5.c.

6.10.F.(2). BASAL CELL CARCINOMA (BCC)

Summary: Single or few; shiny or pearly colored; telangiectasias over surface; depressed center; slowly spreading; usually on light-exposed areas, esp face, neck, forearms; about 80% of skin cancers.

For additional details and rx, see GROWTHS, 11.6.c.

6.10.F.(3). SQUAMOUS CELL CARCINOMA (SCC)

Summary: Usually single; painless; scaly, keratotic, bleeding, friable surface; most are on light-exposed areas but appear on covered areas as well, sometimes adjacent to areas of trauma, ie, chronic leg ulcers, burn scars, or sites of radiation rx; lower lip is frequent location because of chronic sun exposure, as well as chronic tar and heat exposure in smokers.

For additional details and rx, see GROWTHS, 11.6.d.

6.10.F.(4). MELANOMA

Summary: Black or brown, occasionally normal skin color; irregular in outline, may be itchy, bleed, or ulcerate; may have black, white, blue speckles; most common on back; also common on shins of women; whites >> blacks.

For additional details and rx, see GROWTHS, 11.4.b.

7 Feet

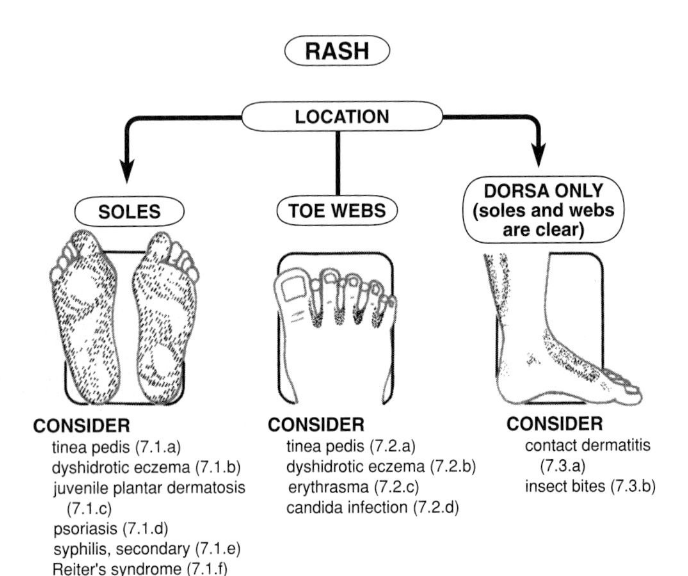

If rash is elsewhere

CONSIDER

psoriasis (3.1.d)
syphilis, secondary (3.1.f)

If rash is of recent (days) onset

CONSIDER

viral exanthems (8.1.b)
Rocky Mountain spotted fever (8.1.m)
erythema multiforme (2.1.b)
syphilis, secondary (3.1.f)
scabies (3.1.e)
drug reaction (8.1.a)

GROWTHS ON SOLE

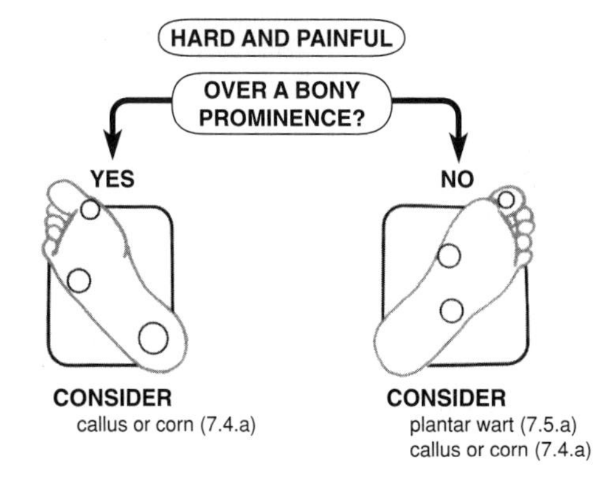

APPEARANCE

(after thin shaving of the surface with a surgical or razor blade)

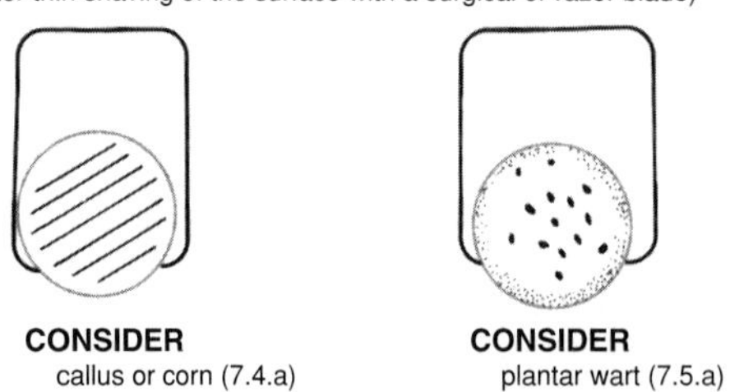

Note: For soft fleshy protruding growths, see section on growths.

RASH CONFINED TO SOLES

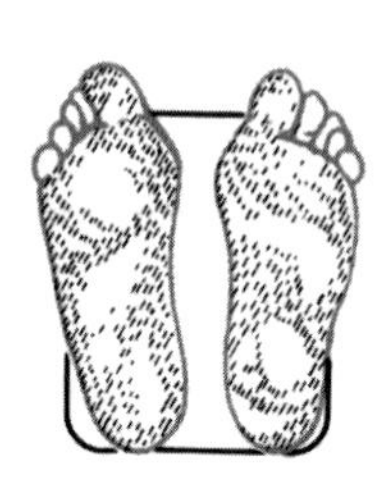

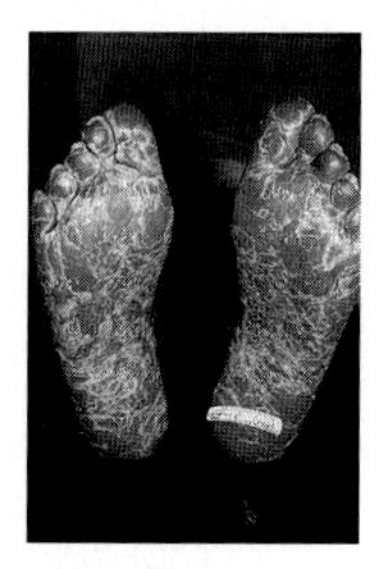

Psoriasis

7.1.A. TINEA PEDIS (ATHLETE'S FOOT)

Cause: Mostly 3 genera of fungi: *Trichophyton* species, esp *T. rubrum*, common dry scaly form; and *Microsporum* and *Epidermophyton* species: acute blistering forms; occlusive footwear, hot weather, sweating support fungal growth.

Epidem: Because fungi are ubiquitous, individual susceptibility, probably inherited, rather than gym or swimming pool exposure, determines who becomes infected.

Sx: Itchy or painful, if skin is cracked or blistered.

Si:

- *Chronic*: scaly and, if moist, malodorous; generally confined to toe webs and plantar surface in "moccasin" distribution.
- *Acute*: soggy, whitish, cracking, deep blisters; both feet usually involved.
- *Both*: toenails almost always infected; yellow, crumbly, thick subungual debris; serve as source for reinfection (see NAILS, 20.3.a.); hands may be involved (see HANDS, 14.7.b.), often only 1 hand is involved along w both feet, the **one hand–two foot syndrome**; *children*: rare, seek other cause, ie, contact dermatitis (see 7.3.a.) or juvenile plantar dermatosis (see 7.1.c.).

Crs: Chronic, unless rx'd; recurrence after rx is typical; often flares in summer.

Lab: *Chronic scaly pattern*: clinical suspicion usually suffices; KOH (DX.3) or submit scale to clinical lab for KOH if not able to do in office; if neg, consider another dx; fungal culture is not necessary before rx; *acute soggy blistering pattern*: KOH often neg.

Rx:

- Chronic: reduce heat and moisture by switching to light, ventilated shoes, to cotton socks, and to foot powders; white socks or boiling of socks offers no advantage; prescribe topical antifungal agent (see RX.10.) bid or hs; if extensive or recalcitrant, add systemic antifungal agent (see RX.11.) for 2 wk and continue w topical rx.
- Acute: compress w dilute acetic acid (1 oz household vinegar to 2 cups warm tap water) for 20 min q 2–6 h (see RX.2.); separate toes w cotton; after a few days when inflammation has subsided, start topical antifungal agent (see RX.10.) bid or hs and a systemic antifungal agent (see RX.11.) for 2 wk; recurrences are common, esp if toenails are infected (see NAILS, 20.3.a.); pts w acute tinea pedis often are referred to a dermatologist or podiatrist.

7.1.B. DYSHIDROTIC ECZEMA (POMPHOLYX)

Cause: Unknown; not a sweat gland disorder; episodes triggered by irritation or trauma.

Sx: *Acute* phase: intensely itchy; *chronic* or dry phase: some discomfort from cracking.

Si: *Acute* phase: soles, interdigital spaces, toes, foot margins are studded w minute, sand grain–sized, deep blisters; feet may be oozing, swollen, painful; may have hyperhidrosis; hands often involved (see HAND, 14.7.a.); *chronic*: dry, cracking skin.

Crs: *Acute* episodes start w severe itching and deep but tiny blisters, redness, oozing, last 1–3 wk; followed by *chronic* dry crusting, scaling; followed by period of relative or complete clearing lasting wks to mos; sometimes new episodes follow immediately.

Compl: 2° infection.

Lab: A search for contact allergies is usually fruitless.

Rx: *Acute blistering phase*: compress w saline (see RX.2.) 20 min qid, then apply TCS (class I) cr (see RX.5.), if severe or resistant add systemic CS (40 mg prednisone for a few d, then taper); *chronic dry, cracked phase*: stop compressing, switch to TCS (class I) oint, which is less drying; pts w frequent or disabling episodes usually are rx'd by a dermatologist.

7.1.C. JUVENILE PLANTAR DERMATOSIS

Summary: Tender; red plantar surface; fissures in toe webs; children only; 2° to irritation and maceration from occlusive boots or tennis shoes; also called "tennis shoe" syndrome; sometimes manifestation of atopic dermatitis; cotton socks and open shoes or sandals often relieve condition.

7.1.D. PSORIASIS

Summary: Either scaly patches as part of widespread psoriasis or pustular patches on sole; pustular form usually on weight-bearing part; most pts w pustular form do not have psoriasis elsewhere, and such pts do not have HLA haplotypes assoc w typical psoriasis, suggesting the 2 forms are unrelated; both forms are resistant to rx; try TCS (class I) oint, topical calcipotriene, or tazarotene (see BODY, 3.1.d.); PUVA often effective; refer recalcitrant cases to a dermatologist.

For additional details and rx, see BODY, 3.1.d.

7.1.E. SYPHILIS, SECONDARY

Summary: Many patterns; most common: widespread, slightly scaly, tan, copper-colored, nonitchy patches, lesions on palms and/or soles; recent or healing genital ulcer; moist, wartlike genital growths (condylomata lata); painless oral erosions and mucous patches; "moth-eaten" scalp hair loss; mild or absent constitutional si and sx; LN↑, esp epitrochlear nodes; no blisters except in newborn; 2° lesions appear few wk after 1° rash disappears.

For additional details, see BODY, 3.1.f.

7.1.F. REITER'S SYNDROME

Cause: Unknown, probably immunologic; some follow urogenital infections, esp mycoplasmal or chlamydial, or GI infections, esp shigella or salmonella; assoc w HLA B-27 (Inf Dis Clin N Am 1994;8:533).

Epidem: Mostly young adult males 9:1 > females.
Sx: Sometimes uncomfortable when thick.
Si: *Keratoderma blennorrhagica*, oyster shell–like, crusty, pustular, single or multiple thick plaques, on soles; 10%–20%; also: nail dystrophy, nail fold swelling, subungual debris; other manifestations: nonsuppurative polyarthritis of axial, sacroiliac, knee, ankle joints; heel pain; conjunctivitis and iritis; balanitis or urethritis; diarrhea; renal insufficiency.
Crs: Generally self-limited; 25% recur; 20% become chronic.
Compl: Arthritis and glomerulitis are major serious sequelae.
Ddx: Other causes of arthritis, urethritis, or conjunctivitis; only 8% present w classic triad (Comp Ther 1994;20:441).
Lab: Path resembles psoriasis; dx is clinical; RA titer neg; ESR often ↑.
Rx: Thick lesions may be softened w propylene glycol hs and TCS (class I) oint; most cases are followed and rx'd by PCP w multiple specialties.

FEET

RASH IN TOE WEBS

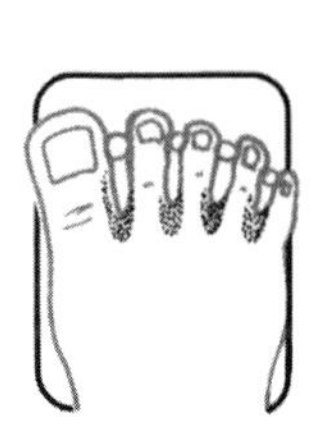

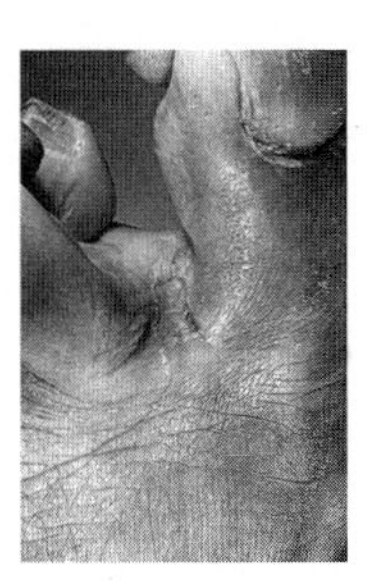

Tinea pedis

7.2.A. TINEA PEDIS

Summary: Toe webs nearly always involved in tinea pedis; itchy; r/o erythrasma (DX.4) if confined to 4th to 5th toe web; topical antifungals (see RX.10.) are sufficient (see 7.1.a.).

7.2.B. DYSHIDROTIC ECZEMA

Summary: Restriction to toe webs occurs in mild or early cases; lesions extend quickly to sides and tops of feet (see 7.1.b.).

7.2.C. ERYTHRASMA

Summary: Scaly dermatitis between toes, esp between 4th and 5th; does not involve soles or dorsum of feet; bacterial infection; dx is by Wood's light (DX.4), if available.

For details and rx, see GROIN RASH, 10.3.a.

7.2.D. *CANDIDA* INFECTION

Summary: Moist; pink-red dermatitis; cheesy surface; assoc w DM; immunosuppression; rx w broad-spectrum topical antifungal (see RX.10.).

RASH ON DORSA OF FOOT ONLY (SOLES AND WEBS ARE CLEAR)

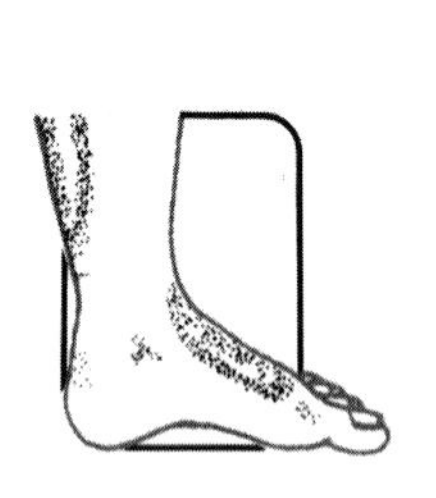

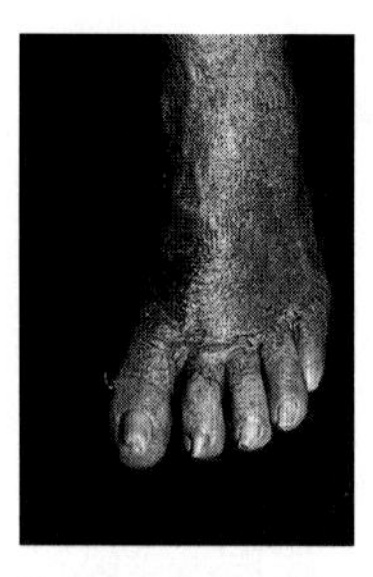

Contact dermatitis

7.3.A. CONTACT DERMATITIS

Cause: Allergic or irritant rxn to ingredient of socks, shoes, foot med; *allergic* rxns: develop slowly, causes include dyes, metal salts, elastic, adhesives, tanning agents, rubber components, medicated foot preparations; *irritant* rxns: develop shortly after exposure, worse w repeated physical trauma, ie, alkaline, gritty cement particles.

Sx: Itch and discomfort.

Si: Scaly, pink to red; worse or restricted to dorsum, tops or tips of toes and ankles; distribution often corresponds to outline of contactant, ie, a shoe tongue, at toe-grip of leather sandals or shower shoes.

Crs: Worse in summer or in a hot workplace.

Lab: Determining the antigen requires specialized allergy patch testing (see DX.6.), which may be performed by some dermatologists, allergists, or occupational medicine specialists.

Rx: TCS (class I–III) cr applied frequently; protect from irritants, ie, cement; change footwear if allergen is suspected; pts w confirmed shoe allergy may purchase footwear manufactured free of identified allergens through local orthopedic specialty supply stores or contact 2 companies that specialize in custom-made shoes: P.W. Minor and Son, Inc (3 Treadeasy Ave, Batavia, NY 14021-0678, 716.343.1500, www.biomech.com/mall/pwminor) and Loveless Orthopedica Appliance (2434 Southwest 29th St., Oklahoma City, OK 73119, 405.631.9731, www.lovelessboots.com).

FEET

7.3.B. INSECT BITES

Summary: Itchy; usually isolated but scratching and superimposed infection may produce a patch; lower legs (fleas) or at constriction from clothing or shoes (chiggers); for additional details, see LEG RASH, 17.2.a.

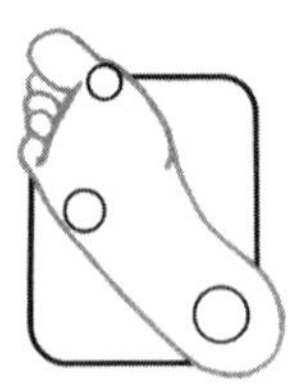

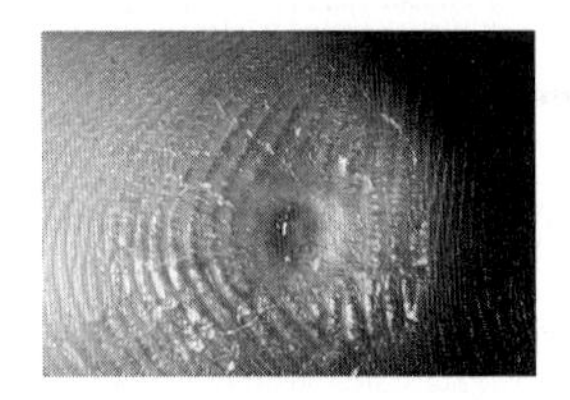

Callus

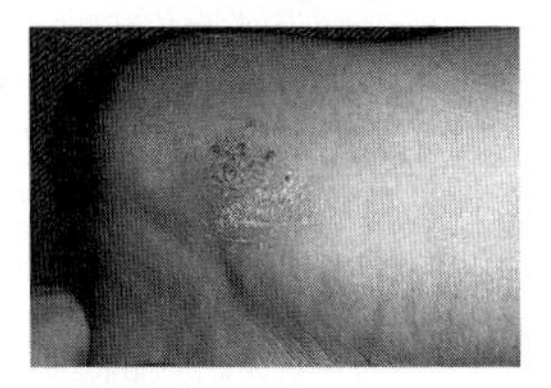

Plantar

7.4.A. CALLUSES AND CORNS

Cause: Mostly improperly fitting footwear; some abn bony foot structure and/or abn gait; pts w DM, vascular insufficiency, or neurologic deficit are esp prone.

Sx: Callus may not hurt; corn is painful w walking.

Si: Thick, round pad of horny material (**callus**) on sole or toes at pressure points; callus may further thicken in center to form a hard "kernel" (**corn**); *moist callus (soft corn)*: in toe web space, esp 4th to 5th, from maceration and pressure.

Crs: Chronic; progressive.

Ddx: Distinguish from plantar wart by paring surface w a surgical or razor blade; look for glistening horny material of callus or corn; plantar warts have light or black specks instead.

Rx: Pt may pare callus or corn w single-edged razor blade, pumice stone, or file (from Dr. Scholl section in pharmacy), most easily done after bathing when skin is soft; change to softer-soled shoe w broader toe; orthopedic or podiatric consultation may be required.

GROWTHS ON SOLE, MAY BE OVER BONY PROMINENCE

7.5.A. PLANTAR WART

Cause: Transmissible DNA human papillomavirus.

Epidem: Contagious; children and young adults >> adults.

Sx: Frequently painful.

Si: Firm to hard, slightly raised, rough surface, deeply seated growths; location: on plantar surface or sides of foot or toes but may occur at pressure points similar to callus; *mosaic wart*: resembles large callus but w fine, black specks on surface, most common on heel or plantar side of toes.

Crs: Persistent; may be painful.

Ddx: Distinguish from callus or corn by paring surface w a surgical or razor blade; look for light or black specks instead of glistening horny material seen w callus or corn; plantar warts occur anywhere on sole or toes, but corns and calluses occur over pressure points; plantar warts are randomly scattered on sole but corns or calluses tend to be symmetric.

Rx: Keratolytics: sometimes effective; most pts have tried, at least for short time; numerous OTC products available, all w salicylic acid (Duofilm, Salactic film, or Viranol), follow package instructions, usually hs; if such rx is not effective within 2 mo, refer to podiatrist for rx that may include LN2, D&C, laser, or excision; goal is to destroy wart w/o producing a scar that may be permanent and painful.

8 Fever

plus RASH

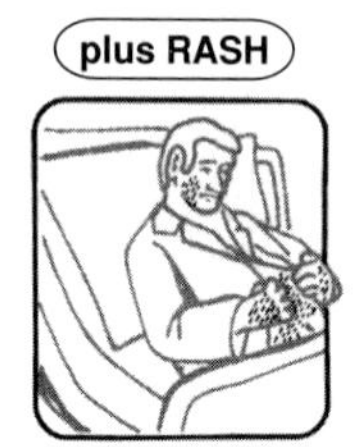

DID THE RASH *FIRST* APPEAR ON THE

TRUNK

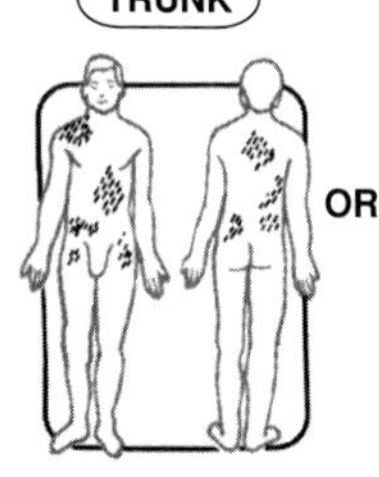

OR

FACE OR EXTREMITIES

CONSIDER (trunk)
- drug reaction (8.1.a)
- viral exanthems (8.1.b)
- bacterial exanthems (8.1.c)
- spirochetal infections (8.1.d)
  - Lyme disease
  - syphilis, secondary
- typhoid (8.1.e)
- rickettsial infections (8.1.f)
  - typhus

CONSIDER (face or extremities)
- septicemia (8.1.l)
  - meningococcus
  - gonococcus
  - *Pseudomonas*
  - *Staphylococcus aureus*
- Rocky Mountain spotted fever (8.1.m)
- vasculitis (8.1.n)
- mucocutaneous lymph node syndrome (8.1.o)

plus BLISTERS

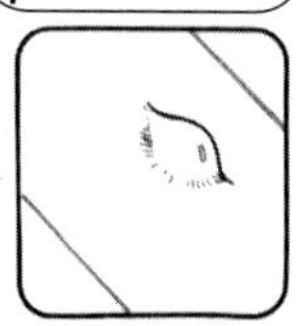

Scrape blister base for

(1) Bacterial (DX.1.), if **positive**

CONSIDER
- impetigo or pyroderma (8.2.a)
- septicemia (8.1.l)

(2) Multinucleated giant cells (DX.2.), if **positive**

CONSIDER
- herpes simplex (8.2.b)
- varicella (8.2.c)
- herpes zoster (8.2.d)

(3) If both (1) and (2) are **negative**

CONSIDER
- erythema multiforme (8.2.l)
- toxic epidermal necrolysis (8.2.m)
- staphylococcal scalded skin syndrome (8.2.n)
- drug reaction (8.2.0)
- pemphigus and pemphigoid (8.2.p)

plus ARTHRALGIA and RASH

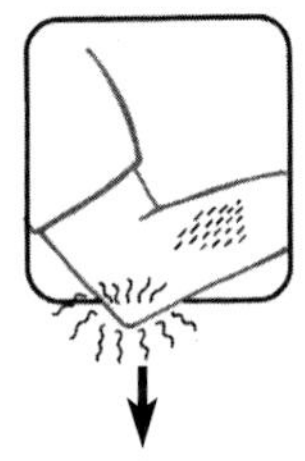

CONSIDER
- systemic lupus erythematosus (8.3.a)
- dermatomyositis (8.3.b)
- scleroderma (8.3.c)
- septicemia (8.1.l)
  - meningococcus
  - gonococcus
- drug-induced eruption (8.1.a) and serum sickness
- vasculitis (8.1.n)
- Rocky Mountain spotted fever (8.1.m)
- typhus (8.1.f)
- viral exanthems (8.1.b)
  - measles
  - enterovirus
- spirochetal infection (8.1.d)
  - Lyme disease
  - secondary syphilis

plus ORAL LESIONS and RASH

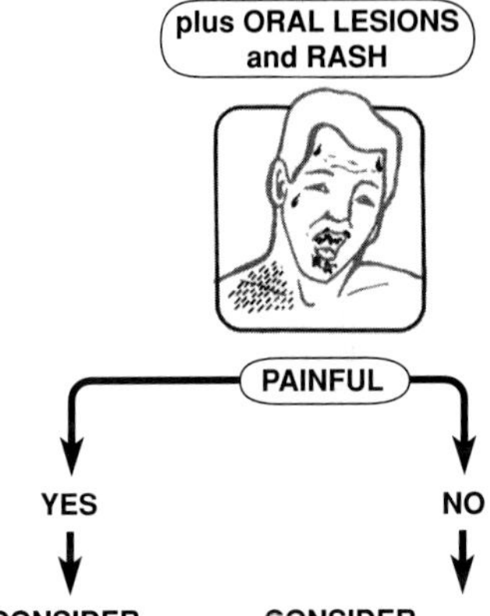

YES → CONSIDER
- erythema multiforme (8.2.l)
- pemphigus and pemphigoid (8.2.p)
- bacterial exanthems (8.1.c)
- toxic epidermal necrolysis (8.2.m)
- herpes simplex (8.2.b)

NO → CONSIDER
- collagen, vascular disease (8.3.a to c)
- viral exanthems (8.1.b)
  - measles
  - rubella
  - erythema infectiosum
  - roseola
  - hand-foot-and-mouth disease
  - infectious mononucleosis
  - acute exanthem of HIV
  - Rocky Mountain spotted fever
- mucocutaneous lymph node syndrome (8.1.o)
- secondary syphilis (8.1.d)

FEVER, RASH, STARTED ON TRUNK

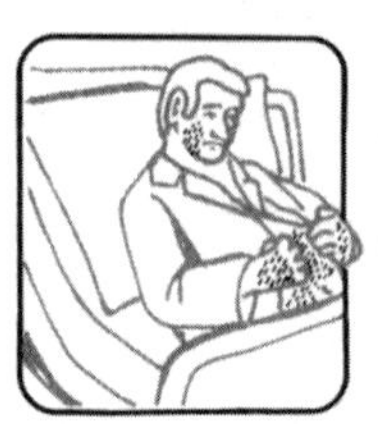

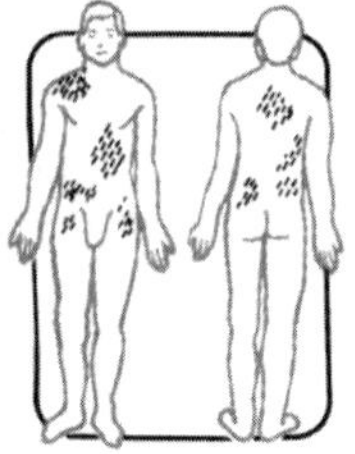

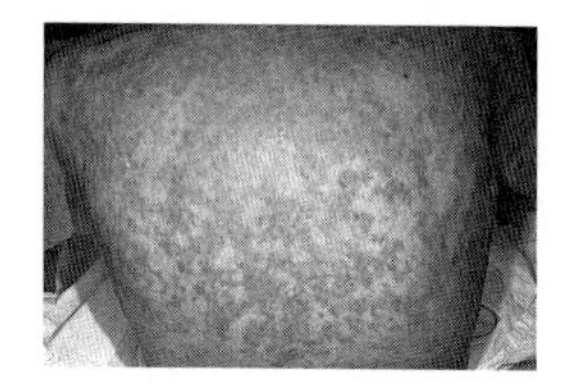

Drug reaction

8.1.A. DRUG REACTION

Cause: Drugs most assoc w febrile rxn: antimicrobials (esp β-lactam), sulfonamides, nitrofurantoin, penicillin, cephalosporin, barbiturates, hydantoins, iodides, isoniazid, procainamide, methyldopa, hydralazine, ethambutol (Review: Arch Derm 2001;137:357).

Si: Many forms: faint pink, evanescent, nonscaly rash, usually on trunk; urticaria (see ITCH, 16.3.a.); blisters (see BLISTERS, 2.); pustules; erythema multiforme (see BLISTERS, 2.1.b.); purpura or serum sickness; arthralgias; vasculitis; temperature may be normal, low grade, or high, may be accompanied by chills.

Crs: Fever usually starts 1–3 wk after start of rx but may start within days; fever usually decreases within 48 h but may last for days or wks, depending on rate of clearance of med.

Ddx: R/o underlying infection for which suspected drug is being used; r/o septic emboli.

Lab: Eosinophilia and/or rash found only in 20% of pts w drug fever.

Rx: Stop drug or drugs suspected of causing rxn; serious systemic rxns, esp renal and liver failure, may develop if an attempt is made to suppress rxn w antihistamines or systemic CS while continuing drug; use both to relieve and speed resolution of eruption once offending drug has been dc'd.

For additional details, see BODY, 3.1.b.

8.1.B. VIRAL EXANTHEMS

Summary: Viral eruptions generally are not distinctive except for blistering eruptions: varicella and HSV/HZ; most consist of flat or barely raised, dime-sized or smaller, pink patches; most begin on face or trunk, rather than extremities; fever, headache, and myalgias precede most exanthems; constitutional si and sx usually outweigh cutaneous signs.

RUBELLA (GERMAN MEASLES)

Cause: RNA togavirus; human is only reservoir; natural infection or immunization confers lifelong immunity.

Epidem: Spreads via respiratory tract; peak incidence: late winter and early spring; contagious several d before rash and up to 2 wk after onset of rash.

Sx: Not itchy; sx only minimal; more severe in adults; usually clears when rash appears.

Si: Pink to red macules and papules; first on face; petechiae appear frequently on soft palate.

Crs: Incubation: 2–3 wk; mild prodrome: 1–4 d, low-grade fever, headache, conjunctivitis, rhinitis, posterior cervical, and postauricular LN↑; rash begins on face and rapidly spreads down trunk; rash gone in 2–4 d.

Compl: Rare encephalitis, neuritis, thrombocytopenic purpura; adult women may get arthritis that may take wks to clear; fetus exposed during 1st trimester has 80%–90% risk for *congenital rubella syndrome*: now only about 4 cases/yr in U.S. (Mmwr 1997;46:350); multiple fetal abn, esp heart, eyes, CNS; women of childbearing age who intend to become pregnant need immune status testing (Mmwr 1994;43:1).

Rx: Sx rx if ill: bed rest, fluids, analgesics; vaccine (Meruvax, Merck (rubella); Biavax, Merck (rubella and mumps)) is available; use for children 12 mo to puberty; nonpregnant adolescents and adult women of childbearing age; postpartum women; international travelers; immunize only if rubella titer is neg; vaccine may be given to immunocompromised pts.

MEASLES (RUBEOLA)

Cause: RNA paramyxovirus; human is main reservoir; natural infection or immunization confers lifelong immunity.

Epidem: Spreads by sneezing and coughing; contagious several d before rash; most late winter and spring.

Sx: Not itchy; sx do not clear when rash appears; asx cases are rare.

Si: *Koplik's spots*: pathognomonic tiny, blue-white spots w red halo on buccal mucosa opposite molars, present during prodrome and 1–2 d w rash; pink, macular, papular rash starting on face and behind ears, generalized LN↑.

Crs: Incubation: 1–2 wk; prodrome: 3–4 d, high fever, malaise, coryza, cough; spreads downward from face and clears in same order; si and sx clear in 1 wk; often followed by branny desquamation; **modified measles syndrome**: mild illness from partial immunization; **atypical measles syndrome**: previously vaccinated 1963–67 w killed virus; rash, edema, pneumonia, high fever, now rare.

Compl: Usually benign; most complications in adults, malnourished children, immunocompromised pts; rash absent in 30% if pt immunocompromised; ↓ platelets w purpura; keratitis; myocarditis; hepatitis; rare encephalitis (5 × > rubella); encephalitis in immunocompromised pt may develop wks to mos after 1° infection (Clin Infect Dis 1993;16:654; Jama 1992;267:1237).

Rx: Symptomatic: bed rest, fluids, analgesics; vaccine (Attenux, Merck (measles); M-R-Vax II, Merck (measles and rubella); M-M-R II, Merck (measles, mumps, and rubella)) is available (made w eggs) (J Infect Dis 1996;173:731) but often underutilized; use for all children >15 mo; may need booster at age 5 yo (CDC) or age 12 yo (American Academy of Pediatrics); international travelers born after 1956; immune globulin (0.25–0.5 mg/kg within 6 d of exposure) may be needed for certain exposed pts: HIV pos; pregnant women; immunocompromised children.

ERYTHEMA INFECTIOSUM (FIFTH DISEASE)

Cause: Parvovirus B19, a small DNA virus (Adv IM 1992;37:431).

Epidem: Most cases winter and spring; not contagious once rash appears.

Sx: Minimal; arthritis, esp in adults.

Si: Bright erythema on face (slapped cheeks) w relative pallor about mouth; 1–4 d later: rash w lacelike pattern extends to trunk and extremities.

Crs: Prodrome: mild or absent; eruption flares and remits over 2 wk before clearing.

Compl: Adults: arthritis, esp women sometimes w/o rash; HIV: chronic anemia and aplastic crisis (Ann IM 1990;113:926); 1st trimester pregnancy: hydrops fetalis or fetal death; sickle cell anemia: transient aplastic crises.

Lab: Confirmed by measuring B19-specific IgM and IgG antibodies.

Rx: Symptomatic; iv IgG if immunosuppressed; no vaccine yet available; protect pregnant health care workers (Peds 1990;85:131).

ROSEOLA (EXANTHEM SUBITUM, SIXTH DISEASE)

Cause: Human herpesvirus 6.

Epidem: Children 6 mo–3 yr.

Sx: Child does not appear sick; febrile until rash appears.

Si: Barley-sized pink macules and papules that remain discrete; rash starts on neck and spreads to trunk; minimal or absent on face and extremities.

Crs: Fever for about 4 d; fever clears as rash develops; rash clears in 2 d.

Compl: Febrile convulsions.

Rx: Symptomatic.

HAND-FOOT-AND-MOUTH DISEASE

Cause: Coxsackievirus A16.

Epidem: Summer and fall; children <10 yo; quickly spreads to close contacts.

Sx: Lesions are tender.

Si: Pinhead to pea sized, red lesions; hands, feet, mouth; evolve into small blisters that quickly ulcerate; transient fever.

Crs: Incubation: 4–6 d; prodrome: fever, malaise; clears in 1 wk.

Rx: Symptomatic.

INFECTIOUS MONONUCLEOSIS

Nejm 2000;243:481; Ann IM 1993;118:45.

Cause: Epstein-Barr virus.

Si: Nonspecific, faint, fine, or papular rash in 5%, but 95% w ampicillin; 1/4 have petechial eruption on palate; other: low-grade fever, malaise, pharyngitis, LN↑, splenomegaly.

FEVER

Crs: Incubation: 4–6 wk; prodrome: mild sx 1–2 wk; illness: 2–4 wk and longer.
Compl: Encephalitis; autoimmune hemolytic anemia; splenic rupture.
Lab: Lymphocytosis w atypical CD8+ lymphocytes; heterophile antibodies.

ACUTE EXANTHEM OF HIV

Summary: Pink-red; morbilliform; trunk and upper arms; 2–4 wk after infection; often subclinical; assoc w flulike syndrome, often severe; antibodies may be evident; bx not specific; highly infectious during acute exanthem (see HIV, 15.3.a.).

SMALLPOX (variola):

Summary: Poxvirus; eliminated from the world except in the lab; potential terrorist weapon; transmission is respiratory; asx for 12–13 d after infection; prodrome of 3 d; then deep papules that vesiculate to cloudy, umbilicated pustules; all lesions in same stage; high mortality; report suspected cases; isolate patient.

OTHER VIRAL EXANTHEMS

Clin Infect Dis 1993;16:199.

Summary: Several viral causes, inc enterovirus, coxsackievirus, and echovirus; generally w prodrome: fever, headache, malaise; rash generally starts on face or trunk and spreads to extremities; *note*: this distribution is distinct from rash of **RMSF** (see 8.1.m.), which starts on hands and feet; determination of viral cause requires special tests not generally available; if such a determination may be needed (ie, start of epidemic): freeze 5 mL of both an acute-phase serum taken early in the illness and a convalescent-phase serum taken 2–4 wk later; if appropriate, obtain throat culture to r/o streptococcal infection.

8.1.C. BACTERIAL EXANTHEMS

J Am Acad Derm 1998;39:383.

SCARLET FEVER

Cause: Erythrogenic toxin of group A β-hemolytic streptococci.
Epidem: Less common in recent yrs; less virulent now than early in 20th century; most are children <10 yo.
Pathophys: Probable hypersensitivity rxn to toxin.
Sx: Sore throat, fever.

Si: Circumoral pallor: face is involved except for area about mouth; body rash feels rough, like fine sandpaper; throat is purulent and in 1/2 the tongue becomes red and swollen w prominent papillae (strawberry tongue); after rash subsides, skin often peels, esp hands and feet.

Crs: Sudden onset of fever, pharyngitis, malaise; fine, pink rash starts 1–3 d later; rash usually begins about neck and body folds (Pastia's lines); extends to trunk and extremities; spares palms/soles; clears in 1 wk.

Compl: Poststreptococcal rheumatic fever, glomerulonephritis, vasculitis.

Ddx: Viral exanthem; staphylococcal erythrotoxin; **streptococcal toxic shock–like syndrome**: multiorgan failure, high mortality esp w HIV infection, rash common (Med 1997;76:238); also see TSS below.

Lab: Throat culture; ↑ ASO titer.

Rx: Penicillin, clindamycin; obtain infectious disease consultation.

TOXIC SHOCK SYNDROME (TSS)

Cause: Exotoxins and enterotoxins of *Staphylococcus aureus* from site of infection; similar pattern also seen w streptococcus.

Epidem: 1/2 assoc w gynecologic problems (tampons, abortion, IUDs); other 1/2 in both sexes and all ages, esp postoperative and postpartum.

Pathophys: Develops in pts w/o protective antibodies.

Sx: High fever.

Si: Severe illness w diffuse erythema, often flexural, during first 2 d of illness; strawberry tongue; desquamation of palms/soles 1–2 wk later; ↓ BP and shock; involves other organ systems, esp GI, kidney, liver, CNS, platelets, mucosa; streptococcal TSS more often has localized soft-tissue infection (Nejm 1989;321:1).

Crs: Fatality: 2.5% for menstrual cases and 6.4% for nonmenstrual cases (CDC).

Compl: Multiorgan system failure.

Ddx: Viral exanthem, streptococcal erythrotoxin, RMSF, meningococcemia, sepsis, drug rxn.

Lab: Find site of infection.

Rx: Supportive; drainage of infected sites; penicillin, clindamycin; obtain infectious disease consultation.

MENINGOCOCCEMIA

Summary: Rash may start on extremities as septic emboli (see 8.1.l.) or on trunk as a macular eruption, often w petechial centers; progresses rapidly to become hemorrhagic and purpuric; pt is febrile, toxic, has headache, arthralgias, malaise; course may be fulminant.

8.1.D. SPIROCHETAL INFECTION

LYME BORRELIOSIS

Ann IM 1991;114:472.

Cause: *Borrelia burgdorferi*, a tick-transmitted spirochete.

Epidem: Transmitted by *Ixodes* tick; tick is size of pinhead; requires vector of white-footed mouse and white-tailed deer.

Sx: Skin lesion not painful or itchy; often has headache w neck stiffness; Bell's palsy; arthralgias; malaise; fatigue (Jama 1993;269:1812).

Si: **Erythema migrans**: usually single, often multiple; warm; often spreads to become large ring; bite usually not evident; rash present in 75%.

Crs: Incubation: 3–30 d; early clinical disease: additional annular skin lesions, musculoskeletal pain, neuritis, carditis; sx often intermittent and changing; mos to yrs later: arthritis, neuropathy, cardiopathy, acrodermatitis.

Ddx: Bites from *Lone Star tick* cause rash identical to rash of Lyme disease, but cause may not be *Borrelia* as Lyme serology does not become pos; more common in south and central U.S.; rx is same (Arch Derm 1998;134:955).

Lab: Serologic tests become pos within several wk of infection; may remain pos after old infection for yrs (Jama 1999;282:62).

Rx: Doxycycline (100 mg bid) (Nejm 1997;337:289); alternatives: amoxicillin (250–500 mg tid), cefuroxime (500 mg bid), ceftriaxone (2 gm iv/im), erythromycin (250 mg qid); duration of rx: 3 wk if only fever, LN↑, rash (Nejm 1997;337:289); 6 wk if neurologic and/or cardiac and/or recurrent polyarthritis (Nejm 1994;330:229); avoid systemic CSs; avoid overzealous dx and rx (Jama 1998;279:206).

SYPHILIS, SECONDARY

Summary: 2° syphilis may be assoc w mild fever and malaise, but rash, sore, or hx of infected sexual contact is more likely reason for pt to come to office; within 12 h of rx w penicillin, >90% develop fever, chills, headache, leukocytosis (*Jarisch-Herxheimer reaction*), which subsides in 24 h and is of no consequence in pts w early stages of syphilis; warn pt that the rxn will occur and suggest aspirin for the discomfort; rxn may be life-threatening in pts w 3° cardiovascular or neurosyphilis.

For additional details, see BODY, 3.1.f.

8.1.E. TYPHOID (ENTERIC FEVER)

Arch IM 1998;158:633.

Cause: Infection w *Salmonella typhi* or related serovar; cultured from stool, blood, skin.

Epidem: Acquired from ingestion of water or food contaminated by human carrier; uncommon in U.S. but increasing w world travel; ↑ frequency if HIV pos.

Sx: Febrile w abdominal pain.

Si: 2/3 develop rash w characteristic "rose spots": slightly raised, pink, nontender papules, appearing in crops of 10–20 lesions on trunk, typically between nipples and umbilicus and absent on back and extremities; also: diarrhea, abdominal distention, disorientation, pneumonia, fever w/o tachycardia.

Crs: Incubation: 1–8 wk; stepwise ↑ in fever.

Compl: Include GI perforation, hemorrhage; mortality if not rx'd: 15%; 3%–5% become asx carriers.

Ddx: Other infections.

Lab: Low or normal wbc counts; organism difficult to culture; serologic tests (Widal) become pos.

Rx: Prompt treatment w chloramphenicol, amoxicillin, or trimethoprim-sulfamethoxazole cures most cases, but some bacteria have become resistant, esp in developing countries.

8.1.F. RICKETTSIAL INFECTION

TYPHUS

Jama 1991;266:1365.

Cause: Rickettsia.

Epidem: *Endemic (flea-borne) typhus*: transmitted from rat fleas; *epidemic "classic" (louse-borne) typhus*: transmitted from human body lice; *scrub (chigger-borne) typhus*: transmitted from mites endemic in Asia and Far East.

Si: *Endemic (flea-borne) typhus*: faint macular and papular rash, not petechial, starts on trunk or axillary folds, rather than hands and feet (RMSF); rash in 1/2; *epidemic (flea-borne) typhus*: rash is common, starts on upper trunk, becomes generalized, except face, palms, soles, may be petechial, photophobia, skin necrosis if severe; *scrub (chigger-borne) typhus*: rash in 1/2.

Crs: *Endemic (flea-borne) typhus*: incubation: 1–3 wk, prodrome 1–3 d; *epidemic or (louse-borne) typhus*: incubation: 1 wk, abrupt-onset severe illness, fatal in 40% w/o rx; *scrub (chigger-borne) typhus*: incubation: 1–2 wk, abrupt-onset fever, GI and pulmonary sx, may have eschar at chigger bite, LN↑.

Compl: Multisystem but endemic less severe than epidemic.

Ddx: RMSF.

Lab: IFA.

Rx: Doxycycline or other antibiotics as w RMSF.

FEVER, RASH, STARTED ON FACE OR EXTREMITIES

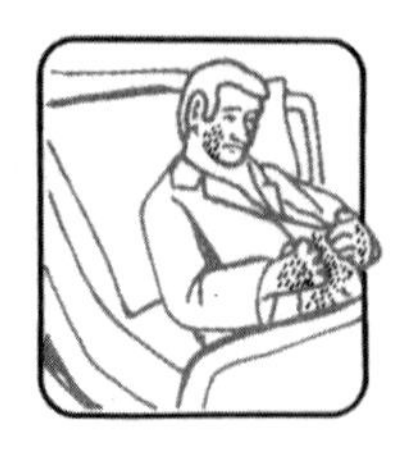

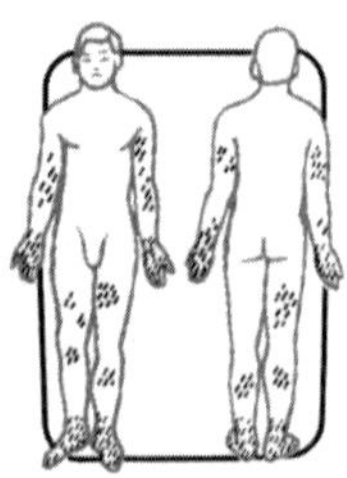

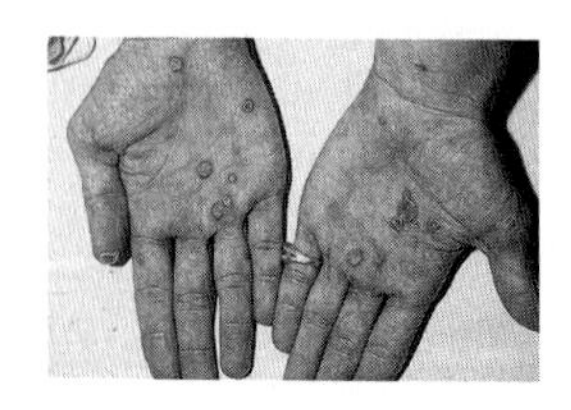

Secondary syphilis

8.1.L. SEPTICEMIA

See color plate section.

Summary: Septic emboli lead to vascular wall necrosis and produce purpuric and palpable lesions; most are at distal parts of extremities, ie, finger and toes, while lesions of vasculitis tend to be worse on lower legs, buttock, and over joints; pts are febrile and toxic; infections usually assoc w septic emboli are *Neisseria meningitidis*, gonococcus, *Pseudomonas* species, and *S. aureus*.

- **Meningococcemia** and **gonococcemia**: both may have septic emboli, but pts w meningococcus are more febrile, sicker, have a more acute onset, and have more hemorrhagic, petechial, and purpuric lesions; skin lesions usually precede meningitis by 1–2 d.

8.1.M. ROCKY MOUNTAIN SPOTTED FEVER (RMSF)

Nejm 1993;329:941. J Infect Dis 1984;150:480.

Cause: *Rickettsia rickettsiae* transmitted from a tick bite: dog tick in eastern U.S. and wood tick in western U.S.; vector is rodent; <0.1% of ticks are infected; several h may be needed to inoculate sufficient numbers of organisms to infect a human.

Epidem: Seasonal, esp early summer, but seen throughout yr; major reservoirs: mid-Atlantic and Rocky Mountain region, but no area is devoid of cases; a single episode confers long-lasting immunity to reinfection.

Pathophys: Damage is from ↑ vascular permeability, rather than DIC.

Sx: Starts w nonspecific viral-like illness: fever, severe headache, muscle and joint discomfort.

Si: Rash: starts by 4th day of fever in 50%; 1st appears on wrists and ankles, then on hands and feet, may include palms and soles (50%); initially light pink and easily blanched; over several days spots become deeper red, even petechial and purpuric; may have edema of hands and feet; rash spreads centrally to genitalia, trunk, extremities; if rash is faint or absent (10%), dx and rx may be delayed; 2/3 recall tick bite, and eschar may be present, look esp in scalp; muscle tenderness.

Crs: Incubation: few d to 2 wk.

Compl: Mortality is low if dx is made early and rx initiated; ↑ fatality rate in males, esp black males w G-6-PD deficiency; w ↑ age, and if rx is delayed >5 d; severe cases: generalized vasculitis, localized gangrene, liver and renal failure, DIC, myocarditis, respiratory failure, splenomegaly, meningitis, seizures, coma; unrx mortality: 50%–80%, but fatal cases occur even w proper rx; postinflammatory desquamation, esp of palms, is common.

Lab: Do not delay rx waiting for lab results; skin bx is diagnostic during early stage if immunofluorescent staining is available, otherwise histology shows only a necrotizing vasculitis w mononuclear infiltrate; serum indirect IFA and enzyme binding assays become pos after 1 wk, too late to wait to initiate rx but tests are specific; also: ↑liver enzymes, ↓ platelets.

Rx: Doxycycline (100 mg bid po or iv) × 7–10 d; tetracycline (25–50 mg/kg/d po) × 7–10 d; or chloramphenicol (50 mg/kg/d available iv only) in divided doses × 7–10 d; 1:30,000 develop aplastic anemia; tetracycline and doxycycline may permanently stain developing teeth in children <8 yo; use iv doxycycline or chloramphenicol if there is CSF pleocytosis; no vaccine is available.

8.1.N. VASCULITIS

J Am Acad Derm 1998;39:667. Med 1998;77:403. Arthritis Rheum 1994;37:187. Ann IM 1978;89:660.

Summary: Various cutaneous lesions: most characteristic lesions are rice grain to dime sized, discrete, palpable, purpuric, petechial; *palpable purpura* results from inflammation of vessel wall w leakage of blood; bx shows inflammatory cells in vessel wall.

Vasculitic disorders are divided into numerous subtypes; classification remains controversial; in most cases, the PCP will obtain a skin bx and seek consultation from dermatology and rheumatology as well as from those specialties dealing w organ systems that seem to be involved.

Cause: Most common precipitating factors (Clin Infect Dis 1995;20:1010):

- Infections: bacterial; viral (hepatitis A, B (up to 30%), C; HSV, influenza virus); fungal (*Candida* species); parasites.
- Drugs: insulin, penicillin and other antibiotics, allopurinol, hydantoins, thiazides, quinine, bcp's, flu vaccine; most drug rxns are not vasculitis.
- Chemicals: insecticides, petroleum products.
- Foods: milk proteins, gluten.

Most common coexistent diseases:

- Connective tissue diseases: SLE, RA, UC, CF, biliary cirrhosis (Rheum Dis Clin N Am 1995;21:1077).
- HIV and AIDS.
- Malignant neoplasms (Med 1998;77:403).

Pathophys: Immune mediators.

Sx: Variable; systemic vasculitis often assoc w low-grade fever, arthralgias, malaise, GI discomfort and melena, renal inflammation and hematuria.

Si: Most important sign to recognize is presence of purpura; typical lesions become palpable, but may not be palpable at onset; patterns characteristic of some subtypes include:

- **Allergic granulomatosis (Churg-Strauss syndrome)**: palpable purpura w asthma, pulmonary infiltrates, ↑ eos.
- **Henoch-Schönlein purpura** (anaphylactoid purpura): arthralgias, abdominal pain w melena, nephritis w hematuria, and occasionally, pulmonary involvement; most common vasculitic disease of children; boys >> girls; often follows URI; ↑ IgA in 50%; usually resolves in few wk; 40% have recurrences; some develop renal insufficiency (Review: Arch Dis Child 1999;80:380); may be assoc w monoclonal gammopathy in adults (Arthritis Rheum 1996;39:698).
- **Hypergammaglobulinemic purpura of Waldenström**: palpable purpura accompanied by polyclonal hypergammaglobulinemia; chronic; worse w standing; may be assoc w Sjögren's syndrome.
- **Lymphomatoid granulomatosis**: rare systemic vasculitis w papular, nodular, and ulcerated skin lesions but w/o purpura; may develop multiple granulomas in lungs and kidneys, which, as they surround small blood vessels, may lead to occlusion; lymphoma develops in up to 50% (pulmonary angiocentric lymphoma).
- **Nodular vasculitis** (erythema induratum): most are women; 30–60 yo; chronic, recurrent, deep, painful nodules; lower legs, esp calves, sometimes arms; often ulcerate; pt usually not febrile (see LEG RASH, 17.4.a.).

- **Pityriasis lichenoides et varioliformis acuta** (PLEVA, Mucha-Habermann's disease): acute and recurrent eruption of hemorrhagic, blistering, necrotic, pea-sized papules; fever and constitutional sx are not common; for additional details, see BODY, 3.1.n.
- **Polyarteritis nodosa**: palpable purpura; segmental necrotizing vasculitis of small and medium muscular arteries; assoc w renal and visceral vasculitis (Arthritis Rheum 1998;41:2100); 20%–30% are hepatitis B pos.
- **Rheumatoid vasculitis**: assoc w severe RA and high titer RF; may get deep vascular occlusion, digital infarcts, cutaneous ulcers (Med 1986;65:365); *rheumatoid nodules* appear in 20% of chronic RA, elbows and hands, persist.
- **Temporal giant cell arteritis**: palpable, thickened temporal artery and scalp pain; fever, polymyalgia, anemia, ↑ ESR, headaches, other arterial occlusions; most >55 yo; women > men; rare in blacks; serious complication: MI, CVA, optic neuritis, and blindness; responds to CS (Rheum Dis Clin N Am 1990;16:399).
- **Urticarial vasculitis**: similar to hives, but lesions persist 2–3 d; sometimes petechial; may feel burning > itching; can become chronic; often assoc w systemic sx (see Sx); note that vasculitis of any cause may be accompanied by hives.
- **Wegener's granulomatosis**: skin lesions in 50%, inc palpable purpura, ulcers; upper and lower respiratory tract granulomatous vasculitis w nephritis; high ANCA (Jama 1995;273:1288).

Crs: Depends on type.

Compl: Drug induced may lead to **Stevens-Johnson syndrome** (see BODY 3.1.b.).

Ddx: R/o systemic vasculitis.

Lab: Bx of involved tissue to confirm is crucial: "vasculitis" is a pathologic dx, not a clinical dx; lab: (Int Angiol 1995;14:188; Arch IM 1989;149:161) wbc may be ↑; eos may be ↑; ESR may be ↑; stool guaiac; may have hepatitis B surface antigen; ANCA often pos (Curr Opin Rheum 1993;5:18); also consider: ANA; RF; chest x-ray; cryoglobulins; HIV test; cardiac evaluation (for underlying endocarditis).

Rx: Depends on type; prognosis may be poor if systemic; watch renal and hepatic function; some types respond to CS, others to CS plus cytotoxic agents; interferon may be useful if hepatitis is present; multiple specialties, esp rheumatology, should be involved.

SWEET'S SYNDROME (ACUTE FEBRILE NEUTROPHILIC DERMATOSIS)

J Am Acad Derm 1994;31:535.

Cause: Unknown; 10% assoc w malignancy; may follow use of granulocyte colony-stimulating factor (Arch Derm 1994;130:77); other drugs (J Am Acad Derm 1996;34:918).

Epidem: Women >> men; 30–60 yo; occas children (Br J Derm 1991;124:203).

Pathophys: Immune complexes assumed.

Sx: Plaques are painful, not itchy.

Si: Raised, red, rapidly expanding, thickened plaques; quarter to palm sized; assoc w fever, neutrophilic leukocytosis.

Crs: Often starts 1–3 wk after URI or flulike illness; severity depends on extent of organ involvement; may be fatal.

Compl: Underlying malignancy, esp leukemia (10%); extracutaneous sites: joints, muscles, eye, kidney, lung.

Ddx: Cellulitis, sepsis, erythema multiforme, erythema nodosum.

Lab: Skin bx (DX.7): dermal neutrophilic infiltrate w/o vasculitis; look for systemic involvement: ↑wbc, ↑ESR.

Rx: Systemic CS; refer to dermatology for confirmation of dx and alternative rx, if needed.

8.1.O. MUCOCUTANEOUS LYMPH NODE SYNDROME (KAWASAKI DISEASE)

Am Fam Phys 1999;59:3093. Jama 1991;265:2699.

Cause: Unknown; presumed infectious and partially immune mediated (Ped Clin North Am 1995;42:1205).

Epidem: Uncommon; 80% <5 yo; boys > girls.

Pathophys: Vasculitis of coronary arteries in fatal cases.

Si: Prodrome: nonspecific febrile illness; diagnostic criteria (American Heart Assoc Guidelines in Am J Dis Child 1990;144:1218): fever of 5 or more d duration plus 4 of the next 5 features: (1) changes in extremities (redness, edema); (2) nonspecific, pink exanthem beginning within 5 d after start of fever; (3) bilateral conjunctival injection; (4) mouth/pharynx inflammation; (5) ↑ cervical LNs (50%–75%); exclude other diseases.

Crs: 80% resolve completely in 2–4 wk w occas arthritis, transient abn RFTs and LFTs; recurrences are rare.

Compl: 20% develop myocardial or coronary artery inflammation w arrhythmias, valvular insufficiency, or aneurysms and 1%–2% have fatal outcome, usually during convalescence; arthritis; aseptic meningitis (Circ 1994;89:916; Circ 1993;87:1776).

Ddx: RMSF because of eruption on hands and feet; measles; TSS; drug rxns; scarlet fever; juvenile rheumatoid arthritis; leptospirosis.

Lab: No specific test available; ↑ ESR, ↑ wbc, ↑ platelets, ↑ C-reactive protein.

Rx: Aspirin (80–100 mg/kg/d) during acute phase until afebrile, then 3–5 mg/kg/d for at least 2 mo w 1 course of iv IgG (Nejm 1991;324:1633); avoid CS; no response to antibiotics; pts generally require pediatric, infectious disease, and cardiac consultations.

FEVER, BLISTERS, POSITIVE GRAM'S STAIN OR VIRAL OR BACTERIAL CULTURE

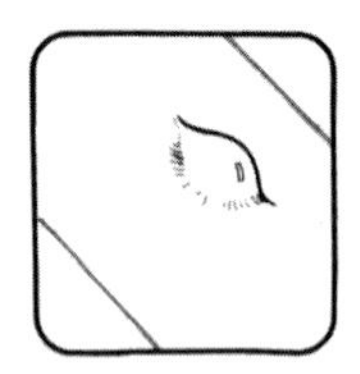

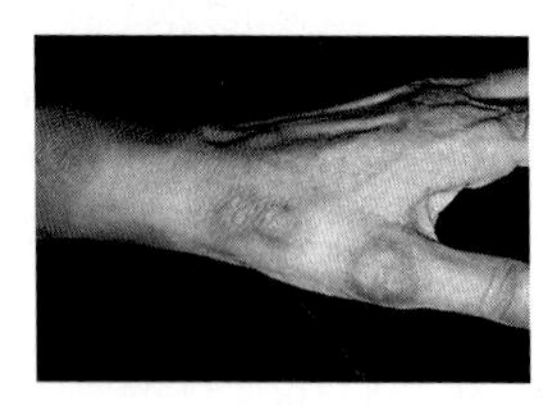

Erythema multiforme

8.2.A. IMPETIGO, PYODERMA

Cause: Crusty form: usually group A β-hemolytic streptococci; blistering form: usually *S. aureus*.

Sx: Mild irritation or pain.

Si: Either honey-colored, stuck-on crusty patches or single or multiple blisters; most commonly on face; most are in young children; LN↑ often present; fever usually absent.

Compl: Most serious: glomerulonephritis following streptococcal impetigo.

Lab: Swab base below crust or aspirate fluid from a blister w small syringe; submit to lab for Gram's stain, bacterial and viral culture.

For additional details and rx suggestions, see FACE, 6.6.a.

8.2.B. HERPES SIMPLEX

Summary: Groups of pinhead-sized blisters on lip, usually at vermilion border; hx of recurrence at same or nearly same site; may be assoc w malaise; LN↑.

For additional details and rx, see BLISTERS, 2.1.a.

8.2.C. VARICELLA (CHICKENPOX)

Summary: An itchy, sick, febrile child w scattered pea-sized blisters and pustules generally has varicella; prodrome is mild w fever and malaise for 1–3 d; fever after new lesions cease appearing: 2° bacterial infection, Reye's syndrome, vasculitis, inflammation of viscera, myocarditis; can be severe or fatal in immunosuppressed persons; systemic complications are more severe in adults than children.

For additional details and rx, see BLISTERS, 2.3.a.

8.2.D. HERPES ZOSTER (SHINGLES)

Summary: Group of vesicles, each w a central dell; sharply demarcated at midline, following distribution of a peripheral nerve; pain >> itch; pt not generally febrile, but may follow a febrile or acute illness; most common in pts w ↓ immunity; varicella may be contracted from pt w active zoster.

For additional details and rx, see BLISTERS, 2.3.d.

FEVER, BLISTERS, NEGATIVE GRAM'S STAIN OR VIRAL OR BACTERIAL CULTURE

8.2.L. ERYTHEMA MULTIFORME

Summary: Abrupt onset w flat, dusky lesions resembling dime- to quarter-sized hives; central part often is darker or blistering, like a bull's-eye or target; pain > itch; usually extensor surfaces; palmar and plantar lesions are tender; individual lesions persist longer than hives; severe cases may be hemorrhagic, peeling, or blistering; mucous membrane erosions are common and often disabling.

For additional details and rx, see BLISTERS, 2.1.b.

8.2.M. TOXIC EPIDERMAL NECROLYSIS (TEN)

Summary: Red, tender rash on face and extremities that quickly becomes confluent, then blisters; blisters become large, rupture easily, and leave large, denuded areas; mucous membranes almost always severely involved; pts are febrile; mortality is high w damage to lung, GI, renal, and eyes.

For additional details and rx, see BLISTERS, 2.3.e.

8.2.N. STAPHYLOCOCCAL SCALDED SKIN SYNDROME (SSSS)

Summary: Sudden onset; starts w purulent eruption of nose, eyes, throat; evolves in 1–2 d into widespread redness, tenderness, and finally, large blisters and shedding of skin in sheets; mucosal surfaces not involved; most cases are young children; course is <1 wk; cause is staphylococcus, often otitis media or occult sinus infection; ddx: TEN (see 8.2.m.); bullous impetigo may be localized SSSS.

For additional details and rx, see BLISTERS, 2.3.f.

8.2.O. DRUG REACTION

Summary: Severe drug rxns may be bullous, esp assoc w barbiturates, halogens, and penicillin; drugs also induce erythema multiforme (see BLISTERS, 2.1.b) and TEN (see 8.2.m.); for additional details, see 8.1.a.

8.2.P. PEMPHIGUS AND PEMPHIGOID

Summary: Large blisters of skin and erosions of mucous membranes are hallmark signs; blistering may start acutely or develop only after mo of oral lesions; pts may be mildly febrile but fever is minor compared to dramatic skin changes.

For additional details and rx, see BLISTERS, 2.4.d.

FEVER

FEVER, RASH, ARTHRALGIAS

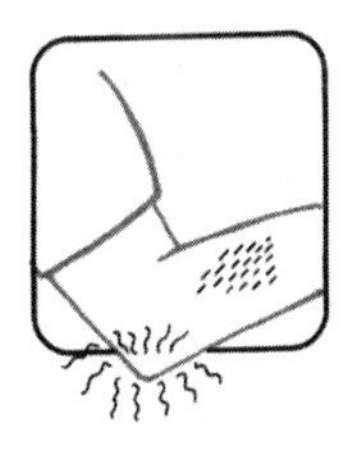

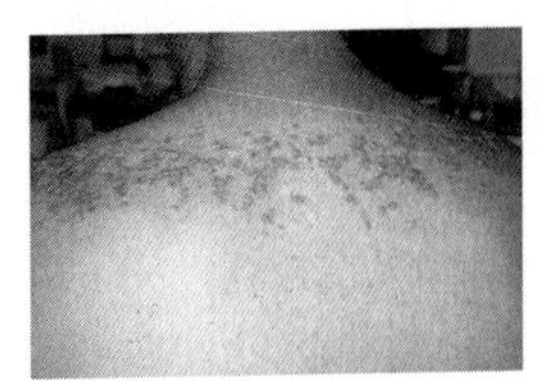

Systemic lupus erythematosus

8.3.A. LUPUS ERYTHEMATOSUS, SYSTEMIC (SLE)

Med Clin N Am 1998;82:1217. Ann IM 1995;122:940. Ann IM 1995;123:42. Nejm 1994;330:1871. Med 1993;72:113.

See color plate section.

Cause: Genetic?; environmental?; hormonal?; immunologic?; viral?; drug induced: procainamide, hydralazine, quinidine, methyldopa, chlorpromazine.

Epidem: Women >> men; blacks > whites.

Pathophys: Tissue damage from immune complexes and autoantibodies.

Sx: Acute or active stage: fatigue, arthralgias, fever (usually is low grade), visual changes.

Si: Pink to red rash w slight local swelling and scale; usually on sun-exposed areas, ie, characteristic malar "butterfly" rash over nose and cheeks in 1/3 (pts w butterfly rash usually have active disease); hands: red raised patches, esp between knuckles and about nails; asx gray-white patches on mucous membranes in 1/4; diffuse hair thinning; about 5% of pts w SLE have discoid LE lesions (see FACE, 6.2.c): coin-shaped plaques that are pink to red, scaly and w areas of atrophy and follicular plugging leading eventually to shiny, depressed, depigmented, and hairless lesions.

- 11 signs of SLE were selected as useful for classification by the American Rheumatism Association (Arthritis Rheum 1982;25:1271): malar rash, discoid rash, photosensitivity, oral ulcers, arthritis involving 2 or more joints, serositis (pleuritis or pericarditis), renal disorder (proteinuria > 0.5 gm/d or cellular casts), neurologic disorder (seizures or psychosis), hematologic disorder (low total wbc or low lymphocyte numbers or low platelet count or hemolytic anemia), immunologic disorder (LE cells or anti-DNA or anti-Sm or biologic false-pos serologic test for syphilis), ↑ ANA titers; Raynaud's phenomenon and alopecia also occur frequently in pts w SLE, but are not on this list of criteria; 4 or more, serially or simultaneously during any interval of observation, confirms dx of SLE for clinical studies (*note*: these criteria are not useful to dx individual cases, as fewer criteria may be at hand at the time that SLE is suspected and rx started); **subacute cutaneous LE**: a subset of SLE w photosensitivity, nonscarring skin lesions, low incidence of systemic vascular, CNS, and renal involvement (J Am Acad Derm 1998;38:405; J Invest Derm 1993;100:2S).

Crs: Variable w periods of flares and remissions; often predictable by pattern set during first 2 yr; renal disease at time of presentation is poor sign; SLE pts w predominant skin lesions generally have milder form than those w/o skin lesions; 5-yr survival has improved from 50% 30 yr ago to >90% now (Med 1999;78:167), presumably because of better rx; sun exposure, pregnancy, and oral bcp's tend to worsen course; poorest survival w high BP and/or nephritis w proteinuria (Rheum Dis Clin N Am 1988;14:67).

Compl: Infections and renal failure cause most deaths in 1st decade after dx; thromboses in 2nd decade; any organ may become involved.

Lab: Skin bx helps establish dx, esp w IFA; obtain ANA as screen for SLE; neg ANA is strong but not absolute evidence against SLE; if ANA titer pos, obtain more specific tests, esp anti-dsDNA (native dsDNA) and anti-ENAs, which detect RNP and Sm; anti-dsDNA and anti-Sm are highly specific for SLE; anti-RNP is present in 100% of pts w *mixed connective tissue disease*; low titer is assoc w better prognosis; **subacute cutaneous LE:** pts w photosensitive dermatitis; often ANA neg w circulating antibodies to cytoplasmic antigens Ro (SS-A) and La and to ssDNA; ↓ C′ assoc w worsening SLE, esp w renal disease; also: ↓ rbc, ↓ wbc, ↓ platelets, ↑ ESR, BFP STS; renal function tests may be abn (renal disease does not occur if *drug-induced SLE*; DNA-histone test pos in most drug-induced SLE); obtain RFTs and LFTs to establish baseline.

Rx: Suppress active disease during flares and reduce or stop rx during remissions; no cure exists; complete permanent remissions are rare.

- Acute: for systemic signs, ie, fever, fatigue, serositis, arthritis, or new rash: bed rest and either enteric-coated ASA or NSAID (avoid NSAID in pts w ↓ renal function, and avoid ibuprofen and tolmetin, as pts w SLE on either have developed aseptic meningitis); si or sx not controlled by NSAID require prednisone, usually 10–20 mg/d; immunosuppressive agents, ie, cyclophosphamide or azathioprine, also are used, but because they produce bone marrow suppression and possibly induce malignancies, they are generally reserved for more severe or refractory manifestations, ie, nephritis (Ann IM 1995;122:940) or vasculitis; watch for sudden clinical change that may be caused by a bacterial infection to which pt is predisposed by both SLE and its rx.

- Long-term: antimalarials for only skin and joint involvement (hydroxychloroquine 200–400 mg/d, pt needs yrly eye exams for visual field monitoring); reduce dose of all meds during periods of remission; avoid sun exposure and use sunscreens; avoid bcp's and estrogens.

Most pts w SLE have multisystem disease and several specialties usually become involved in their care.

Contact Lupus Foundation of America (1300 Picard Drive, Suite 200, Rockville, MD 20850; 800.558.0121 or 301.670.9292; www.lupus.org/lupus) for pt education materials.

8.3.B. DERMATOMYOSITIS

J Am Acad Derm 1998;39:899. Med Clin N Am 1998;82:1217. Miller OF, Newman ED, Dermatomyositis and polymyositis, in Cutaneous medicine and surgery, WB Saunders, Philadelphia, 1996:283.

Cause: Immune mediated?; environmental?; genetic?; controversial ↑ w systemic malignancy, esp for pts >40 yo (J Rheum 1995;22:1300; Nejm 1992;326:363); drug induced (penicillamine, NSAIDs, hydroxyurea, provastatin, zidovudine).

Epidem: Uncommon; women > men; most 45–55 yo; some juvenile cases.

Sx: Proximal symmetric muscle weakness and soreness; leading to difficulty w combing hair, rising from a chair, and climbing stairs; difficulty swallowing; fatigue.

Si: Violaceous discoloration and edema of eyelids (50%), frequently w red to purple scaly patches and swelling of face; patches and plaques over joints, including elbows and knees; violaceous papules over joints (70%), esp finger joints (*Gottron's papules*); induration and calcification of subcutaneous tissues and muscle; telangiectasia, atrophy, pigmentation, skin thickening, scalp rash and alopecia, Raynaud's phenomenon, photosensitivity; erythema (30%), and periungual telangiectasia.

Crs: Acute and fulminant, or slowly progressive, or recurrent; few remit permanently; skin and muscle signs usually coexist, skin usually

1st, but either can exist alone; SLE may coexist (**mixed connective tissue disease** or **overlap syndrome**); overall mortality: 20% 5-yr from disease or complications of rx; ↓ survival: age >45 yo; malignancy; heart or lung involvement; children: generally good prognosis; calcification is more common.

Compl: No correlation between severity of skin and muscle disease activity; cutaneous calcium deposition may be troublesome and does not respond to present rx.

Ddx: Consider trichinosis; limit w/u for internal malignancy in pts >40 yo to hx, ROS, and evaluation of suspicious areas (J Am Acad Derm 1982;6:235).

Lab: Skin bx: only nonspecific changes; muscle bx: may show inflammation, but such changes are also present in SLE and scleroderma; EMG often abn, esp if clinically abn muscle is tested; ↑ enzymes assoc w muscle, esp serum creatine kinase, aldolase, AST, ALT, esp during exacerbations; creatine kinase levels correlate w disease activity (Arthritis Rheum 1987;30:213); obtain sera prior to EMG or muscle bx as procedures ↑serum muscle enzyme levels; RF and ANA: may be ↑ but at low titer; not specific for myositis; many pos pts have features of SLE or scleroderma; more myositis-specific antibodies are assoc w specific clinical syndromes:

1. *Anti–aminoacyl-tRNA synthetase antibodies*: **antisynthetase syndrome**: rash w palmar hyperkeratosis (mechanic's hands); interstitial lung disease; nonerosive arthritis; Raynaud's phenomenon; fever; severe crs; onset in spring; accounts for 25% of pts w myositis.
2. *Anti-SRP antibodies*: severe myositis; cardiac involvement; mostly in black women; onset usually in fall; 5% of pts w myositis.
3. *Anti–Mi-2 antibodies*: prominent rash, esp upper back (shawl sign); Gottron's papules; periungual thickening; 5%–10% of pts w myositis.

Rx: Initial: systemic CS (prednisone 0.5–1.5 mg/kg/d); follow serum creatine kinase levels; alternatives and adjuvants include MTX, cyclophosphamide, or azathioprine; cyclosporine: beneficial effects may be dramatic (J Rheum 1994;21:381); most pts require a multidisciplinary approach and usually are referred to university medical centers.

8.3.C. SCLERODERMA (MORPHEA, SYSTEMIC SCLEROSIS)

Curr Opin Rheum 1996;8:473. Rheum Dis Clin N Am 1995;21:203. J Rheum 1992;19:673.

Cause: Autoimmune?
Epidem: Women >> men; systemic sclerosis: 40–70 yo; morphea: 2–20 yo.
Pathophys: Sclerosis, fibrosis, and vascular thickening w occlusion.
Sx: Depends on organs involved.
Si:

- **Systemic sclerosis**: progressive sclerosis of skin (sclerodactyly, loss of forehead and finger skin wrinkling, ↓ diameter of mouth opening) and other organs: esophagus (dysphagia), lung (dyspnea), vessels of kidneys (renal failure), and heart (arrhythmias and failure); also Raynaud's phenomenon (see below), joint stiffness, periungual telangiectasia, hyperpigmentation.
- **Morphea**: lesions are 1 to few; initially pink; gradually become firm, hairless, and ivory colored, like a thick or depressed scar; rare pts develop multiple lesions or bizarre linear patterns.
- **Raynaud's disease and phenomenon**: cold-induced finger or toe tip vasospasm leading to blanching (white), cyanosis (blue), and rubor (red) color changes; women >> men; 20–40 yo; *Raynaud's disease*: mild, self-limited; *Raynaud's phenomenon*: underlying assoc cause, esp collagen/vascular disease, smoking, drug rxn (ergots, β-blockers, bleomycin, vinblastine, and cisplatin); ANA-neg pts have only 10% progression in 2–5 yr (Scand J Rheum 1998;27:319); capillary nail fold microscopy has a pos predictive value of 47% (Arch IM 1998;158:595); technique: use +20 diopter lens of an ophthalmoscope to examine capillary pattern at nail fold just proximal to fingernail after area has been covered w a drop of immersion or mineral oil and a coverslip; look for avascular areas or irregular dilated capillary loops.
- **CREST syndrome**: *c*alcinosis cutis, *R*aynaud's phenomenon, *e*sophageal dysfunction, *s*clerodactyly, and *t*elangiectasia; ↑anticentromere antibodies; assoc w fewer systemic complications.

- **Fasciitis with eosinophilia**: sudden onset of swelling and erythema of arms/legs plus ↑blood eos, ↑ESR, various hematologic abn; bx of indurated skin and fascia: inflammation, thickening of skin and fascia w eos; rx: systemic CS; multiple specialties usually involved.

Crs:

- *Systemic sclerosis*: 10-yr survival is 65% (Ann IM 1993;118:602), but many stabilize at an ambulatory plateau.
- *Morphea*: probably never becomes systemic; eventually 1/2 clear or improve spontaneously.

Compl: *Systemic sclerosis*: most serious consequences: renal insufficiency, hypertension, pulmonary and heart failure.

Lab: Skin bx; ANA pos (95%), esp w speckled pattern (Int Rev Immunol 1995;12:145); C′ normal; ↑RF (25%); ↑ESR.

Rx: No specific rx is available (Semin Arth Rheum 1993;23:22); systemic CS often used for acute changes but not chronically; D-penicillamine of unproven value; ACE blockers for high BP; nifedipine for heart and Raynaud's; pts w systemic sclerosis require multidisciplinary approach and usually are referred to medical centers.

Contact Scleroderma Foundation (89 Newberry Street, Suite 201, Danvers, MA 01923; 800.722.HOPE or 978.750.4499; www.scleroderma.org and www.srfcure.org) for pt education materials.

FEVER

FEVER, RASH, ORAL LESIONS, PAINFUL

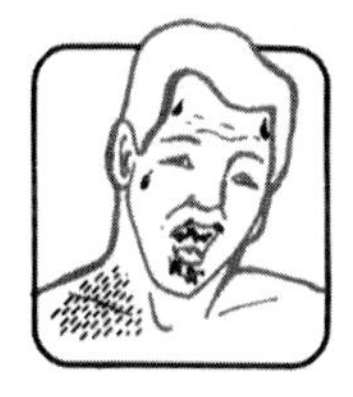

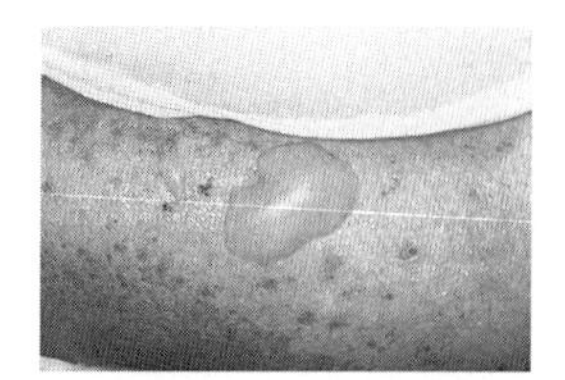

Toxic epidermal necrolysis

Erythema multiforme, see 8.2.l.
Pemphigus/pemphigoid, see 8.2.p.
Scarlet fever, see 8.1.c.
TEN, see 8.2.m.
Herpes simplex, see 8.2.b.

FEVER, RASH, ORAL LESIONS, PAINLESS

Collagen vascular disease, see 8.3.a.–c.
Enterovirus infections, see 8.1.b.
Mucocutaneous lymph node syndrome, see 8.1.o.
Syphilis, secondary, see 8.1.d.

9 Genital

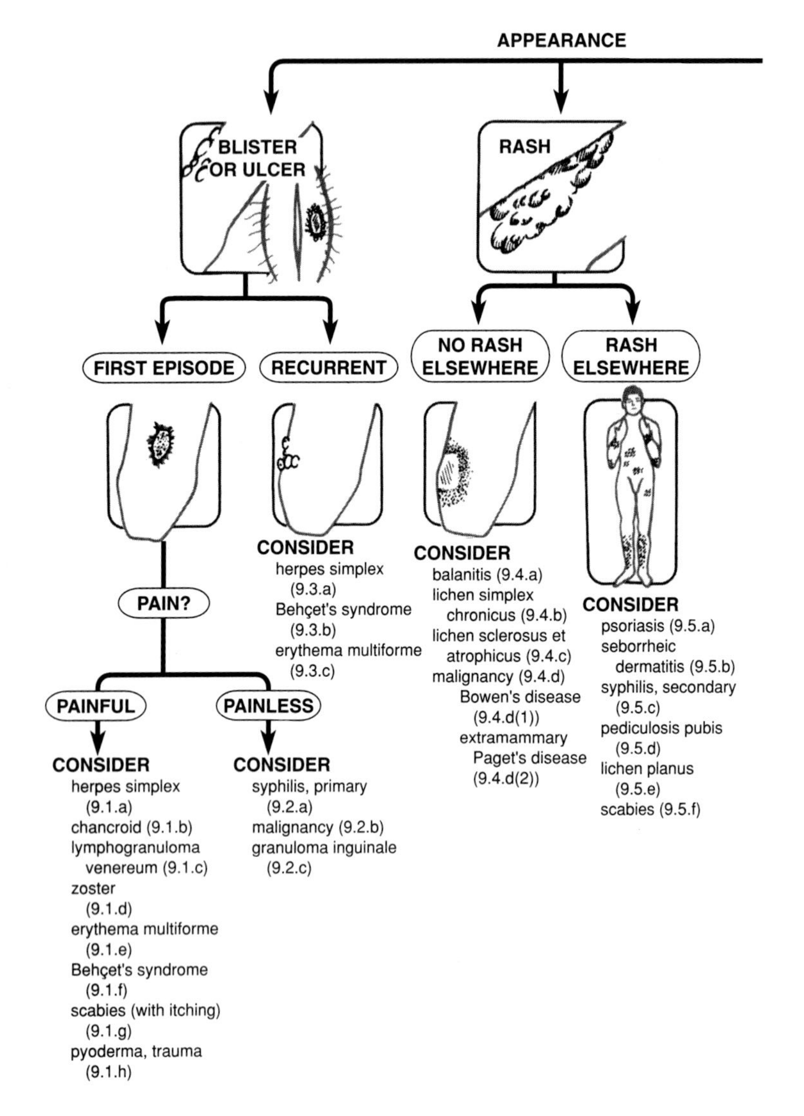

APPEARANCE
BLISTER OR ULCER
RASH
FIRST EPISODE
RECURRENT
NO RASH ELSEWHERE
RASH ELSEWHERE
PAIN?
PAINFUL
PAINLESS
CONSIDER
herpes simplex (9.1.a)
chancroid (9.1.b)
lymphogranuloma venereum (9.1.c)
zoster (9.1.d)
erythema multiforme (9.1.e)
Behçet's syndrome (9.1.f)
scabies (with itching) (9.1.g)
pyoderma, trauma (9.1.h)
CONSIDER
syphilis, primary (9.2.a)
malignancy (9.2.b)
granuloma inguinale (9.2.c)
CONSIDER
herpes simplex (9.3.a)
Behçet's syndrome (9.3.b)
erythema multiforme (9.3.c)
CONSIDER
balanitis (9.4.a)
lichen simplex chronicus (9.4.b)
lichen sclerosus et atrophicus (9.4.c)
malignancy (9.4.d)
Bowen's disease (9.4.d(1))
extramammary Paget's disease (9.4.d(2))
CONSIDER
psoriasis (9.5.a)
seborrheic dermatitis (9.5.b)
syphilis, secondary (9.5.c)
pediculosis pubis (9.5.d)
lichen planus (9.5.e)
scabies (9.5.f)

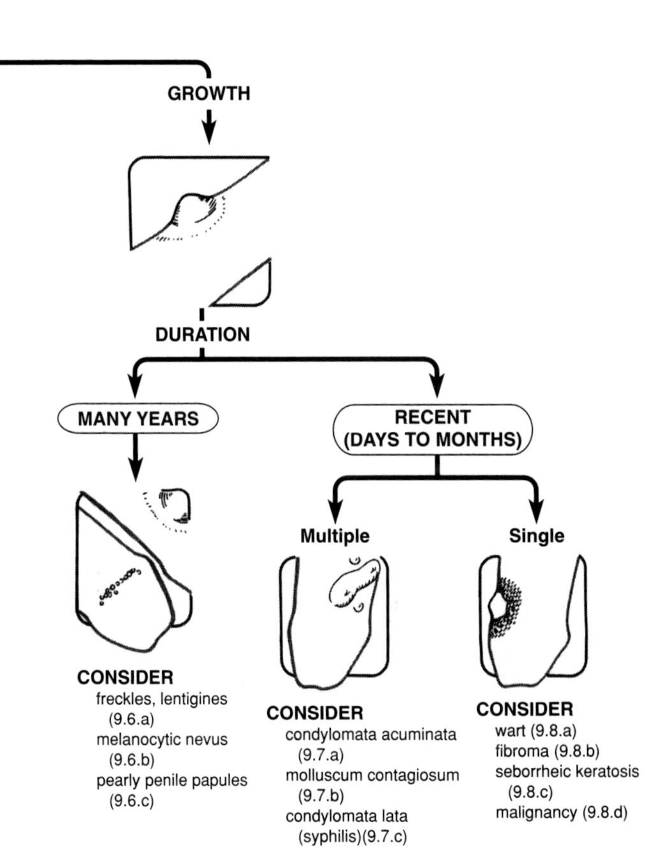
GROWTH
DURATION
MANY YEARS
RECENT
(DAYS TO MONTHS)
Multiple
Single
CONSIDER
freckles, lentigines
(9.6.a)
melanocytic nevus
(9.6.b)
pearly penile papules
(9.6.c)
CONSIDER
condylomata acuminata
(9.7.a)
molluscum contagiosum
(9.7.b)
condylomata lata
(syphilis)(9.7.c)
CONSIDER
wart (9.8.a)
fibroma (9.8.b)
seborrheic keratosis
(9.8.c)
malignancy (9.8.d)

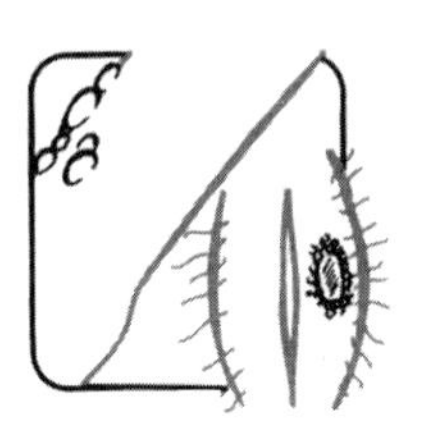

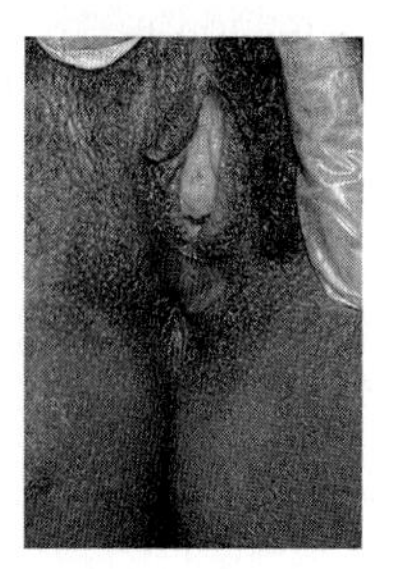

Herpes simplex—vulva

9.1.A. HERPES SIMPLEX

Summary:

- Primary: initial infection; often w fever, malaise, tender LN↑; small blisters, often in groups; may be pyoderma; resolves in 1–3 wk; no scarring.
- Recurrent: groups of pinhead-sized blisters on lip, usually at vermilion border; hx of recurrence at same or nearly same site; may be assoc w malaise; LN↑; usually resolves within 1 wk.

For additional details and rx, see BLISTERS, 2.1.a.

9.1.B. CHANCROID

Jaad 1999;41:511; Mmwr 1998;No. RR-1:47:18. Med Clin N Am 1998;82:1081. J Am Acad Derm 1991;25:287.

Cause: Gram-neg intracellular and extracellular bacillus, *Haemophilus ducreyi.*

Epidem: Transmitted through sexual contact; females are often asx carriers.

Si: 1° lesion is a small but enlarging and ulcerated papule, resembling syphilis, but unlike syphilis is ragged, dirty, purulent, painful, and often multiple; tender inguinal LN ↑ (buboes) after days or wks in 1/2; mostly males.

Crs: 1° starts 3–5 d after exposure; inguinal lymph nodes become painful and swollen.
Compl: 10% have coinfection w syphilis or HSV.
Lab: Difficult to culture; special media required; aspirate from LN may be submitted for culture and smear; dx is made on combination of painful ulcer, tender adenopathy, neg HSV culture, and neg RPR at least 7 d after onset of ulcer.
Rx: Azithromycin 1 gm po in single dose or ceftriaxone 250 mg im in a single dose or ciprofloxacin 500 mg po bid for 3 d (not in pregnant and lactating women or if <18 yo) or erythromycin base 500 mg po qid for 1 wk; does not respond to penicillin; treat sexual partners.

9.1.C. LYMPHOGRANULOMA VENEREUM (LGV)

Jaad 1999;41:511; Mmwr 1998;No. RR-1:47:27. Med Clin N Am 1998;82:1081. J Am Acad Derm 1991;25:287. Prim Care 1990;17:153.

Cause: Chlamydial organism, *Chlamydia trachomatis*.
Epidem: Rare in U.S.; sexual transmission, often from asx females.
Sx: Fever and myalgias w painful adenopathy.
Si: 1° : small, nontender papule erodes then heals in days, ulcer may not be recalled; 2° : inguinal LNs that enlarge, mat, rupture, and drain.
Crs: 1° occurs few days to wks after exposure; LNs enlarge within a few wks; if untreated 1° and LNs appear to heal in 2–3 mos.
Compl: Mos to yrs later, lymphatic blockage, edematous thickening of genitalia, and rectal stricture may develop.
Lab: LGV complement fixation becomes pos a mo after infection; cross-reacts w *psittacosis*, bx is not specific; culture is difficult.
Rx: Doxycycline 100 mg bid × 3 wk; alternative: erythromycin base 500 mg qid × 3 wk; penicillin is not effective.

GENITAL

9.1.D. ZOSTER

Summary: Grouped small blisters, each w a central dimple; unlikely to be restricted to genitals, but in ddx of HSV.
For additional details and rx, see BLISTERS, 2.3.d.

9.1.E. ERYTHEMA MULTIFORME

Summary: Abrupt onset w flat, dusky lesions resembling dime- to quarter-sized hives; central part often is darker or blistering, like a bull's-eye or target; pain > itch; usually extensor surfaces; palmar and plantar lesions are tender; individual lesions persist longer than hives; severe cases may be hemorrhagic, peeling, or blistering; mucous membrane erosions are common and often disabling.

For additional details and rx, see BLISTERS, 2.1.b.

9.1.F. BEHÇET'S SYNDROME

Summary: Genital ulcers are size of pencil eraser to quarter, painful and recurrent; associated w oral ulcers, uveitis, cutaneous vasculitis, arthritis, diarrhea, and/or a variety of neurologic changes.

For additional details and rx, see MOUTH, 19.1.h.

9.1.G. SCABIES

Summary: Excoriated, red papules, some w a thin "burrow"; numerous scratch marks, lichenified patches; genital lesions include pea-sized lumps on penis and scrotum or vulva; look for excoriated lesions or scratch marks at finger webs, elbows, areolae, umbilicus, lower abdomen, wrists, antecubital fossae, and gluteal cleft; itching worse at night; conjugal partners are involved.

For additional details and rx, see BODY, 3.1.e.

9.1.H. PYODERMA/TRAUMA

Summary: Single or multiple superficial erosions; eliminate other causes.

BLISTER OR ULCER, FIRST EPISODE, PAINLESS

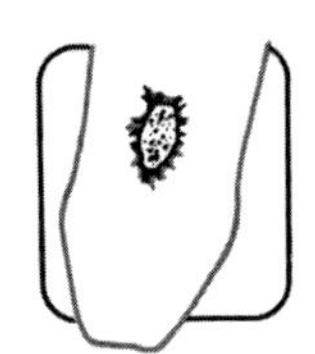

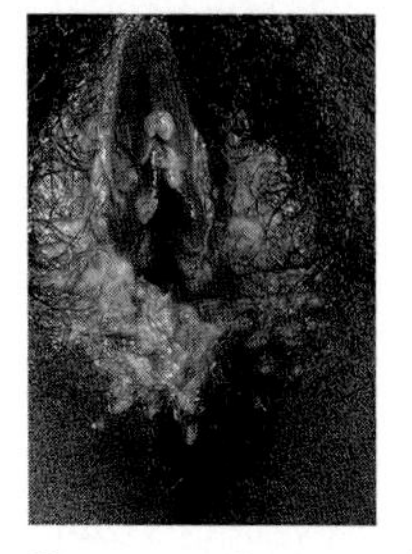

Chancre—primary syphilis

9.2.A. SYPHILIS, PRIMARY (CHANCRE)

Jaad 1999;41:511; Am Fam Phys 1999;59:2233. Mmwr 1998;No. RR-1:47:31. Med Clin N Am 1998;82:1081.

Cause: *Treponema pallidum*, a spirochete; incidence of syphilis is now highest since 1949 (Am Fam Phys 1994;50:1013).

Si: Starts as a single small papule; develops into a nearly painless relatively clean erosion over thickened "button" of skin; diameter: 0.5–2 cm is typical; usual sites: penile shaft, labia; atypical sites: lips, fingers, within anus or vagina; also multiple erosions, balanitis, phimosis, urethral discharge; no 1° in 1/4; nontender inguinal LNs (Clin Infect Dis 1997;25;292).

Crs: Appears 2–4 wk after infection; may be delayed up to 3 mo; untreated ulcer disappears spontaneously in 3–6 wk w thin scar.

Lab:

- **Nonspecific antibodies** against lipoidal antigens: VDRL or RPR test; pos when 1° is present in 30%–50%; nearly always pos in secondary syphilis; obtain 1 mo and 3 mo after suspicious chancre; nonreactive tests for 3 mo excludes syphilis; inexpensive, sensitive, and can be quantitated: if pos, repeat and obtain FTA: if pos, pt has or has had a treponemal disease.
- **Specific antibodies:** FTA or FTA-ABS test; pos when 1° is present in 75%–90%.

GENITAL

- **Darkfield:** rapid and reliable but now only rarely performed
- **BFP rxn** to VDRL/RPR is common; FTA almost always neg; BFP rxns of <6 mo: infections, esp viral infections, vaccinations, malignancy, narcotic abuse, or even pregnancy; chronic BFP rxns of >6 mo: collagen vascular disease, leprosy (see BODY, 3.3.q.).
- All pts w syphilis should be tested for HIV (J Infect Dis 1989;160:530).

Rx:

- Benzathine penicillin G, 2.4 million units im in a single dose for 1° or 2° and syphilis of <1-yr duration; if allergic to penicillin use tetracycline 500 mg qid po for 2 wk or doxycycline 100 mg bid po for 2 wk; if neither can be used, erythromycin 500 mg qid po for 2 wk is a less effective alternative; for pregnant and penicillin allergic, desensitization is necessary as erythromycin does not cure an infected fetus (Mmwr 1998;No. RR-1:47:40); *WARNING*: chills, fever, myalgias, headache, exacerbation 6–8 h after rx (Jarisch-Herxheimer rxn); benzathine penicillin G is not rx for gonorrhea.
- Treat sexual partners exposed to 1° or 2° syphilis or syphilis of <1-yr duration; esp if f/u is uncertain; transmission is less likely if syphilis is present for >1 yr.
- F/u: obtain quantitative VDRL/RPR at 6 and 12 mo after rx; titers generally become neg if syphilis is <1-yr duration; if titers do not become neg or decline 4 × by 6 mo, consider rx failure, HIV infection, and/or CNS infection; such cases generally are referred for specialty care; also refer if titer ↑ 4 x, rx has failed or pt was reinfected.

9.2.B. MALIGNANCY

Summary: Painless ulcer, esp >6 wk; bx suspicious lesions.

For additional details, see 9.8.d.

9.2.C. GRANULOMA INGUINALE

Summary: Rare outside of tropics; inguinal or perianal; vegetative, friable, ulcerated dirty plaque resembling infected granulation tissue; organism is a gram-neg intracellular encapsulated human parasite, *Calymmatobacterium (Donovania) granulomatis*; responds to trimethoprim-sulfamethoxazole, double-strength tab bid × 3 wk or doxycycline 100 mg bid × 3 wk; does not respond to penicillin (Jaad 1999;41:511; Mmwr 1998;No. RR-1:47:26; Med Clin N Am 1998;82:1081; Clin Infect Dis 1997;25:24; J Am Acad Derm 1991;25:287); consider concomitant HIV infection.

BLISTER OR ULCER, RECURRENT

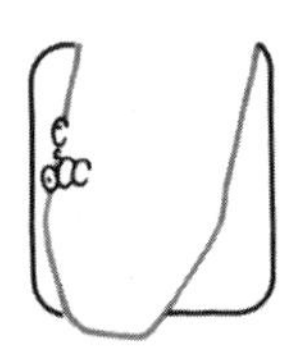

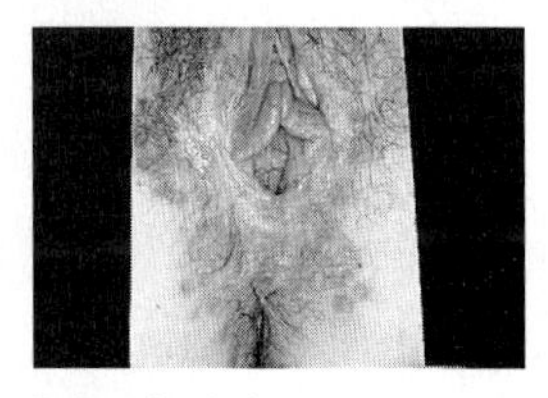

Behçet's circinata

9.3.A. HERPES SIMPLEX

Summary: Groups of pinhead-sized blisters; hx of recurrence at same or nearly same site; may be assoc w malaise; LN↑.

For additional details and rx, see BLISTERS, 2.1.a.

9.3.B. BEHÇET'S SYNDROME

Summary: Genital ulcers are size of pencil eraser to quarter, painful and recurrent; associated w oral ulcers, uveitis, cutaneous vasculitis, arthritis, diarrhea, and/or a variety of neurologic changes.

For additional details and rx, see MOUTH, 19.1.h.

GENITAL

9.3.C. ERYTHEMA MULTIFORME

Summary: Abrupt onset w flat, dusky lesions resembling dime- to quarter-sized hives; central part often is darker or blistering, like a bull's-eye or target; pain > itch; usually extensor surfaces; palmar and plantar lesions are tender; individual lesions persist longer than hives; severe cases may be hemorrhagic, peeling, or blistering; mucous membrane erosions are common and often disabling.

For additional details and rx, see BLISTERS, 2.1.b.

RASH ON GENITALS, NO RASH ELSEWHERE

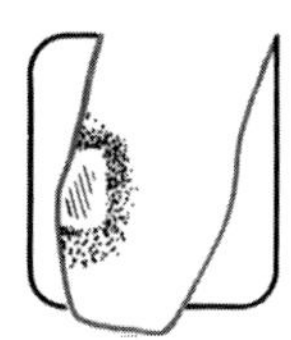

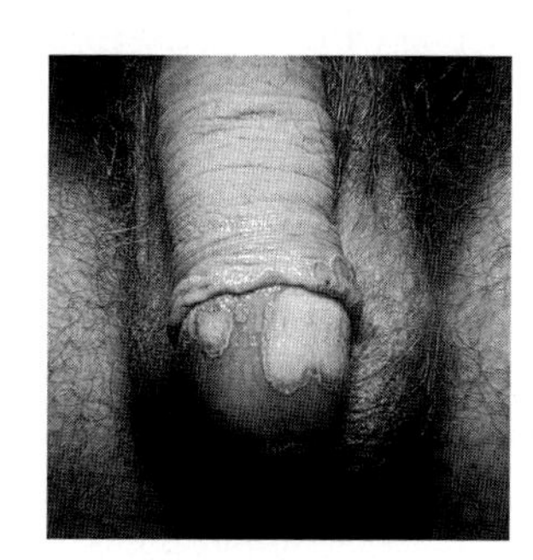

Balanitis circinata

9.4.A. BALANITIS

Si: Glans penis is reddened and painful or irritating.

Ddx: If accompanied by white, cheesy debris loosely adherent to glans, consider candidal infection (see GROIN RASH, 10.2.a.); circular reddened patch, consider Reiter's disease (see FEET, 7.1.f.), Bowen's disease, squamous cell carcinoma in situ (see 9.4.d.), or plasma cell balanitis, which is benign; or a white, depressed, shiny patch, consider lichen sclerosis et atrophicus (see 9.4.c.); most cases are in uncircumcised males.

9.4.B. LICHEN SIMPLEX CHRONICUS (LOCALIZED NEURODERMATITIS)

Summary: Skin, esp vulva, scrotum, and/or perianal area, is thickened, often w a rough, tree barklike surface, lichenification; itches more during unoccupied evening hrs and at times of emotional stress; pts tend to be "high strung" and intense; usually has been present for many mos to yrs; waxes and wanes; bx not diagnostic; pts often wrongly rx for psoriasis or tinea.

For additional details and rx, see GROIN RASH, 10.4.d., and LEG RASH, 17.1.a.

9.4.C. LICHEN SCLEROSIS ET ATROPHICUS

J Am Acad Derm 1995;32:393

Cause: Unknown; some cases in Europe, but not in U.S., may be due to *Borrelia burgdorferi* (J Am Acad Derm 1995;33:617).

Sx: Often itchy and irritating.

Si: Transient initial inflammatory phase; later atrophic smooth, whitish, thinned, cigarette paper–like, nonscaly patches; may cover a large area of vulva, glans penis, perianal region, esp in women; may swell and blister.

Crs: Chronic.

Compl: Atrophy can lead to sclerosis w vaginal stenosis and pain; uncommonly, leukoplakia and SCC develop.

Lab: Skin bx; KOH and culture to r/o *Candida* infection.

Rx: Suppress inflammatory phase w TCS or IL triamcinolone acetonide (Kenalog, 10 mg/mL) diluted to 4 mg/mL w saline (see RX.7.); TCS worsens atrophic stage.

9.4.D MALIGNANCY

9.4.D.(1). BOWEN'S DISEASE

Summary: Single, thickened, sharply defined, dull red, scaly plaque; when in a moist area, ie, groin, it is brighter red and nonscaly; resembles psoriasis (see BODY, 3.1.d.) but only 1 patch can be found; Bowen's disease is a persistent, slowly growing neoplasia w potential to become invasive SCC, particularly in groin; dx is confirmed by skin bx (see DX.7.).

For additional details and rx, see GROWTHS, 11.5.c.

9.4.D.(2). EXTRAMAMMARY PAGET'S DISEASE

Cause: Intraepidermal carcinoma; may be cutaneous sign of rectal or abdominal carcinoma.

Si: Plaque >2 mo in groin or perianal area may be malignancy.

Lab: Skin bx.

Rx: Refer for confirmation of dx and rx, usually to dermatologist or gynecologist; rx is topical chemotherapy, surgery, or x-radiation.

RASH ON GENITALS, RASH ELSEWHERE

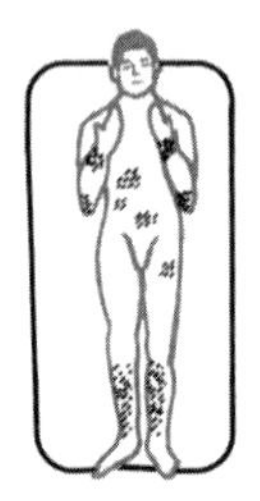

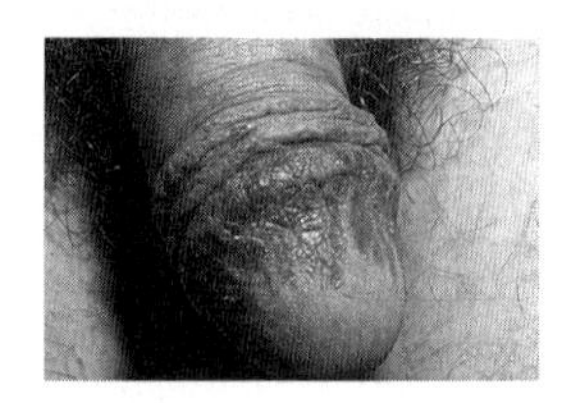

Psoriasis

9.5.A. PSORIASIS

Summary: Because of moist location, silvery scale typical of psoriasis is replaced by a red and glistening rash involving both hairy and nonhairy parts; irritating and itchy; look for typical psoriasis elsewhere, esp scalp, to confirm dx; some pts have concomitant seborrheic dermatitis; groin psoriasis is cause of considerable discomfort and embarrassment; rx w low-potency TCS (class VI–VII), ie, 1%–2.5% HC cr, as more potent fluorinated TCSs may lead to atrophy and striae (see RX.5.).

For additional details and rx, see BODY, 3.1.d.

9.5.B. SEBORRHEIC DERMATITIS

Summary: Usually diffuse but may be patchy; hairy areas most involved; yellowish greasy scale; mild redness and itching; similar scale and itching usually present at scalp, ear canals, retroauricular areas, eyebrows, nasolabial folds; look for si of psoriasis elsewhere; consider candidal infection if pustules are present; rx: TCS (class VI–VII) cr; avoid stronger TCSs, which may cause atrophy and striae in flexural areas.

For additional details and rx, see FACE, 6.2.a., and SCALP, 24.3.b.

9.5.C. SYPHILIS, SECONDARY

Summary: Many patterns; most common: widespread, slightly scaly, tan, copper-colored, nonitchy patches, lesions on palms and/or soles; recent or healing genital ulcer; moist, wartlike genital growths (condylomata lata); painless oral erosions and mucous patches; "moth-eaten" scalp hair loss; mild or absent constitutional si and sx; LN↑, esp epitrochlear nodes; no blisters except in newborn; 2° lesions appear few wk after 1°; rash disappears.

For additional details, see BODY, 3.1.f.

9.5.D. PEDICULOSIS PUBIS

Epidem: Mostly sexual contact, but transmission by bedding or toilets occurs.

Sx: Itching, often severe.

Si: Hairy areas are infested w dark brown, flat lice whose wide crablike bodies "plastered" on skin look like large freckles; areolae, umbilicus, axillae, eyebrows, eyelashes often involved; scratching leads to excoriations and 2° infections in groin, scrotal, labial area.

For additional details and rx, see GROIN RASH, 10.5.a.

9.5.E. LICHEN PLANUS

Summary: Multiple pink to purple, flat-topped, itchy papules, often tightly grouped into plaques; look on wrists, lower legs, ankles and for a lacy white patch on buccal mucosa.

For additional details and rx, see BODY, 3.3.n.

9.5.F. SCABIES

Summary: Excoriated, red papules, some w a thin "burrow"; numerous scratch marks, lichenified patches; pea-sized lumps on penis, scrotum, vulva; excoriations at finger webs, elbows, areolae, umbilicus, lower abdomen, wrists, antecubital fossae, gluteal cleft; itching worse at night; conjugal partners are involved.

For additional details and rx, see BODY, 3.1.e.

GROWTH, MANY YEARS' DURATION

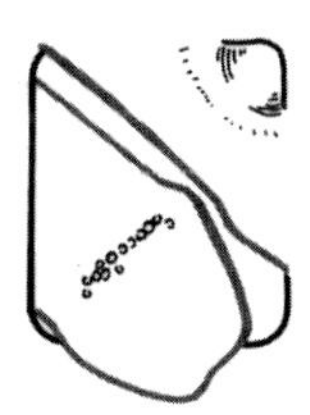

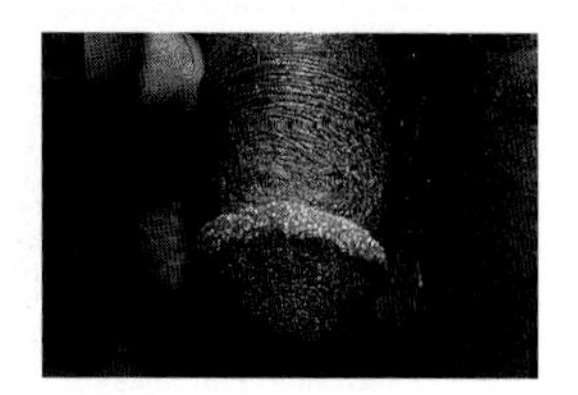

Pearly penile papules

9.6.A. FRECKLE/LENTIGO

Summary: *Freckle*: common; 1–3 mm; multiple; brown; flat; genetically determined on face; presence on trunk and arms indicates past intense sun exposure; not premalignant; rx not necessary or practical; *lentigo*: smaller and darker than freckle; fewer in number; not confined to sun-exposed areas; bx occasionally warranted to r/o melanoma.

For additional details and rx, see GROWTHS, 11.7.a.

9.6.B. NEVUS, MELANOCYTIC (MOLE)

Summary: Round; tan to dark brown; sharply outlined, present since young adulthood; average white adult has 20; prophylactic removal of all nevi is neither possible nor necessary; excise or bx a nevus that has changed, bled, or is irregular or black.

For additional details and rx, see GROWTHS, 11.1.a.

9.6.C. PEARLY PENILE PAPULES

Summary: Pearly white, pinhead- to BB-sized, painless growths about corona of glans penis; 10%–20% of males; appear by age 20; need no rx; viral warts have a rough surface, are fewer in number, and are of recent onset.

GROWTH, RECENT (DAYS TO MONTHS), MULTIPLE

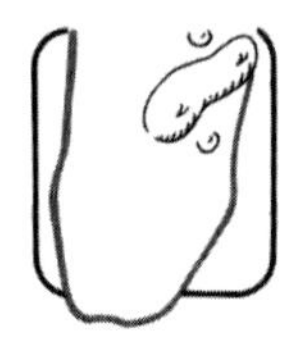

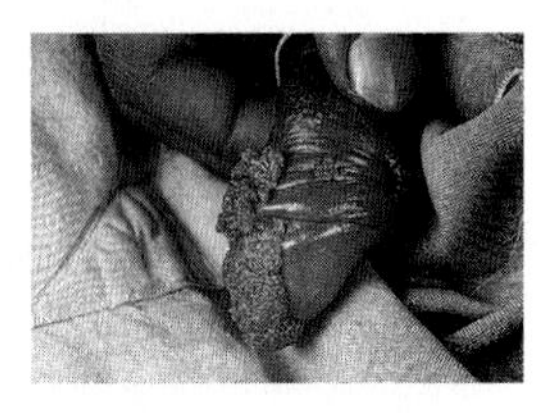

Condylomata acuminata

9.7.A. CONDYLOMATA ACUMINATA (VENEREAL WARTS)

Jaad 1999;41:661; Mmwr 1998;No. RR-1:47:88. Med Clin N Am 1998;82:1081. Am J Med 1997;102:1. J Am Acad Derm 1991;25:287

Cause: Transmissible HPV of numerous subtypes; different subtypes from common warts.

Epidem: More contagious than other warts, probably because of moist surface; acquired through sexual contact.

Sx: Asx to irritating; subclinical infection is frequent.

Si: Anogenital area; roughened, cauliflower-like surface; pinhead to marble in size; moist in moist areas, ie, glans, labia, or anus, dry on penile shaft; perianal warts common in homosexual men.

Crs: Persist, multiply, or resolve on their own.

Compl: Some HPV subtypes assoc w cervical dysplasia.

Ddx: Consider condyloma of 2° syphilis if lesions are of short duration, and Bowen's disease and extramammary Paget's disease if single, eroded, and spreading.

Lab: R/o other STDs in pt w multiple partners; if warts recur, source may be intraurethral, intravaginal, or anal.

Rx: Several options are available applied by pt or physician; rx should remove visible and sx warts; it is unproved that any rx eradicates HPV infection.

- Podofilox (podophyllotoxin) (Condylox, Rx, $$$, gel (3.5 gm) or soln (3.5 mL)); applied by pt at home; apply bid w an applicator or fingers to visible warts for 3 consecutive d followed by a rest for 4 d w/o rx; repeat up to 4 wkly cycles before re-examination (Arch Derm 1998;134:33); podophyllin resin (25% podophyllin compounded in tincture of benzoin, $), applied in physician's office; best for large verrucous moist warts, apply only to wart; pt washes area well after 4 h; reapply q 2 wk until warts are just nubs; a smooth wart remnant often remains beyond which podophyllin does not work; electrocautery or LN2 is needed to complete rx; avoid in pregnant and nursing mothers.

- LN2, electrocautery, or 85% TCA, usually w/o local anesthesia, is best for a few small warts.
- Topical 5-FU (see RX.19.), apply 1–3 ×/wk, wash off after 3–10 h (Am J Med 1997;102:28); assoc w irritation; do not use in vaginal area.
- Imiquimod (Aldara cr; Rx, $$$, box of 12 packets), mechanism unknown, applied by pt at home; apply to wart area 3 ×/wk, not on consecutive d; wash off 6–10 h later, repeat up to 16 wk, expect irritation, discontinue for a wk if severe, then restart (Arch Derm 1998;134:25; J Am Acad Derm 1998;38:230).

9.7.B. MOLLUSCUM CONTAGIOSUM

Cause: DNA poxvirus, generally restricted to humans (Jaad 1999;41:661).

Epidem: Contagious; adults: usually sexual; children: close person-to-person contact, ie, nursery school or school wrestling; large numbers of lesions in HIV-pos persons (J Am Acad Derm 1992;27:583).

Sx: Asx unless traumatized.

Si: Pale to pink, shiny, elevated bump or papule; white central dimple; size: pinhead to bean size; 5–20 are typical but may be hundreds; look for others on abdomen of adults and face of children.

Crs: Appear within a few wk of exposure; 2° bacterial infection is common.

Compl: Rarely SCC in long-standing large lesions.

Lab: Skin bx confirms but not usually necessary; dx also can be confirmed w a removed core sent between glass slides to pathology; consider other STDs and HIV infection.

Rx: Removal of core is simple and effective; can be done w sharp toothpick or toothpick-like splinter from twisted tongue blade; twist toothpick until central core is pried out; teach pt or parent to continue rx at home if lesions are numerous; other methods: topical retinoid; light curettage; LN2; laser; cantharidin (Jaad 2000;43:503); imiquimod (Aldara cr; Rx, $$$, box of 12 packets) 3 ×/wk for 4 wk (J Derm 1998;25:309); no antiviral or vaccine available.

9.7.C. CONDYLOMATA LATA (SECONDARY SYPHILIS)

Summary: Moist warty growths of recent onset in genital area may be 2° syphilis; obtain VDRL/RPR.

For details, see 9.2.a. and BODY, 3.1.f.

GROWTH, RECENT (DAYS TO MONTHS), SINGLE

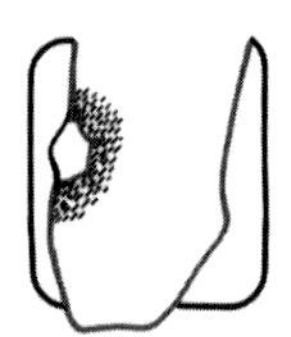

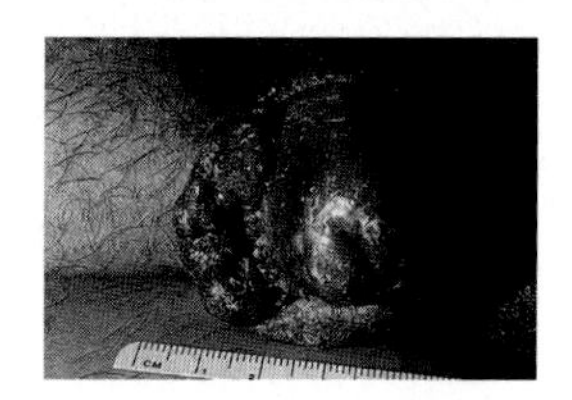

Squamous cell carcinoma

9.8.A. VERRUCA VULGARIS (COMMON WART)

Summary: Single lesion on genitals of recent duration probably is a wart; surface is raised, rough, cauliflower like; pinhead to a pencil eraser in size; painful but easily traumatized and bleed.

For additional details and rx, see 9.7.a. and HANDS, 14.1.a.

9.8.B. FIBROMA

Summary: Fleshy, skin-colored growth; smooth surface; also consider intradermal nevus, FEPs, neurofibroma; easily irritated by friction.

For additional details and rx, see GROWTHS, 11.3.c. and 11.9.a.

9.8.C. SEBORRHEIC KERATOSIS

Summary: Common benign growths, tan to dark brown, slightly roughened, waxy, crumbly; feels "stuck on" surface; usually fhx of similar lesions; most >40 yo.

For additional details and rx, see GROWTHS, 11.10.b.

9.8.D. MALIGNANCY

Summary:

- SCC: most common; single, painless, firm, and irregular growth w a scaly, keratotic, bleeding, friable surface.
- Bowen's disease (intraepithelial SCC): single, barely thickened, sharply defined, dull red plaque, nonscaly in moist groin area.
- BCE: rare on genitals.
- Melanoma: uncommon; usually black or brown but may have normal skin color; tend to be irregular in outline; outward spreading of pigment, may be itchy, bleed, or ulcerate; have a poor prognosis in genital area.
- Extramammary Paget's disease: persistent, moist, scaly patch on genitals, groin, or perianal skin; about 1/2 have underlying intestinal cancer (see 9.4.d.(2).).

Lab: Bx or refer for bx any suspicious lesion or one that does not clear during a mo of topical care.

For additional ddx, see the chapter: GROWTHS.

10 Groin Rash

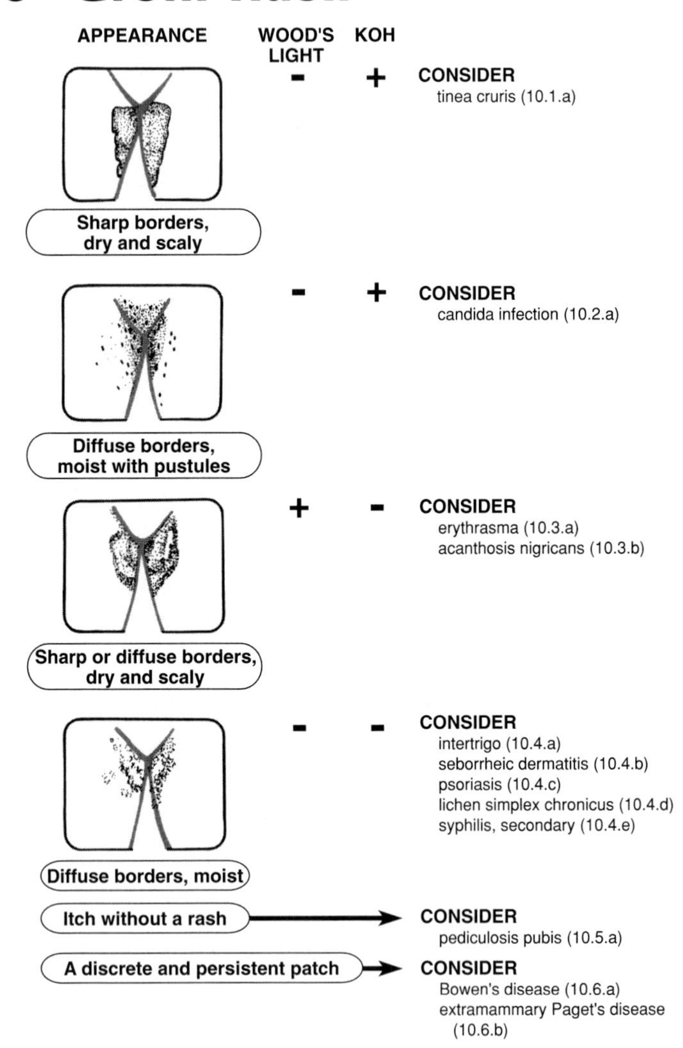

Note: When rash also involves genitals, see section Genital. For growth in the groin or a persistent patch, see sections Genital and Growths.

SHARP BORDERS, DRY/SCALY, WOOD'S LIGHT NEGATIVE, KOH POSITIVE

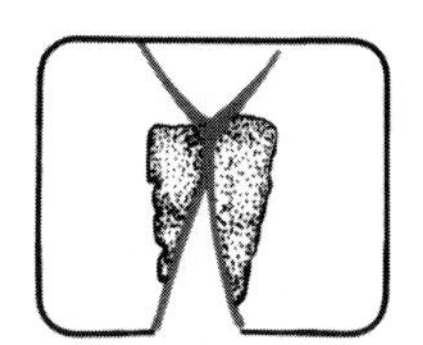

Tinea cruris

10.1.A. TINEA CRURIS

Cause: Usually *Trichophyton* species.

Epidem: Men >> women; more common in summer, in persons working in hot environments, and obese.

Sx: Itchy.

Si: Scaly, reddened border w partial or complete clearing in center; most common sites: inner thighs, buttocks, and lower abdomen; scrotum and labia are spared in tinea cruris but not in candidal infection; if pustules are present, see 10.2.a.

Crs: Chronic unless treated; may improve in winter; frequently recurs.

Lab: KOH exam (see DX.3.) confirms dx when pos; Wood's light exam (see DX.4.) is neg; fungal culture is not necessary.

Rx: Topical antifungal agents (see RX.10.) used sparingly bid; measures to ↓ moisture in area, ie, talc and cotton instead of polyester underwear and trousers; if extensive or severe, add systemic antifungal (itraconazole 100 mg bid for 1 wk) or terbinafine (not effective for *Candida* species) 250 mg qd for 1 wk or fluconazole 100 mg qd for 3 d (see RX.11.).

DIFFUSE BORDERS, MOIST WITH PUSTULES, WOOD'S LIGHT NEGATIVE, KOH POSITIVE

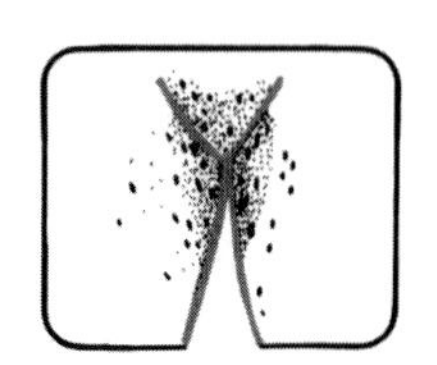

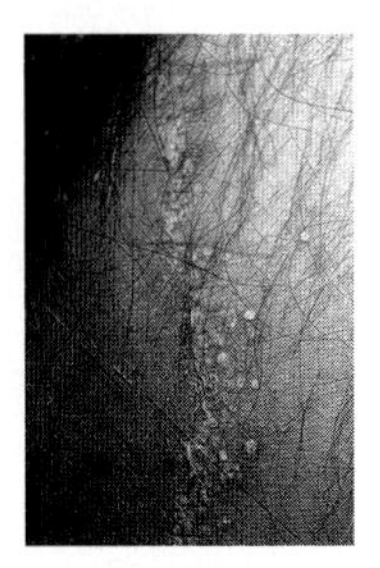

***Candida* infection**

10.2.A. *CANDIDA* INFECTION

Cause: A yeast, usually *Candida albicans*.

Epidem: Common in obese, diabetic persons, those taking broad-spectrum antibiotics, or immunosuppressed pts (esp HIV infection).

Sx: Tender > itchy.

Si: Moist, red; edge is indistinct and edge and adjacent normal skin are often studded w tiny pustules, so-called "satellite" pustules; other areas: inframammary and axillary regions in women and glans penis in men (balanitis).

Crs: Onset tends to be acute and uncomfortable.

Lab: KOH (see DX.3.): *Candida* organisms appear as short hyphae and spores in clumps and chains; culture is not useful; if DM is contributing, glycosuria usually is present.

Rx:

- Acute and tender: compress w cool saline (1 tsp salt/pint tap water) 20 min tid (see RX.2.), thoroughly dry w a towel or fan, then apply sparingly nystatin cream, nystatin powder, or a broad-spectrum antifungal cream (see RX.10.), cover rash w a thick layer of ZnOx paste or oint (see RX.4.), remove excess ZnOx w mineral oil on a cotton ball, compresses and paste usually can be stopped after 3 d, but continue topical antifungal for 2 wk.

- Chronic or unresponsive to topical rx: use systemic antifungal: itraconazole, ketoconazole, or fluconazole (preferred); (see RX.11); if perianal: consider chronic GI candidal infection: add oral nystatin suspension (100,000 units/mL, 60 mL, $) 1 tsp qid po × 3 d or fluconazole (Diflucan, Rx, $$$$) 100 mg po × 3 d; if vaginal or groin in women: miconazole cream, clotrimazole tablets, or nystatin vaginal suppositories following package instructions; or fluconazole (Diflucan, Rx, $$) 150 mg po × 1 tab.

SHARP OR DIFFUSE BORDERS, DRY/SCALY, WOOD'S LIGHT POSITIVE, KOH NEGATIVE

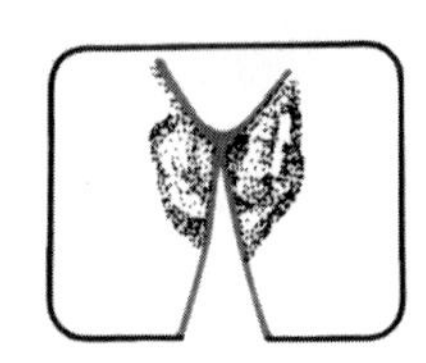

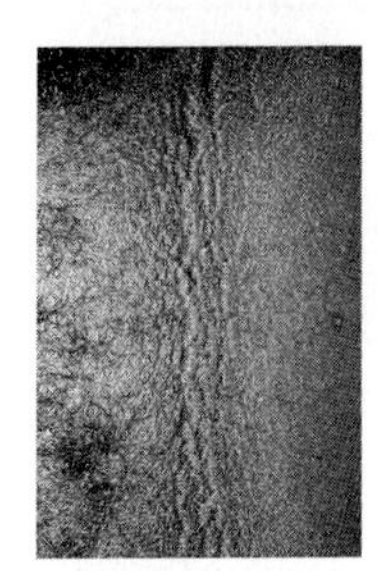

Acanthosis nigricans

GROIN RASH

10.3.A. ERYTHRASMA

Cause: Gram-pos bacteria, *Corynebacterium minutissimum*, which produces a fluorescent porphyrin pigment.

Sx: Minimally itchy, not painful.

Si: Dirty to reddish brown, finely scaly, demarcated, superficial patches; groin most common location, but also toe webs and axillae.

Crs: Chronic and persistent unless rx'd; relapses after rx are common.

Lab: Salmon-red fluorescence under Wood's light (see DX.4.); if no Wood's light is available, consider erythrasma in cases not responsive to topical antifungal agents; culture is not practical.

Rx: Topical 2% erythromycin soln bid × 2 wk, repeated w recurrences; systemic erythromycin (250 mg qid × 7 d) is an alternative.

10.3.B. ACANTHOSIS NIGRICANS

Summary: Brown to black; velvety texture; asx; also look for same change in axillae and neck; benign form: obese adults w pigmentation for mos to yrs; malignant form: thin adult >40 yo; recent onset; may be assoc w underlying malignancy.

For additional details, see PIGMENT INCREASE, 22.2.b.

DIFFUSE BORDERS, MOIST, WOOD'S LIGHT NEGATIVE, KOH NEGATIVE

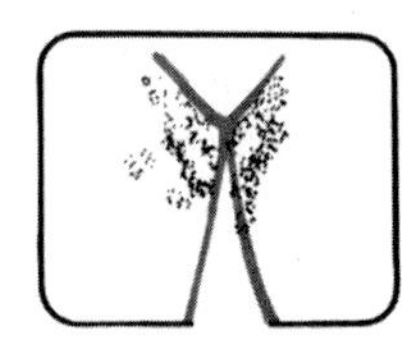

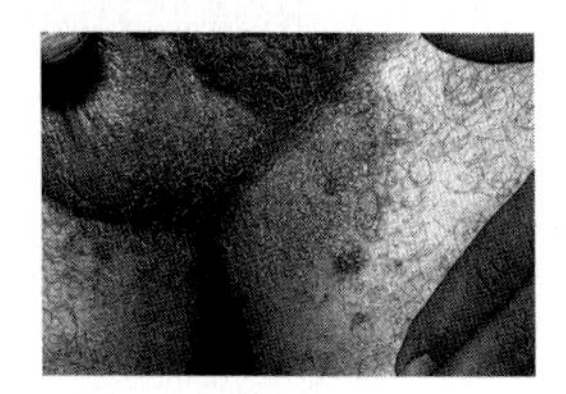

Contact dermatitis

See color plate section.

10.4.A. INTERTRIGO

Cause: Heat, moisture, friction between rubbing skin surfaces results in macerated and inflamed skin w superimposed mixed bacterial or yeast infection; DM or incontinence may be underlying.

Epidem: Most pts are obese; most cases in summer or in a hot, moist environment.

Sx: Sore and itchy, interferes w normal walking.

Si: Shiny, red, macerated, moist; involved area is sharply separated from normal skin and generally restricted to folds where skin rubs skin.

Crs: Onset is acute.

Lab: KOH (see DX.3.) and Wood's light (see DX.4.) results are neg.

Rx: Reduce maceration and friction: lighter, looser clothing w cotton instead of polyester fabrics, adsorbent dusting powder, ie, talc, and temporary use of a protective paste, ie, ZnOx; if inflammation is severe: add 1% HC cr qid; superinfection usually clears when underlying dermatitis resolves.

10.4.B. SEBORRHEIC DERMATITIS

Summary: Red, glistening skin w a yellowish greasy scale; never isolated to groin; other seborrheic areas involved, esp scalp, ear canals, eyebrows, nasolabial folds, and/or axillae; look for signs of psoriasis elsewhere; consider candidal infection if pustules are present; rx: TCS (class VI–VII) cr; avoid stronger TCSs, which may cause atrophy and striae in flexural areas (see RX.5.).

For additional details and rx, see FACE, 6.2.a., and SCALP, 24.3.b.

10.4.C. PSORIASIS

Summary: Because of moist location, silvery scale typical of psoriasis is replaced by a red and glistening rash involving both hairy and nonhairy parts; irritating and itchy; look for typical psoriasis elsewhere, esp scalp, to confirm dx; some pts have concomitant seborrheic dermatitis; groin psoriasis is cause of considerable discomfort and embarrassment; rx w low-potency TCS (class VI–VII), ie, 1%–2.5% HC cr, as more potent fluorinated TCSs may lead to atrophy and striae (see RX.5.).

For additional details and rx, see BODY, 3.1.d.

10.4.D. LICHEN SIMPLEX CHRONICUS (LOCALIZED NEURODERMATITIS)

Summary: Skin, esp vulva, scrotum, and/or perianal area, is thickened, often w a rough, tree bark–like surface (lichenification); itches more during unoccupied evening hrs and at times of emotional stress; pts tend to be "high strung" and intense; usually has been present for many mos to yrs; waxes and wanes; bx not diagnostic; pts often wrongly rx for psoriasis or tinea; Rx: reduce itching and protect area from scratching: mild TCS (class VI–VII) bid (see RX.5.), then cover w ZnOx paste applied thickly, like frosting a cake; advise pt to stay fully dressed until bedtime as many change into shorts or pajamas during evening and make area all too accessible; consider nortriptyline (10–100 mg at dinner) or a serotonin-uptake inhibitor; reassure pt that condition is not STD.

For additional details, see LEG RASH, 17.1.a.

10.4.E. SYPHILIS, SECONDARY

Summary: Many patterns; most common: widespread, slightly scaly, tan, copper-colored, nonitchy patches, lesions on palms and/or soles; recent or healing genital ulcer; moist, wartlike genital growths (condylomata lata); painless oral erosions and mucous patches; "moth-eaten" scalp hair loss; mild or absent constitutional si and sx; LN↑, esp epitrochlear nodes; no blisters except in the newborn; 2° lesions appear few wk after 1°; rash disappears.

For additional details, see BODY, 3.1.f.

ITCH WITHOUT RASH

10.5.A. PEDICULOSIS PUBIS (PUBIC LICE)

Jaad 1999;41:661; Mmwr 1998;No. RR-1:47:105.

Cause: *Phthirus pubis*, the pubic or "crab" louse, so named because of its broad body and large pincer-like legs.

Epidem: Most acquired through sexual contact although they occas may be transmitted by bedding or toilets; crab lice affect only humans; may survive 24–72 h off their host.

Sx: Itching, often severe.

Si: Hairy portions of groin are infested w dark brown, flat lice whose wide crablike bodies, "plastered" on skin, look like large freckles; also often infested: areolae, umbilicus, axillae, eyebrows, and eyelashes.

Crs: Itching starts 1–4 wk after infestation; persists until rx'd.

Compl: Itching leads to excoriations and frequent 2° infections in groin, scrotal, or labial area.

Lab: Use an inverted microscope eyepiece or hand lens to look for crablike lice, the size of a printed capital letter "O," flattened on skin among pubic hair; consider other STDs as well.

Rx: Permethrin 1% cr rinse applied to affected areas and washed off after 10 min; lindane (γ benzene hexachloride lotion or shampoo) applied to affected areas and washed off after 4 min; lindane is neurotoxic and should be avoided in children <2 yo and pregnant or lactating women; if lice are found elsewhere than genital region, entire body including scalp should be rx'd, except for eyelashes as all agents are too irritating to use about eyes; except for permethrin, which kills eggs, repeat rx in 1 wk; all bed or sexual partners should be rx'd; bedding and clothing should be washed, machine dried using the heat cycle, dry-cleaned, or removed from body contact for >72 h.

DISCRETE AND PERSISTENT PATCH

10.6.A. BOWEN'S DISEASE

Summary: Single, thickened, sharply defined, dull red, scaly plaque; when in a moist area, ie, groin, it is brighter red and nonscaly; resembles psoriasis (see BODY, 3.1.d.), but only 1 patch can be found; Bowen's disease is a persistent, slowly growing neoplasia w potential to become invasive SCC, particularly in groin; dx is confirmed by skin bx (see DX.7.).

For additional details and rx, see GROWTHS, 11.5.c.

10.6.B. EXTRAMAMMARY PAGET'S DISEASE

Summary: A persistent plaque >2-mo duration may be malignancy; extramammary Paget's disease is an intraepidermal carcinoma that may be cutaneous sign of rectal or abdominal carcinoma; dx is confirmed by skin bx.

For additional details and rx, see GENITALS, 9.4.d.(2).

11 Growths

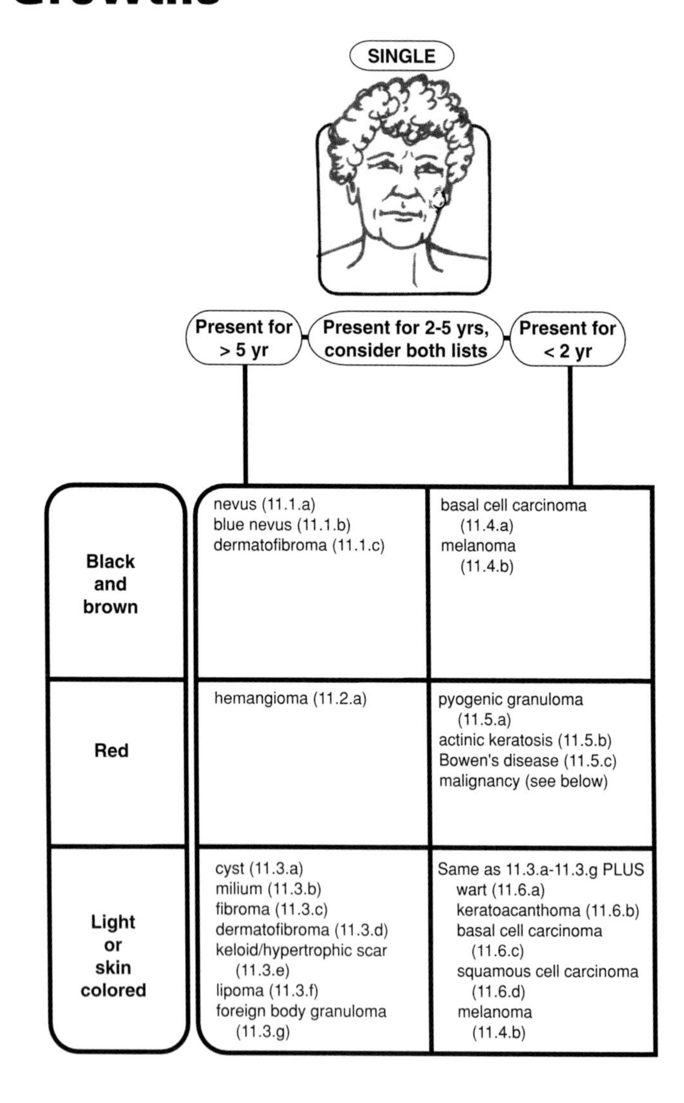

	Present for > 5 yr	Present for < 2 yr
Black and brown	nevus (11.1.a) blue nevus (11.1.b) dermatofibroma (11.1.c)	basal cell carcinoma (11.4.a) melanoma (11.4.b)
Red	hemangioma (11.2.a)	pyogenic granuloma (11.5.a) actinic keratosis (11.5.b) Bowen's disease (11.5.c) malignancy (see below)
Light or skin colored	cyst (11.3.a) milium (11.3.b) fibroma (11.3.c) dermatofibroma (11.3.d) keloid/hypertrophic scar (11.3.e) lipoma (11.3.f) foreign body granuloma (11.3.g)	Same as 11.3.a-11.3.g PLUS wart (11.6.a) keratoacanthoma (11.6.b) basal cell carcinoma (11.6.c) squamous cell carcinoma (11.6.d) melanoma (11.4.b)

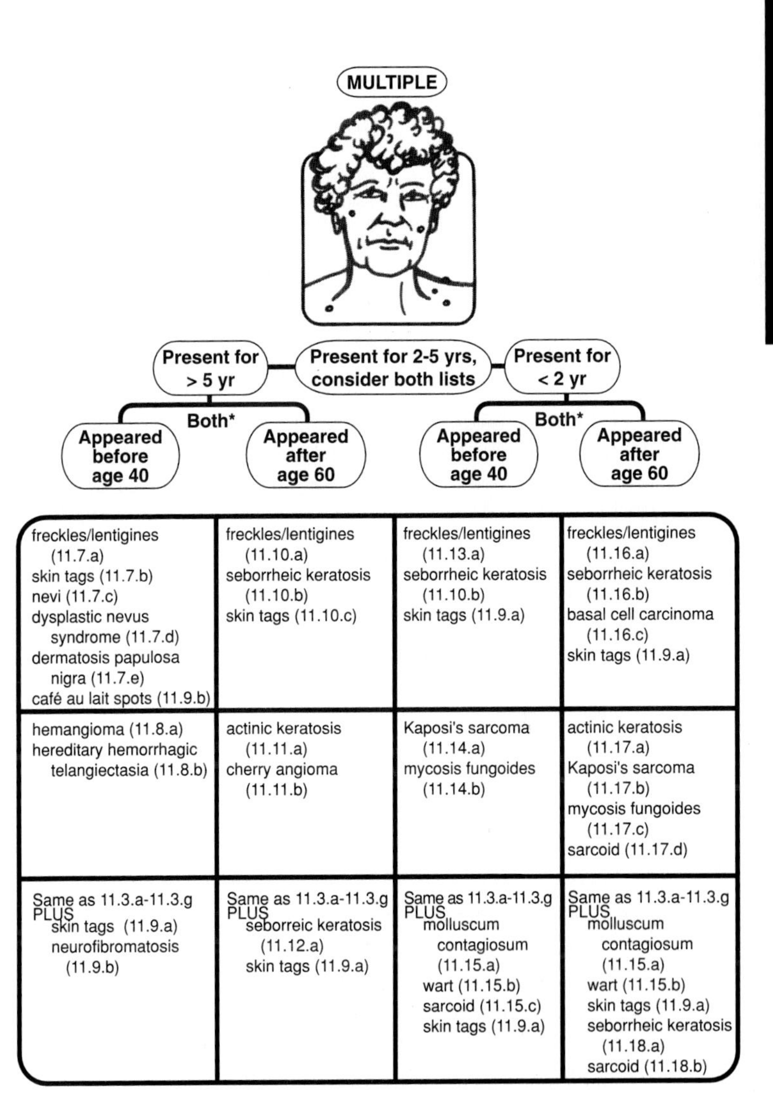

freckles/lentigines (11.7.a) skin tags (11.7.b) nevi (11.7.c) dysplastic nevus syndrome (11.7.d) dermatosis papulosa nigra (11.7.e) café au lait spots (11.9.b)	freckles/lentigines (11.10.a) seborrheic keratosis (11.10.b) skin tags (11.10.c)	freckles/lentigines (11.13.a) seborrheic keratosis (11.10.b) skin tags (11.9.a)	freckles/lentigines (11.16.a) seborrheic keratosis (11.16.b) basal cell carcinoma (11.16.c) skin tags (11.9.a)
hemangioma (11.8.a) hereditary hemorrhagic telangiectasia (11.8.b)	actinic keratosis (11.11.a) cherry angioma (11.11.b)	Kaposi's sarcoma (11.14.a) mycosis fungoides (11.14.b)	actinic keratosis (11.17.a) Kaposi's sarcoma (11.17.b) mycosis fungoides (11.17.c) sarcoid (11.17.d)
Same as 11.3.a-11.3.g PLUS skin tags (11.9.a) neurofibromatosis (11.9.b)	Same as 11.3.a-11.3.g PLUS seborreic keratosis (11.12.a) skin tags (11.9.a)	Same as 11.3.a-11.3.g PLUS molluscum contagiosum (11.15.a) wart (11.15.b) sarcoid (11.15.c) skin tags (11.9.a)	Same as 11.3.a-11.3.g PLUS molluscum contagiosum (11.15.a) wart (11.15.b) skin tags (11.9.a) seborrheic keratosis (11.18.a) sarcoid (11.18.b)

***If appeared between 40 and 60 years of age, consider both lists.**

SINGLE, >5 YEARS, BLACK OR BROWN

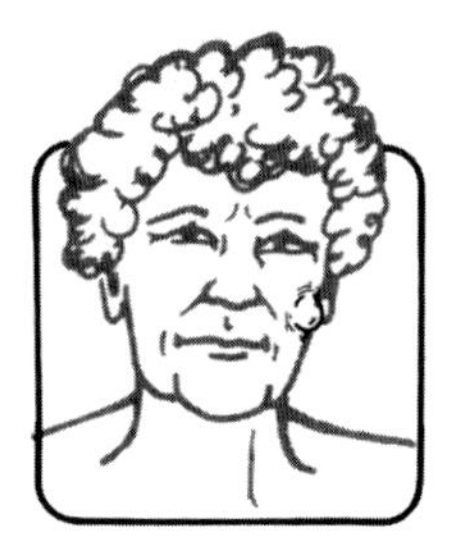

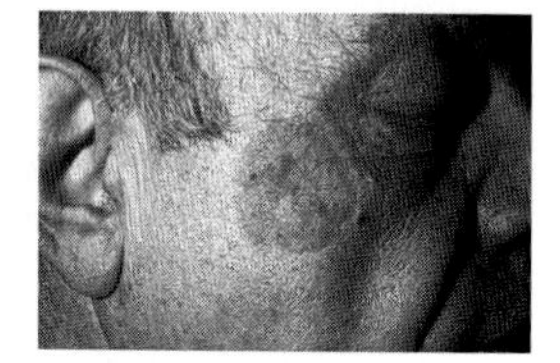

Seborrheic keratosis

11.1.A. NEVUS, MELANOCYTIC (MOLE—JUNCTIONAL, COMPOUND, AND INTRADERMAL)

Cause: Nevus cells are closely related to melanocytes; subtypes depend on dominant location of nevus cells: *junctional* are flat or nearly flat w nests of cells at dermal-epidermal junction; *intradermal* or *compound* are dome shaped or on a stalk w cells within dermis or in both epidermal and dermal locations; in children, nevi tend to be junctional; in adults, they tend to be compound or intradermal; junctional and compound nevi have highest potential for transformation into melanoma.

Sx: None unless irritated.

Si: Most are round, tan to dark brown, sharply outlined, present since young adulthood; may be skin colored, irregular in outline, have a light-colored halo; may be found anywhere on body; the average white adult has about 20.

Crs: Present at birth in about 1% of infants; most develop between late childhood and early adulthood; seldom appear during adulthood, except during pregnancy and in dysplastic nevus syndrome (see 11.7.d.); tend to disappear in old age; some develop a depigmented halo (**halo nevus**) (see PIGMENT DECREASE, 21.4.c.); only 30% of melanomas arise from preexisting nevi, the rest from normal-appearing skin; perhaps 1:100,000 nevi develops into melanoma.

Lab: Bx suspicious lesions; experience is required to determine which of numerous pigmented lesions requires bx or removal.

Rx: Prophylactic removal of all nevi is neither possible nor necessary; nevi present from birth carry a higher risk; large nevi (>2 cm) should be carefully followed, perhaps yrly or when a change is detected; routine avoidance of midday sun and use of protective clothing, esp in light-complexioned persons and those w many nevi; artificial sunblocks may be assoc w ↑ nevi and even melanoma (J Natl Cancer Inst 1998;90:1873); those w irregular pigmented areas that are difficult to assess should be removed, if possible; questionable lesions may require referral to a dermatologist experienced in assessment of pigmented lesions.

11.1.B. BLUE NEVUS

Cause: Melanocytes in dermis produce melanin that appears blue due to its depth.

Sx: None.

Si: Blue-black; raised; split pea size or smaller; typically on back of forearms or hands, head, or lower legs; no irregularity of pigment or ulceration.

Crs: Most date from childhood; persist unchanged; not premalignant.

Ddx: Looks like melanoma because of its blue-black color.

Lab: Bx usually not necessary.

Rx: Excise questionable lesions or refer to a dermatologist who can confirm dx.

11.1.C. DERMATOFIBROMA

Cause: Uncertain, but possibly a rxn to an old insect bite or foreign body.

Epidem: Common.

Sx: Painless but tender if squeezed.

Si: Firm; slightly raised; brown yellowish; pea to bean size; usually on lower legs or forearms; single to several; sideways compression causes a dimple (pinch sign).

Crs: Stable once final size is reached; benign.

Lab: Bx usually not necessary.

Rx: None necessary if confident of dx; does not respond to LN2; excision is usually for cosmetic purposes; excise questionable lesions or refer to a dermatologist who can confirm dx.

SINGLE, >5 YEARS, RED

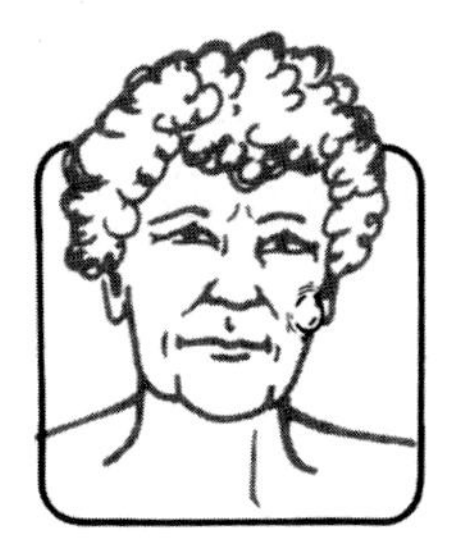

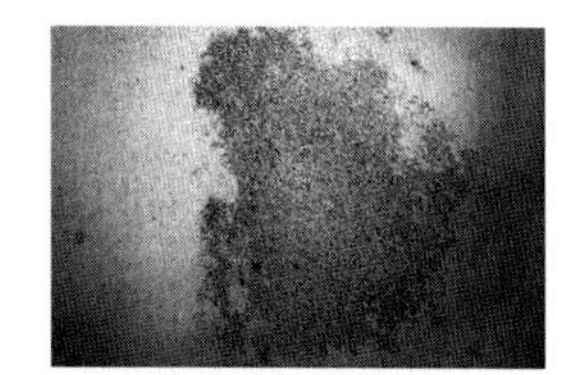

Hemangioma

11.2.A.(1). HEMANGIOMA, CAPILLARY AND CAVERNOUS

Nejm 1999;341:173.

Cause: Developmental anomaly of blood vessels.

Epidem: Congenital but not hereditary; present in 5%–10% of 1 yo children; girls >> boys.

Sx: Usually none unless impinges on structures.

Si: *Strawberry hemangioma*: red-purple; nearly flat to raised; often resembles a strawberry; usually single and dime size or smaller; may be multiple, visceral, or form a large mutilating structure; may have a deep large blood vessel component (*cavernous*) that appears dusky or blue; may bleed or ulcerate but major hemorrhage is unlikely; multiple cutaneous hemangiomas may be accompanied by internal hemangiomas often w complications:

GI bleeding, kidney obstruction, platelet deficiency, interference w visceral organ functions.

Crs: About 55% are present at birth; rest appear within wks; usually grows during 1st yr; if large may interfere w a vital structure; spontaneous involution usually begins in 6–12 mo and is complete by age of 5 yr; generally leaving slight scar or wrinkling; regression of cavernous component is less complete.

Compl: Ulceration is most frequent; blood component consumption in large lesions: **Kasabach-Merritt phenomenon** (J Peds 1997;130:631).

Lab: Consider visceral involvement; consider neurologic and audiometric exam.

Rx: Pts usually are seen by a dermatologist and/or pediatrician to confirm dx and outline rx plan; rx usually not necessary as single strawberry hemangioma usually resolves spontaneously w minimal scarring; surgery, laser destruction, or cryotherapy may be considered if hemangioma impinges on vital structure; oral CS or alpha interferon has been used for rapidly growing or symptomatic multiple hemangiomas (J Am Acad Derm 1997;37:631).

11.2.A.(2). NEVUS FLAMMEUS (PORT-WINE STAIN)

Cause: Developmental anomaly of blood vessels.

Epidem: Congenital but not hereditary.

Sx: None.

Si: *Port-wine stain*: flat; purple-red; sharply demarcated; irregularly shaped patch; most common on face or nape; *salmon patch*: in majority of newborns on nape, glabella, or eyelids; pink rather than dark red-purple; occasionally facial hemangiomas assoc w vascular abnormalities of ipsilateral eye, underlying portion of brain, adjacent soft tissue, or bone; brain involvement is evidenced by intracranial calcifications, seizures, and/or mental retardation (**Sturge-Weber syndrome**) (J Am Acad Derm 1999;41:772).

Crs: Present since birth; *salmon patch*: tends to disappear during childhood, but can be permanent, esp on nape; *port-wine stain*: usually persists and later often develops pebbly surface; neither enlarges after newborn period except in proportion to growth.

Lab: If hemangioma is extensive, esp if it involves upper eyelid, examine both eyes and consider evaluation by ophthalmology and neurology.

Rx: No entirely satisfactory rx exists; consider concealing w opaque cosmetics or suggest removal with lasers; refer to dermatologist, laser center, or plastic surgery.

SINGLE, >5 YEARS, LIGHT OR SKIN COLORED

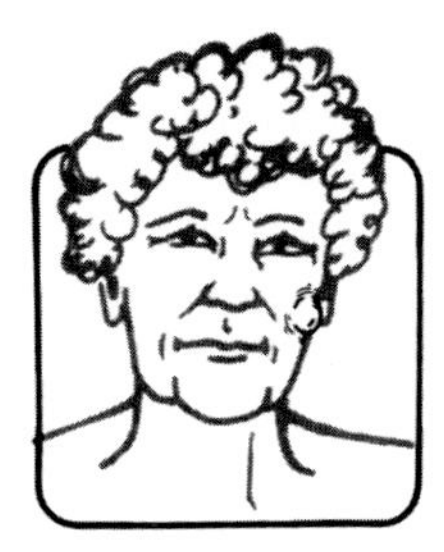

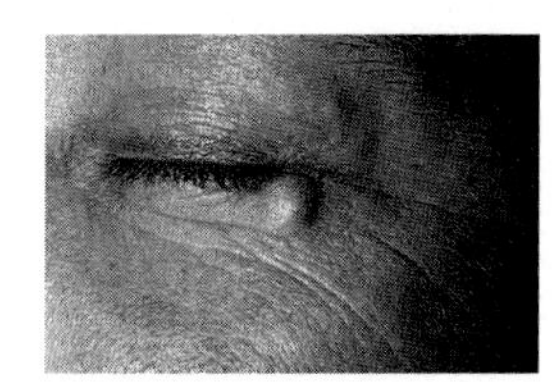

Epidermal inclusion cyst

11.3.A. CYST

Cause: Most are *epidermal inclusion cysts*, in which epidermis invaginates into dermis; *pilar cysts*: common on scalp, composed of expanded outer root sheath of a hair follicle; *sebaceous cysts* w wall composed of sebaceous glands are uncommon.

Sx: Asx unless ruptured.

Si: Movable; firm to soft; dome shaped; pea to cherry tomato in size; skin colored but may have a central, horny punctum; single or multiple; most are on head and upper part of torso; pts w multiple cysts often have or had nodular cystic acne vulgaris.

Crs: Usually stable in size; not premalignant.

Compl: "Infection" is due to escape of irritating cyst contents into surrounding tissue leading to a brisk foreign body rxn, usually sterile; rxn subsides or drains w or w/o I&D, cyst may then scar and disappear or it may return to its previous size.

Ddx: Multiple cysts, usually in pts w other skin growths as well, may be **nevoid basal cell carcinoma syndrome** (multiple basal cell cancers and bony, neurologic, eye, and reproductive abnormalities) or **Gardner's syndrome** (cysts plus colonic polyposis).

Rx: Small asx cysts do not require excision; pts may request removal of an asx cyst that is unsightly or irritating; removal is complicated because of scarring if cyst had been inflamed or ruptured; an inflamed cyst may be allowed to resolve if small or rx'd by I&D if painful; consider referral to a dermatologist or surgeon for evaluation and rx.

11.3.B. MILIUM

Summary: Pinhead to rice grain in size; yellow to white; firm to hard; common on face, esp cheeks, forehead, and around eyes; women > men; persistent; small epidermal keratin inclusion cyst.

For additional details and rx, see FACE, 6.9.c.

11.3.C. FIBROMA

Summary: Fleshy, skin-colored, normal-appearing, noneroded surface; almost certainly benign; ddx: nevus, neurofibroma, FEP.

11.3.D. DERMATOFIBROMA

Summary: Firm; slightly raised; brown yellowish; pea to bean in size; usually on lower legs or forearms; single to several; sideways compression causes a dimple (pinch sign); painless but tender if squeezed (see 11.1.c.).

11.3.E. KELOID OR HYPERTROPHIC SCAR

Cause: Keloids and hypertrophic scars follow injury to skin, ie, burns, surgery, ear piercing, infection, ie, acne cysts; mechanism is unclear.

Epidem: Keloids are esp common in blacks.

Sx: May be tender.

Si: *Hypertrophic scar*: restricted to scar; *keloid*: extends beyond edge of scar, can become unsightly; soft to firm to hard; surface may appear normal, but may be taut, shiny, darkened; more common at certain sites: nape, mid chest.

Crs: Usually expand over a few mo, then persist.

Rx: Existing keloids tend to recur if excised; hypertrophic scars heal w generally good results if excised; both become softer, less tender, and shrink w IL CS injection (see RX.7.) w undiluted triamcinolone acetonide (Kenalog, 10 mg/mL); surgical excision followed by IL CS is an option, usually performed by a dermatologist or plastic surgeon.

11.3.F. LIPOMA

Cause: Unknown; multiple lipomas may be genetic; may be a component of neurofibromatosis (see 11.9.b.) or Gardner's syndrome.

Sx: Asx; painful w vascular (angiolipoma) component.

Si: Soft lump; bean to fist size; 1 or 2 but multiple in some pts; deep within sc fat; overlying skin may be elevated in a dome but usually no surface changes; edge less defined than epidermal inclusion cyst.

Crs: Most develop during adulthood and persist indefinitely; do not become inflamed like epidermal inclusion cysts.

Compl: Malignant degeneration is rare; most liposarcomas arise de novo, not in preexisting lipomas.

Lab: Bx is rarely necessary; bx or excision of one lesion may be necessary to confirm dx.

Rx: Removal is not necessary unless suddenly growing, tender, or interfering w function; lesions are deep and generally are removed by a dermatologist or, if large, by a general surgeon.

11.3.G. FOREIGN BODY GRANULOMA

Summary: Raised lump; may be slightly pink and slightly tender; located on exposed part, ie, face, scalp, arms, or legs; presumed rxn to embedded foreign material, ie, insect biting part, or spicule of glass or sand; summer >> winter; slowly resolve over mos; bx (see DX.7.) confirms dx and may speed resolution if foreign material is removed.

SINGLE, <2 YEARS, BLACK OR BROWN

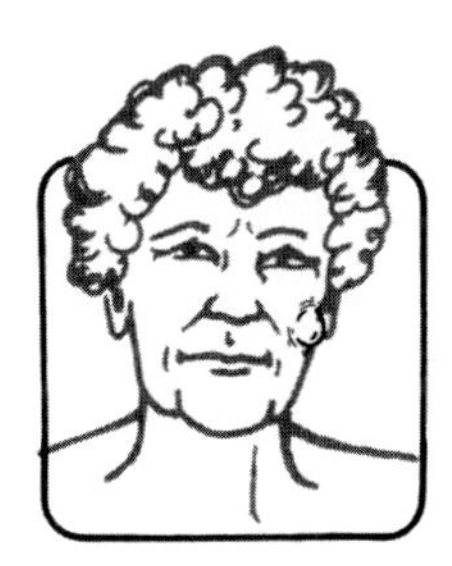

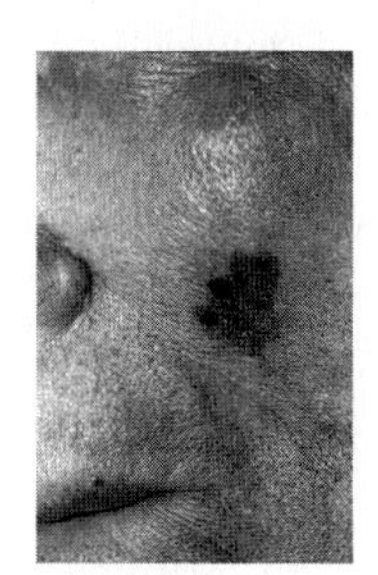

Melanoma

11.4.A. BASAL CELL CARCINOMA (BCC)

Summary: Single or few; shiny or pearly colored; telangiectasias over surface; depressed center; slowly spreading; usually on light-exposed areas, esp face, neck, forearms; about 80% of skin cancers.

For additional details and rx, see 11.6.c.

11.4.B. MELANOMA

Nejm 1999;340:1341. J Am Acad Derm 1995;32:689. Nejm 1991;325:171.

Cause: Melanomas are derived from melanocytes, present throughout epidermis and concentrated in nests in nevi; 30% arise from preexisting nevi, the rest from normal-appearing skin; melanomas are assoc w hx of intense, intermittent UV exposure rather than total cumulative exposure seen w more common skin cancers (J Natl Cancer Inst 1986;76:403); ↑ in posttransplantation pts (J Am Acad Derm 1999;40:177).

Epidem: About 40,000 new cases of melanoma are now dx'd in U.S. each yr w about 7000 deaths; incidence is increasing; risk factors (Jama 1987;258:3146): light complexion, hx of >3 severe sunburns, hx of working as a lifeguard, multiple nevi, dysplastic nevi, fhx of melanoma; rare in blacks.

Sx: Usually asx, but may be itchy initially and later may bleed or ulcerate; ask about si and sx of metastatic disease, ie, bone pain, weight loss, headaches, visual changes.

Si: Usually black or brown, occasionally normal skin color; tend to be irregular in outline w outward spreading of pigment; may appear at any body site but upper back most common site in men, upper back and shins in women; **lentigo maligna**: melanoma in situ; many mos to yrs duration; tan to black; slowly spreads laterally; most are on face, ear, dorsum of hand; elderly person; potential to invade deeper tissue or metastasize as a melanoma.

Crs: Only 3% of all skin cancers are melanomas but they cause 2/3 of skin cancer deaths.

Lab: Histologic depth and growth patterns are prognostic factors assoc w survival; further lab studies in pts w localized melanoma, even up to 4.0 mm in thickness, inc chest x-ray (false-pos rate = 15%) and LFTs, are not justified except to establish a baseline; CT scans and MRIs have too low a yield to be cost-effective unless ROS or px suggests spread to a specific organ (Arch Derm 1998;134:569).

Rx: Although melanomas have a high potential to recur, metastasize, and kill, the majority of pts w melanoma can be cured if dx is made in early stage and lesion is completely excised w appropriate margins (Ann Surg 1993;218:262; Arch Surg 1991;126:438); thin melanomas (<1 mm) have no substantial effect on survival and pts should not be penalized by insurance companies; however, survival is diminished w deeper melanomas, esp if LNs are involved; 5-yr survival is <50% w LN involvement and <5% if metastatic beyond regional LNs; refer pts suspected of having a melanoma to a dermatologist or surgeon for bx or excision; sentinel node bx aids in the determination of prognosis, but as its value in the selection of rx and the care of pts has yet to be proven by randomized trials, it should be considered experimental at this time (BMJ 2000;321:3).

SINGLE, <2 YEARS, RED

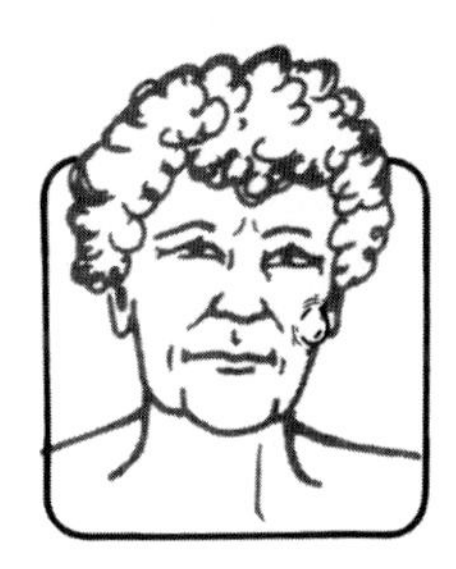

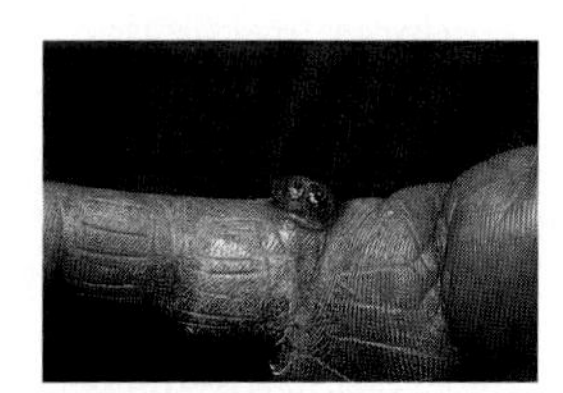

Pyogenic granuloma

11.5.A. PYOGENIC GRANULOMA

Cause: Capillary hemangioma, not "pyogenic" as lesion does not have an infectious origin; may follow injury or surgery, but most appear spontaneously.

Epidem: Any age; common in children.

Sx: None.

Si: Single; bright red; raspberry like; pea to bean in size; often is friable and bleeds easily when traumatized; most are on exposed parts, esp arms, legs, hands, fingers.

Crs: Appears and enlarges rapidly, within wks; does not become malignant.

Ddx: Melanoma is a serious look-alike (see 11.4.b.).

Rx: Excision is best; LN2 is not curative and may only lead to bleeding.

11.5.B. ACTINIC KERATOSIS

Summary: Discrete; persistent; scaly, pink to red; esp in light-complexioned persons >40 yo; hx of excessive sun exposure; considered premalignant but few become SCC (see 11.11.a.).

11.5.C. BOWEN'S DISEASE

Cause: Bowen's disease is an intraepidermal SCC; not assoc w ↑ risk of visceral malignancy (Arch Derm 1999;135:790).

Sx: Usually asx.

Si: Single; thickened; sharply defined; dull red; scaly plaque; 1–6 cm; resembles psoriasis (see BODY, 3.1.d.), but only 1 patch generally present; usual location is covered part of trunk; in a moist area, ie, groin: brighter red and nonscaly.

Crs: Persistent; slowly growing.

Compl: Invasive SCC may arise, esp in groin area.

Lab: Confirm dx by bx (see DX.7.).

Rx: Rx is complicated by sometimes large size and awkward location of many; after bx confirmation, alternative rxs: topical 5-FU (see DX.19.), D&C (RX.7), or cryosurgery (RX.18); total excision is excessive as lesion usually is confined to epidermis; consider referral to dermatology for confirmation of dx and rx.

SINGLE, <2 YEARS, LIGHT OR SKIN COLORED

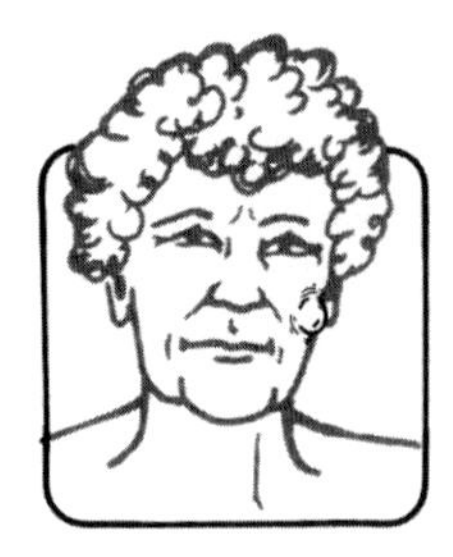

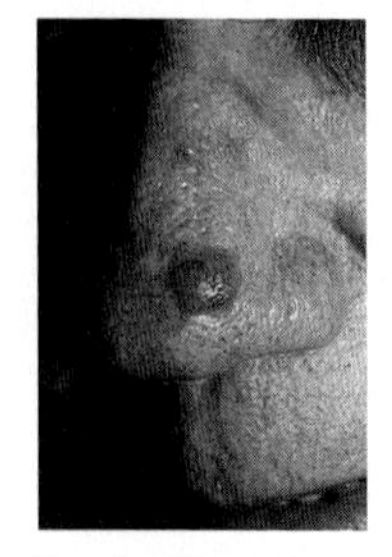

Basal cell carcinoma

- The ddx includes **single, >5 yr, light or skin colored**:
  Cyst (11.3.a.)
  Milium (11.3.b.)
  Fibroma (11.3.c.)
  Dermatofibroma (11.3.d.)
  Keloid/hypertrophic scar (11.3.e.)
  Lipoma (11.3.f.)
  Foreign body granuloma (11.3.g.)
- In addition to:

GROWTHS

11.6.A. VERRUCA VULGARIS (COMMON WART)

Summary: Single to multiple; surface is raised, rough, cauliflower like; pinhead to dime sized; most are on hands, feet, face; usually painless unless periungual or fingertip; may be easily traumatized.

For additional details and rx, see HANDS, 14.1.a.

11.6.B. KERATOACANTHOMA

Cause: Unknown, but sun exposure and environmental tars and oil products may play a role; rare hereditary forms exist.

Sx: Tender or irritating.

Si: Single growth; pea to bean size; hard, umbilicated, or ulcerated center; most are on exposed areas; men > women; most >50 yo; ↑incidence in immunosuppressed pts.

Crs: Often ↑ in size dramatically, in wks to 2 mo; may heal spontaneously in 4–12 mo; some are aggressive leading to extensive tissue destruction, esp on face.

Compl: May have underlying SCC.

Lab: Bx or excise to r/o SCC (see DX.7.).

Rx: Generally excise, as waiting for spontaneous remission is uncertain; recurrences are uncommon; because of dramatic onset and ulceration, most cases are referred early to a dermatologist.

11.6.C. BASAL CELL CARCINOMA (BCC)

Cause: Most are induced by UV light, usually chronic from work or recreational exposure.

Epidem: 80% of all skin cancers; most occur in persons w light complexions, esp northern European origin; whites >> Asians >> blacks.

Sx: Asx or may be irritating.

Si: Single to few; shiny or pearly colored; telangiectasias over surface; depressed center; slowly spreading; usually on light-exposed areas, esp face, neck, forearms.

Crs: Grow slowly over mos to yrs; untreated, they can invade deeply, but rarely metastasize.

Lab: Dx is confirmed by bx; shave bx may suffice; bx not necessary prior to surgery if typical appearance.

Rx: Removal by D&C (see RX.17.); surgical excision has lower recurrence rate than D&C (Arch Derm 1999;135:1177); x-radiation; *superficial type*: LN2 (see RX.18.), topical 5-FU (see RX.19.); imiquimod cr (Aldara, Rx, $$$), qd until clear or 4 mo (Jaad 2000;136:774); extensive, recurrent, or problem areas may need Mohs surgery (microscopic margin control).

11.6.D. SQUAMOUS CELL CARCINOMA (SCC)

Cause: Most appear induced by chronic UV exposure and other sources of chronic irritation and trauma, ie, ulcers, burns, x-radiation, tar and smoking exposure; most occur in persons w light complexions, esp northern European origin; whites >> Asians >> blacks.

Epidem: 15% of skin cancers; potential to metastasize >>> BCE; ↑ freq w immunosuppression, ie, HIV infection, post–organ transplantation (J Am Acad Derm 1999;40:177).

Sx: Asx or may be irritating.

Si: Usually single; firm and irregular; scaly, keratotic, bleeding, friable surface; usually on sun-exposed areas, but on covered areas > BCE; lower lip is common site because of chronic sun exposure as well as irritation from tar and heat in smokers; look for LN↑.

Crs: Grow faster than BCEs; more likely to be friable and bleed.

Lab: Deep bx, not shave, confirms dx in suspicious lesions.

Rx: Surgical excision preferred over D&C; x-radiation sometimes used in elderly; pts w suspected or proved SCC usually are referred to dermatologist or surgeon.

MULTIPLE, >5 YEARS, APPEARED <40 YEARS OLD, BLACK OR BROWN

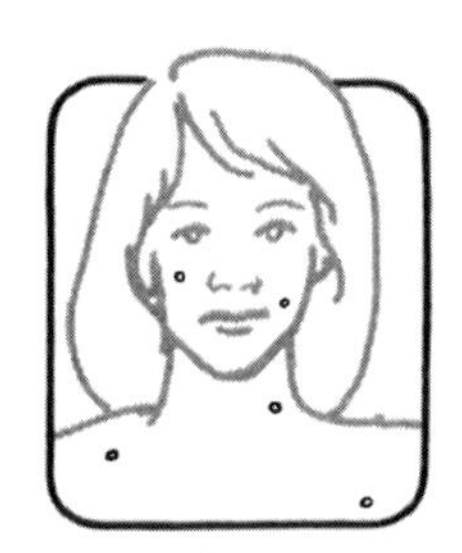

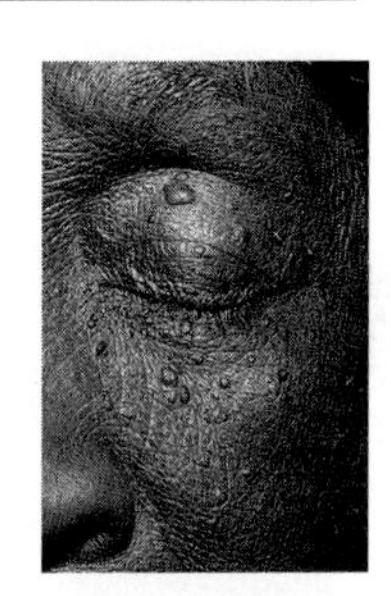

Dermatosis papulosa nigra

11.7.A.(1). FRECKLE (EPHELIDES)

Summary: Common; 1–3 mm; multiple; brown; flat spots; genetically determined on face; presence on trunk and arms indicates past intense sun exposures or sunburns; not premalignant.

11.7.A.(2). LENTIGO

Summary: Similar to a freckle but darker, even black, fewer in number, and not confined to sun-exposed areas; flat surface; < rice grain size; larger pigmented lesions may be melanoma or lentigo maligna (see 11.4.b.); *solar lentigines* (liver spots): flat brown patches on sun-exposed parts of older persons, not assoc w liver disease; **Leopard syndrome**: rare individuals w hundreds of lentigines scattered over face, trunk, and extremities and assoc w EKG, ocular, pulmonary and genital abn, growth retardation, and deafness; **Peutz-Jeghers syndrome**: lentigines on lips and dorsa of fingers assoc w small bowel polyposis; rx of lentigo is not necessary but occas bx is warranted if lesion is suspicious for melanoma; consider referral to a dermatologist for confirmation of dx.

11.7.B. SKIN TAGS (FIBROEPITHELIAL POLYPS, FEPS)

Summary: Common, esp >30 yo; pinhead to BB size; tan to skin colored; also at groin, neck, eyelids; rx w electrocautery w or w/o local anesthetic or prior EMLA cr (see 11.9.a.).

11.7.C. NEVI, MELANOCYTIC (MOLE—JUNCTIONAL, COMPOUND, AND INTRADERMAL)

Summary: Round; tan to dark brown; sharply outlined, present since young adulthood; average white adult has about 20; prophylactic removal of all nevi is neither possible nor necessary; excise or bx a nevus that has changed, has bled, or is an irregular or black area of pigment; suspicious lesions are often referred to a dermatologist.

For additional details and rx, see 11.1.a.

11.7.D. DYSPLASTIC NEVUS SYNDROME

Cause: Multiple dysplastic nevi occur in families, inherited as autosomal dominant, or sporadically; UV light is not an inducing factor.

Epidem: Examine family members.

Si: Large, often 1 cm; few to hundreds; irregular in shape, often w a central papule surrounded by a flat pigmented margin w irregularly pigmented and scattered dark regions.

Crs: New dysplastic nevi often continue to appear in adulthood; manyfold ↑ risk of developing melanoma; perhaps 10% of pts w melanoma are members of high-risk families; >50% of pts w syndrome will develop melanoma.

Lab: Controversial histologic dx; interpretation depends on clinical pattern as well.

Rx: Melanoma may be prevented by 6-mo exams and removal of suspicious lesions; photography of lesions allows comparisons over time; most pts w this uncommon disorder are followed by a dermatologist or medical centers w a special interest in pigmented lesions.

11.7.E. DERMATOSIS PAPULOSA NIGRA

Cause: Unknown; often familial.

Epidem: Blacks >> whites.

Sx: None.

Si: Resemble raised freckles; pinhead to rice grain in size.

Crs: Appear 1st in teens, then ↑ in number for yrs; not premalignant.

Lab: Bx not necessary; resembles seborrheic keratoses.

Rx: Cosmetic importance only; electrocauterization usually satisfactory, but a test area allowed to heal for a mo is prudent to see if hypopigmentation develops.

11.7.F. CAFÉ AU LAIT SPOTS

See 11.9.b.

MULTIPLE, >5 YEARS, APPEARED <40 YEARS OLD, RED

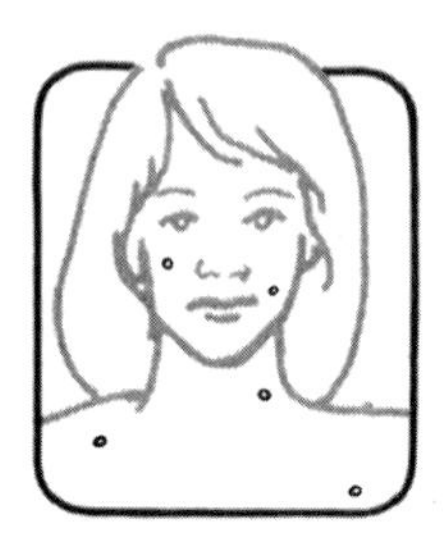

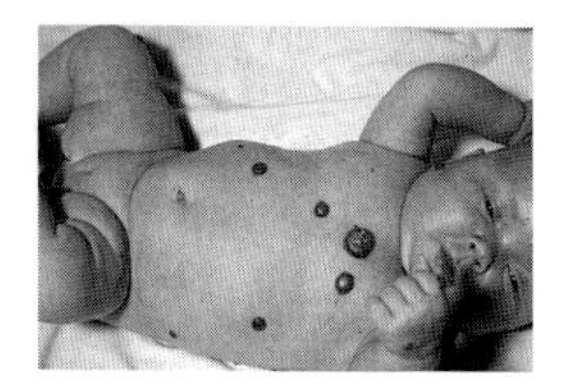

Hemangiomas

11.8.A. HEMANGIOMAS

Summary: Hemangiomas are far more likely to be single than multiple; blue to red vascular lesions that are present from birth or shortly afterward; some assoc w neurologic complications; lesions that appear in adulthood usually follow trauma.

For additional details and rx, see 11.2.a.

11.8.B. HEREDITARY HEMORRHAGIC TELANGIECTASIA (OSLER-WEBER-RENDU SYNDROME)

Cause: Inherited; autosomal dominant.

Si: Deep red to purple mat of blood vessels; flat or raised; pinhead to BB in size; single or grouped into lines or patches; located on lips, tongue, hands, nasal mucosa, upper trunk; bleeds easily after minor trauma, unlike cherry angiomas, which do not.

Crs: Lesions appear or ↑ at puberty.

Compl: Common: epistaxis, bleeding after tooth extraction, GI bleeding, heavy menstruation; assoc w glaucoma and arteriovenous shunts in internal organs.

Lab: Some pts are anemic from internal bleeding; occas coagulation defects add severity to bleeding; pts need evaluation for arteriovenous malformations in liver, kidneys, lungs, and for glaucoma.

Rx: Pts w this rare condition require care from multiple specialties, depending on organs involved; awareness of syndrome and early dx forestall complications.

MULTIPLE, >5 YEARS, APPEARED <40 YEARS OLD, LIGHT OR SKIN COLORED

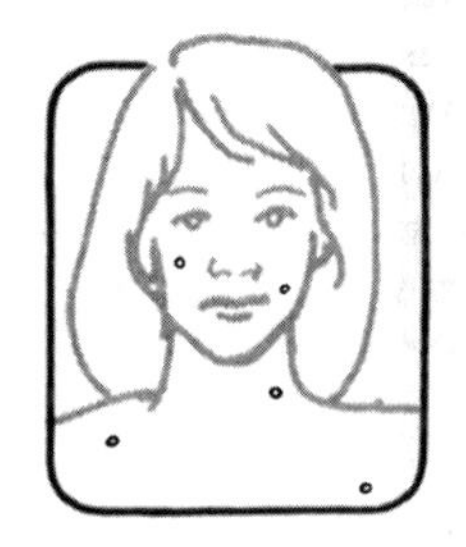

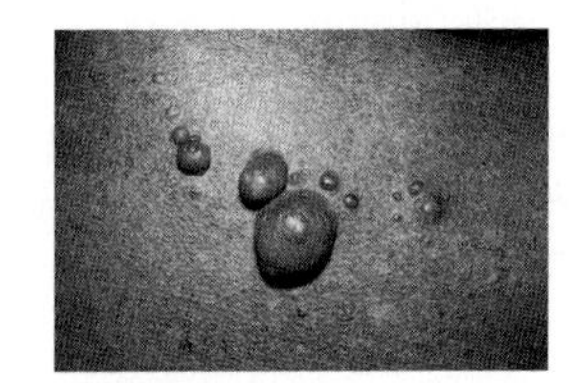

Neurofibromas

- The ddx includes **single, >5 yr, light or skin colored**:
  Cyst (11.3.a.)
  Milium (11.3.b.)
  Fibroma (11.3.c.)
  Dermatofibroma (11.3.d.)
  Keloid/hypertrophic scar (11.3.e.)
  Lipoma (11.3.f)
  Foreign body granuloma (11.3.g.)
- In addition to:

11.9.A. SKIN TAGS (FIBROEPITHELIAL POLYPS, FEPS)

Cause: Epidermal covered outgrowths that appear at sites of chronic "wear and tear."

Epidem: Common, esp >30–40 yo; esp w obesity.

Sx: Irritating when rubbed.

Si: Minute flaps or balls of skin; pinhead to BB in size; skin colored to tan; most common at axilla, groin, neck, eyelids.

Crs: Continue to appear over time.

Lab: None; not assoc w colonic polyps.

Rx: Electrocautery w or w/o injected local anesthetic or after topical EMLA, applied q 15 min for 2 h before procedure.

11.9.B. NEUROFIBROMATOSIS (NF, VON RECKLINGHAUSEN'S DISEASE)

Jama 1997;278:51. J Am Acad Derm 1997;37:625. J Am Acad Derm 1993;29:376.

Cause: NF1: inherited; autosomal dominant; 1/2 are new mutations; highly variable expression; NF2: assoc w acoustic schwannomas.

Epidem: Affected: both sexes, all races.

Pathophys: Tumors are composed of proliferating Schwann cells, fibroblasts, and nerves.

Si: Multiple; fleshy; skin colored; pea- to bean- to egg-sized growths; anywhere on body; *café au lait spots*: not diagnostic of NF1 unless multiple as 1–5 are present in 25% of schoolchildren (Arch Dis Child 1982;57:631); smooth edges, may be present at birth, 6 or more (each >1.5 cm) in an adult or 5 or more (each >0.5 cm) in a child (J Peds 1990;116:845) are diagnostic, but 1/4 pts w neurofibromatosis have fewer lesions; other disorders w café au lait spots: Albright's syndrome (irregular edges like "coast of Maine"), tuberous sclerosis, ataxia-telangiectasia, Hunter's syndrome, Turner's syndrome; freckling in apex of axillae is nearly diagnostic, unless pt is redhead w general body freckling (Derm Clin 1995;13:105); other than skin lesions: bone lesions (scoliosis, localized hypoplasia or hypertrophy, vertebral anomalies); neurologic lesions (variable mental retardation, seizures, acoustic nerve deafness, optic gliomas, brain and spinal cord tumors); endocrine lesions (pheochromocytoma, precocious puberty, functioning adenomas of thyroid, pituitary, hypothalamus); eye lesions, esp hamartomas of iris (*Lisch nodules*).

Crs: Variable; tumors develop after birth, but usually are obvious by puberty, multiply rapidly at puberty and w pregnancy; occas lesions become sarcomas.

Compl: Multiple, depending on organ involved (Jaad 2000;42:939).

Lab: Bx of a neurofibroma or café au lait spot is not diagnostic.

Rx: Genetic counseling is warranted; prenatal testing is available; extent of disorder in pt does not forecast severity in offspring; rapid change in size of a tumor is an indication for bx or removal; multiple specialties are involved depending on organs affected.

MULTIPLE, >5 YEARS, APPEARED >60 YEARS OLD, BLACK OR BROWN

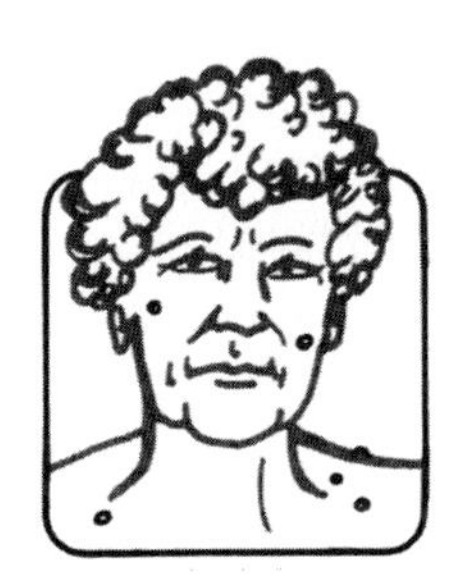

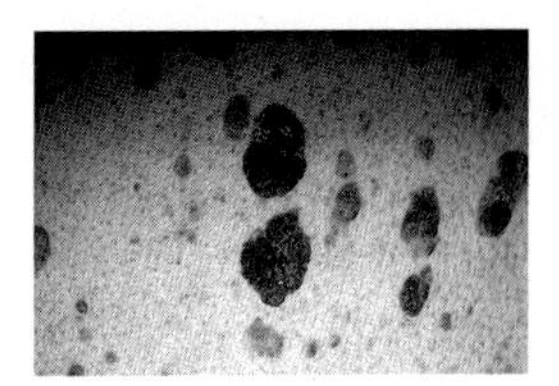

Seborrheic keratosis

11.10.A. FRECKLE/LENTIGO

Summary: *Freckle*: common; 1–3 mm; multiple; brown; flat; genetically determined on face; presence on trunk and arms indicates past intense sun exposure; not premalignant; rx not necessary or practical; *lentigo*: smaller and darker than freckle; fewer in number; not confined to sun-exposed areas; bx occasionally warranted to r/o melanoma (see 11.7.a.).

11.10.B. SEBORRHEIC KERATOSIS

Cause: Unknown; not UV light related; benign neoplasm of keratinocytes; sebaceous glands are not involved.

Epidem: Multiple lesions most common in pts w strong fhx of same; most >40 yo; women = men.

Sx: Sometimes irritating or bleed when traumatized.

Si: Roughened greasy surface feels waxy, hence the term *seborrheic*; common; tan to dark brown; feel stuck on surface, crumbly, partially scraped away w a fingernail; most common on face, upper part of trunk, and legs.

Crs: Darken and ↑ in number over yrs.

Compl: Not premalignant.

Ddx: Commonly confused w nevi, warts, pigmented BCE, melanoma.

Lab: Bx is not necessary for dx in most cases.

Rx: Reassurance that lesions are harmless usually is sufficient; occas lesions that are irritating, bleeding, interfere w function may need removal; methods: D&C, LN2, 50%–75% TCA applied just to lesion w cotton-tip applicator (do not use near eyes); all methods may leave a hypopigmented patch.

11.10.C. SKIN TAGS (FIBROEPITHELIAL POLYPS, FEPS)

Summary: Common, esp >30 yo; pinhead to BB size; tan to skin colored; also at groin, neck, eyelids; rx w electrocautery w or w/o local anesthetic or prior EMLA cr (see 11.9.a.).

MULTIPLE, >5 YEARS, APPEARED >60 YEARS OLD, RED

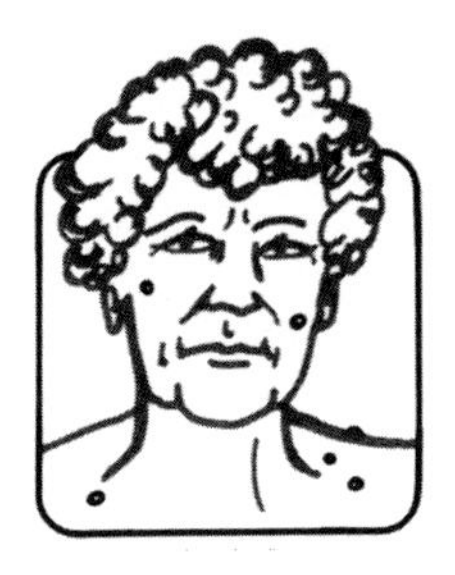

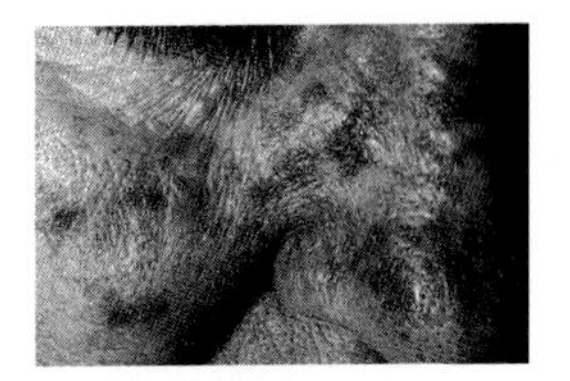

Actinic keratosis

GROWTHS

11.11.A. ACTINIC KERATOSIS

Cause: UV light.

Epidem: Uncommon in darker-complexioned persons.

Sx: Usually asx, but may be irritating.

Si: Discrete; persistent; pink to red; crusty; restricted to light-exposed areas, esp face, bald scalp, tops of ears, nape, back of hands. **Cutaneous horn**: name for particularly thickened, keratotic projection; pathology of base may show underlying hypertrophic actinic keratosis or well-differentiated SCC.

Crs: Controversial: some regard these lesions as SCC in situ (J Am Acad Derm 1999;41:443), while others regard them as simply a hallmark of excess actinic exposure w few, perhaps 1:1000 (Lancet 1988;1795), evolving into SCC; note that SCCs on light-exposed parts often appear on a background of actinic keratoses.

Compl: SCCs that arise in actinic keratoses have a 3% likelihood of metastasis.

Lab: May require bx to r/o skin cancer if lesion is thick or eroded.

Rx: Local destruction: D&C after local anesthesia (see RX.17.) or cryotherapy w LN2 (see RX.18.); excision is not necessary; for pts w numerous actinic keratoses consider a course of topical 5-FU (see RX.19.); discuss use of protective clothing, sun avoidance, and sunscreens; pts need re-examination on a regular, perhaps yrly basis, depending on skin cancer hx and number of lesions; pts w multiple actinic keratoses, esp w a hx of skin cancer, generally are followed by a dermatologist.

11.11.B. CHERRY ANGIOMA (SENILE HEMANGIOMA, CHERRY OR RUBY SPOT)

Cause: Capillary hemangioma.

Sx: None.

Si: Pinhead to rice in size; cherry red; smooth surface; usually above waist, but can be anywhere; do not blanch w pressure.

Crs: Appears in midlife in most persons; slowly ↑ in number w age; not premalignant.

Compl: Bleeding is unlikely.

Lab: None.

Rx: Not necessary.

MULTIPLE, >5 YEARS, APPEARED >60 YEARS OLD, LIGHT OR SKIN COLORED

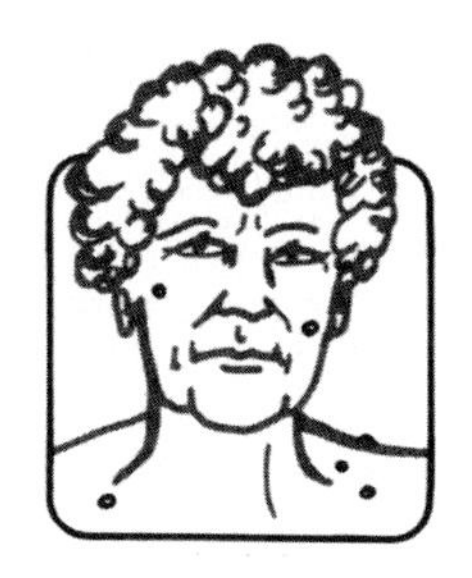

- The ddx includes **single, >5 yr, light or skin colored**:
  - Cyst (11.3.a.)
  - Milium (11.3.b.)
  - Fibroma (11.3.c.)
  - Dermatofibroma (11.3.d.)
  - Keloid/hypertrophic scar (11.3.e.)
  - Lipoma (11.3.f)
  - Foreign body granuloma (11.3.g.)
  - Skin tags (11.9.a.)
- In addition to:

11.12.A. SEBORRHEIC KERATOSIS

Summary: Common benign growths, tan to dark brown, slightly roughened, waxy, crumbly; feels "stuck on" surface; usually fhx of similar lesions; most >40 yo.

For additional details and rx, see 11.10.b.

MULTIPLE, <2 YEARS, APPEARED <40 YEARS OLD, BLACK OR BROWN

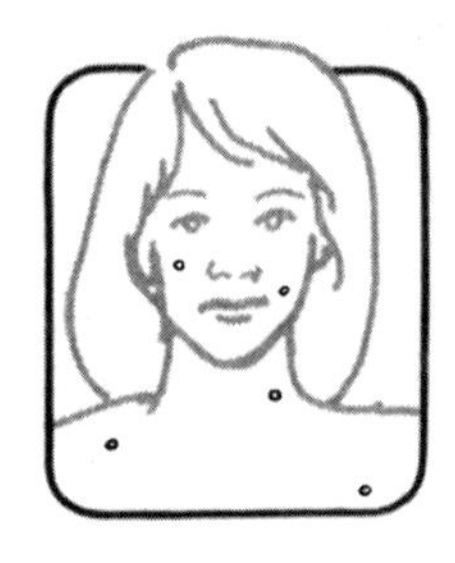

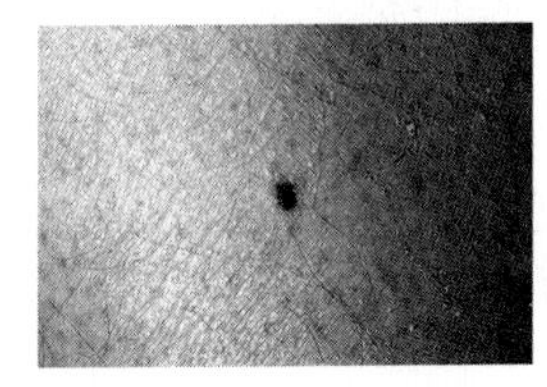

Lentigo

- The ddx includes:
  - Seborrheic keratosis (11.10.b.)
  - Skin tags (11.9.a.)
- In addition to:

11.13.A. FRECKLE/LENTIGO

Summary: *Freckle*: common; 1–3 mm; multiple; brown; flat; genetically determined on face; presence on trunk and arms indicates past intense sun exposure; not premalignant; rx not necessary or practical; *lentigo*: smaller and darker than freckle; fewer in number; not confined to sun-exposed areas; bx occas warranted to r/o melanoma (see 11.7.a.).

MULTIPLE, <2 YEARS, APPEARED <40 YEARS OLD, RED

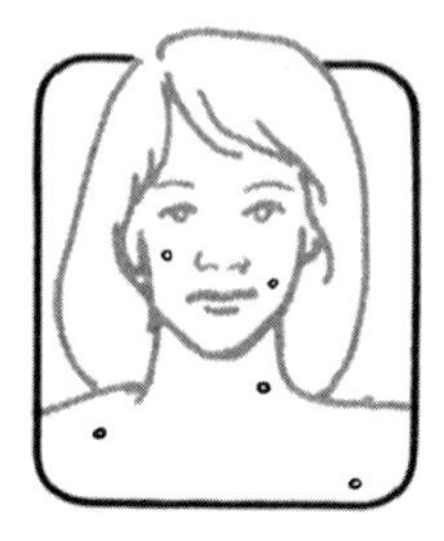

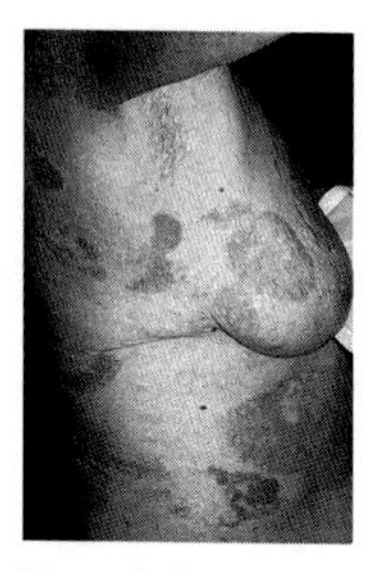

Mycosis fungoides

11.14.A. KAPOSI'S SARCOMA (KS, MULTIPLE IDIOPATHIC HEMORRHAGIC SARCOMA)

Med 1993;72:245. Lancet 1990;335:123.

Cause: Vascular tumor induced by infection w human herpesvirus type 8 (Nejm 1998;338:948); ↑ in immunocompromised persons, ie, after transplantation (J Am Acad Derm 1999;40:177).

Epidem: *Classic* type: rare, mainly in elderly men of eastern European and Mediterranean origin; *homosexual* type: previously higher but now in 10%–15% of HIV-pos persons, nearly all cases in homosexual men or female partners of bisexual men; occasionally seen in HIV-neg men at high risk for HIV infection and after organ transplantation; whites >> blacks.

Sx: Painless to painful.

Si: *Classic* type: feet, legs, hands most common sites; reddish to deep purple patches to plaques to tumors; nonpitting swelling; *homosexual* type: any site, esp common at sites of trauma; isolated or grouped; deep pink to purple; may look like bruise at onset.

Crs: *Classic* type: chronic and slowly expand, often for yrs; *homosexual* type: grow rapidly; ↑ in number and size over wks to mos.

Compl: May involve GI tract w blockage or bleeding, LNs w edema, lungs w shortness of breath, liver, other viscera.

Lab: Bx may be necessary to confirm dx and r/o look-alikes; occurrence not strictly assoc w depressed CD4+ T-cell count.

Rx: Options: alitretinoin gel (Panretin, 60 gm, Rx, $$$$) bid–qid; LN2; local x-radiation; systemic chemotherapy (Ann IM 1985;102:200); interferon (J Invest Derm 1990;95S:166); IL vincristine/vinblastine; often resolves w rx of HIV infection w protease inhibitors; most pts are treated and followed by a dermatologist, oncologist, radiation oncologist, and physicians w a special interest in AIDS.

11.14.B. MYCOSIS FUNGOIDES (MF, CUTANEOUS T-CELL LYMPHOMA, CTCL)

Curr Probl Cancer 1990;14:295. Ann IM 1984;100:187.

Cause: Lymphoma, generally of a helper T-cell subset of lymphocytes; appears to start in skin.

Epidem: Men > women; peak incidence age 55 yo.

Sx: Pruritus in early stages; painful tumors later.

Si: Usually begins as 1 or more itchy thickened patches; may resemble a benign eruption at outset, ie, psoriasis or seborrheic dermatitis; later thickening to form plaques and tumors; **Sézary syndrome**: erythrodermic, exfoliative, most have LN↑, and circulating atypical T cells.

Crs: If lesions remain few and thin, course is prolonged, over yrs, and may not affect longevity; progression to more lesions, esp if >10% of body surface, and to thickened plaques and tumors decreases survival significantly (Arch Derm 1999;135:26); appears to be confined to skin early in its course w later spreading to LNs and internal organs, but T-cell receptor gene analysis shows that the disease may be systemic early in its course (Arch Derm 1998;134:158).

Compl: Most are cutaneous; internal organ compromise occurs late.

Lab: Dx established by skin bx w confirmation by T-cell receptor gene cloning analysis; bx is problematic in early patch stage; evaluation may include LN bx, exam of blood for atypical lymphocytes; CT scans not useful in early stages.

Rx: Optimal rx has not yet been determined (Ann IM 1994;121:592); early-stage options: PUVA, topical nitrogen mustard (J Am Acad

Derm 1995;33:234), topical carmustine (BCNU), or topical CS; later-stage options: same plus interferon, extracorporeal photopheresis, or systemic chemotherapy; evaluation and rx generally are managed by a dermatologist and oncologist.

MULTIPLE, <2 YEARS, APPEARED <40 YEARS OLD, LIGHT OR SKIN COLORED

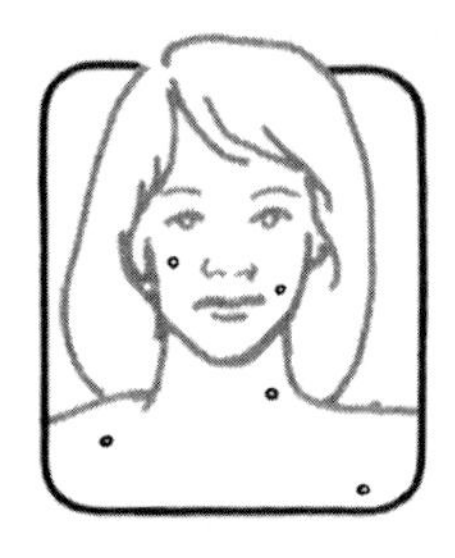

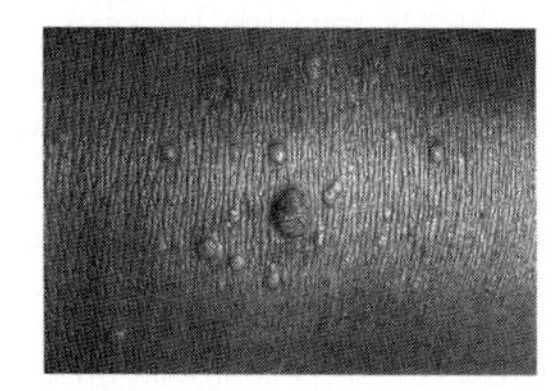

Verruca vulgaris

- The ddx includes **single, >5 yr, light or skin colored**:
  Cyst (11.3.a.)
  Milium (11.3.b.)
  Fibroma (11.3.c.)
  Dermatofibroma (11.3.d.)
  Keloid/hypertrophic scar (11.3.e.)
  Lipoma (11.3.f)
  Foreign body granuloma (11.3.g.)
  Skin tags (11.9.b.)
- In addition to:

11.15.A. MOLLUSCUM CONTAGIOSUM

Summary: DNA poxvirus; pale to pink, shiny, elevated bump or papule w light-colored dimple in center; common on face in children; large numbers on face w HIV infection; look for lesions about genitals and lower abdomen in adults; asx unless traumatized; DNA poxvirus; transmission is by close person-to-person contact.

For additional details and rx, see GENITAL, 9.7.b.

11.15.B. VERRUCA VULGARIS (COMMON WART)

Summary: Single to multiple; surface is raised, rough, cauliflower like; pinhead to dime sized; most are on hands, feet, face; usually painless unless periungual or fingertip; may be easily traumatized.

For additional details and rx, see HANDS, 14.1.a.

11.15.C. SARCOID

Summary: Mimics other eruptions; most are pink to yellow; firm papules or plaques; pinhead to pea size or larger; usually nape, face, extensor surfaces; minimal itching; may develop within preexisting scars; sometimes severe and may distort facial features; may be deep; may ulcerate; may lead to local hair loss; blacks >> whites.

For additional details and rx, see BODY, 3.3.o.

MULTIPLE, <2 YEARS, APPEARED >60 YEARS OLD, BLACK OR BROWN

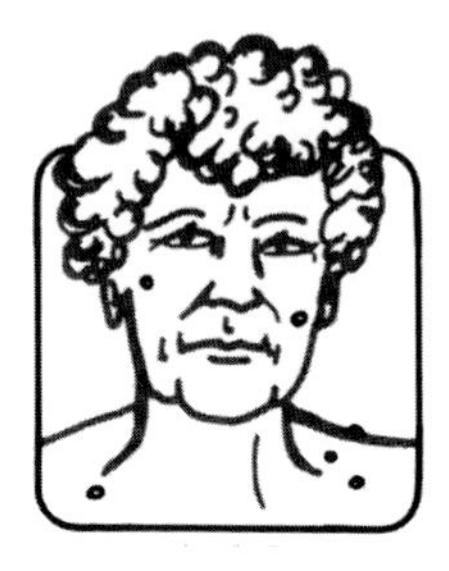

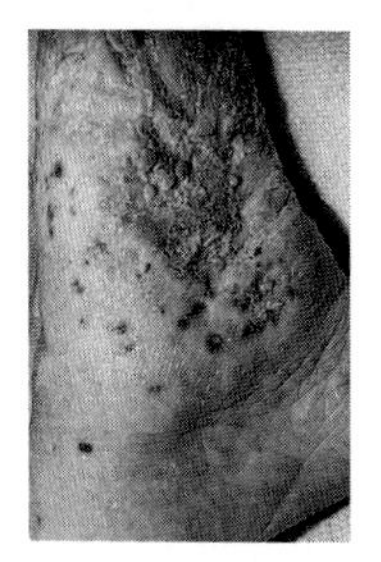

Melanoma

- The ddx includes:
  Skin tags (11.9.b.)
- In addition to:

11.16.A. FRECKLE/LENTIGO

Summary: *Freckle*: common; 1–3 mm; multiple; brown; flat; genetically determined on face; presence on trunk and arms indicates past intense sun exposure; not premalignant; rx not necessary or practical; *lentigo*: smaller and darker than freckle; fewer in number; not confined to sun-exposed areas; bx occas warranted to r/o melanoma (see 11.7.a.).

11.16.B. SEBORRHEIC KERATOSIS

Summary: Common benign growths, tan to dark brown, slightly roughened, waxy, crumbly; feels "stuck on" surface; usually fhx of similar lesions; most >40 yo.

For additional details and rx, see 11.10.b.

11.16.C. BASAL CELL CARCINOMA (BCC)

Summary: Single or few; shiny or pearly colored; telangiectasias over surface; depressed center; slowly spreading; usually on light-exposed areas, esp face, neck, forearms; about 80% of skin cancers.

For additional details and rx, see 11.6.c.

GROWTHS

MULTIPLE, <2 YEARS, APPEARED >60 YEARS OLD, RED

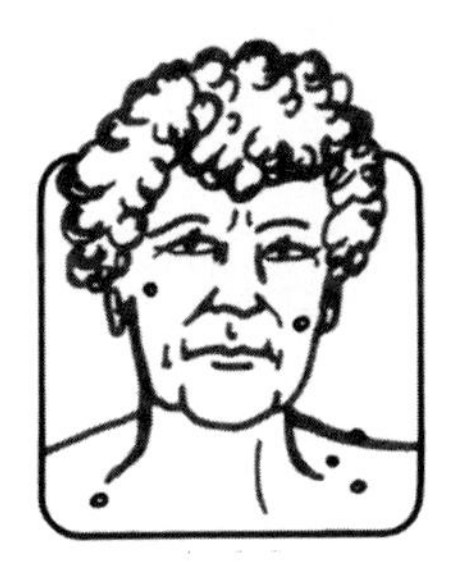

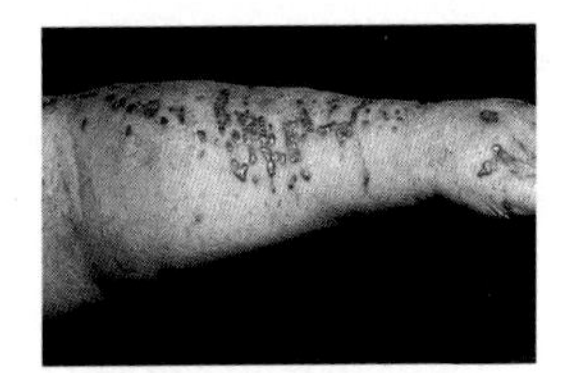

Kaposi's sarcoma

11.17.A. ACTINIC KERATOSES

Summary: Discrete; persistent; scaly, pink to red; esp in light-complexioned persons >40 yo; hx of excessive sun exposure; considered premalignant but few become SCC (see 11.11.a.).

11.17.B. KAPOSI'S SARCOMA (KS, MULTIPLE IDIOPATHIC HEMORRHAGIC SARCOMA)

Summary: Two types: *classic* type: rare, mainly in elderly men of eastern European and Mediterranean origin; feet, legs, hands most common sites; reddish to deep purple; patches to plaques to tumors; nonpitting swelling; *homosexual* type: nearly all cases in homosexual men or female partners of bisexual men; any site, esp common at sites of trauma; isolated or grouped; deep pink to purple; may look like bruise at onset (see 11.14.a.).

11.17.C. MYCOSIS FUNGOIDES

Summary: T-cell lymphoma usually starting as itchy thickened patches; may remain stable or progress to thickened plaques, tumors, and exfoliative erythroderma; appears to start in skin and progress to viscera; men > women; average age 55 yo (see 11.14.b.).

11.17.D. SARCOID

Summary: Mimics other eruptions; most are pink to yellow; firm papules or plaques; pinhead to pea size or larger; usually nape, face, extensor surfaces; minimal itching; may develop within preexisting scars; sometimes severe and may distort facial features; may be deep; may ulcerate; may lead to local hair loss; blacks >> whites.

For additional details and rx, see BODY, 3.3.o.

MULTIPLE, <2 YEARS, APPEARED >60 YEARS OLD, LIGHT OR SKIN COLORED

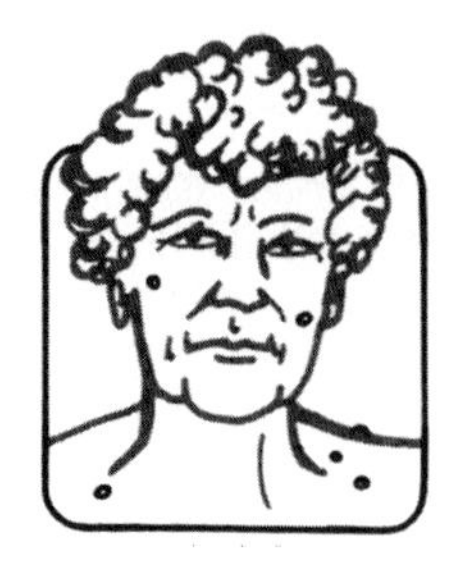

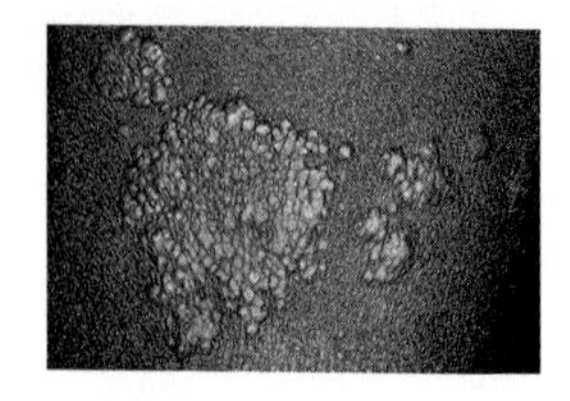

Sarcoid

- The ddx includes **multiple, <2 yr, appeared <40 yo, light or skin colored**:
  - Cyst (11.3.a.)
  - Milium (11.3.b.)
  - Fibroma (11.3.c.)
  - Dermatofibroma (11.3.d.)
  - Keloid/hypertrophic scar (11.3.e.)
  - Lipoma (11.3.f)
  - Foreign body granuloma (11.3.g.)
  - Molluscum contagiosum (11.15.a.)
  - Skin tags (11.9.a.)
  - Verruca vulgaris (common wart) (11.15.b.)
- In addition to:

11.18.A. SEBORRHEIC KERATOSIS

Summary: Common benign growths, tan to dark brown, slightly roughened, waxy, crumbly; feels "stuck on" surface; usually fhx of similar lesions; most >40 yo.

For additional details and rx, see 11.10.b.

11.18.B. SARCOID

Summary: Mimics other eruptions; most are pink to yellow; firm papules or plaques; pinhead to pea size or larger; usually nape, face, extensor surfaces; minimal itching; may develop within preexisting scars; sometimes severe and may distort facial features; may be deep; may ulcerate; may lead to local hair loss; blacks >> whites.

For additional details and rx, see BODY, 3.3.o.

12 Hair Decrease

SCALP APPEARS NORMAL

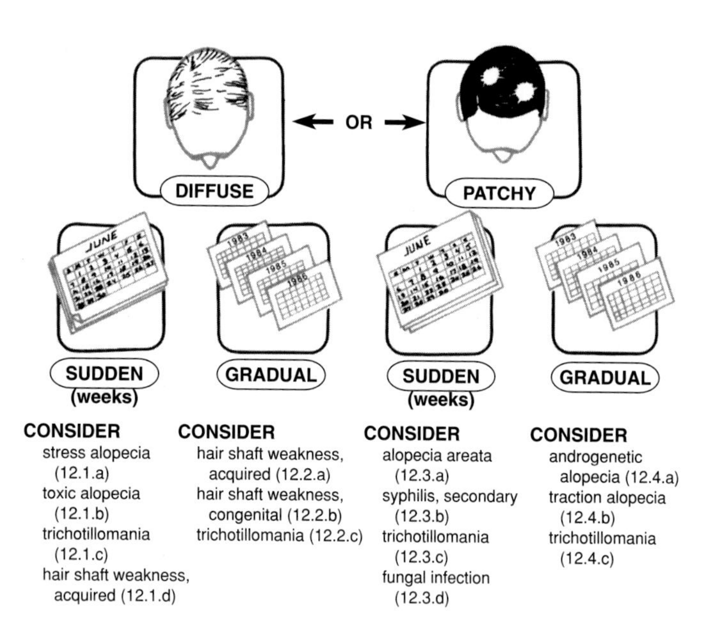

Note: If scalp is scaly, lumpy, or inflamed, see Scalp section.

Summary of hair physiology: Human scalp hair growth proceeds in cycles. The period of active growth, *anagen*, lasts 2–7 yr; the resting phase, *telogen*, lasts 2–4 mo. Anagen and telogen hairs are intermingled w about 80% of scalp hairs in anagen (growing) and 20% in telogen (resting). Once hairs have entered telogen, they do not grow again. Instead, 2–4 mo later, when the hair follicle re-enters the growing phase, a new hair forms below the resting hair, and the resting hair is shed. Hence, some shedding is normal, averaging 25–100 hairs/d. When growing, the hair follicle, which is only 1–2 mm long, produces 10–15 mm of hair every mo.

Med Clin N Am 1998;82:1155. Olsen EA, Disorders of hair growth, McGraw-Hill, New York, 1994.

DIFFUSE SCALP HAIR LOSS, SUDDEN (WEEKS)

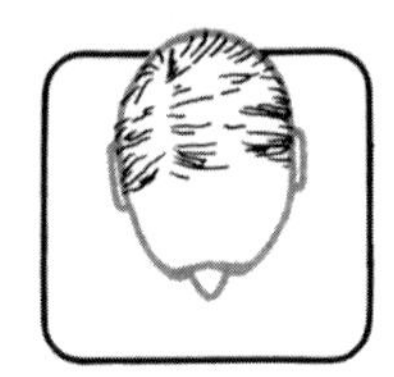

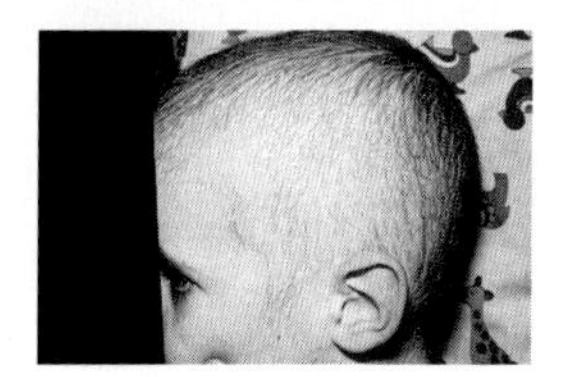

Toxic alopecia

12.1.A. STRESS (TELOGEN) ALOPECIA

J Am Acad Derm 1996;35:899.

Cause: Physical, chemical, and emotional events are registered sensitively by fluctuations in hair growth and, if severe enough, may turn off growth temporarily; when growth resumes 2–4 mo later, quantities of hair are shed; known triggers of stress (telogen) hair loss include:

- Fever, generally >41° C.
- Certain meds, including:
  Allopurinol (Lopurin, Zyloprim)
  Amitriptyline (Amitril, Elavil, Endep)

Amphetamines
Antibiotics: gentamicin
Anticoagulants: coumarin, heparin, phenindione
Anticonvulsants: pheny/hydantoin, diones, valproic acid
Arthritis drugs: all "-profens," indomethacin, Naproxen, Piroxicam, gold
β-Blocking agents
Blood pressure meds: captopril, enalapril, most others
Cancer treatment drugs: most
Carbamazepine (Tegretol)
Cholesterol-lowering agents: clofibrate, nicotinic acid, triparanol, cholestyramine
Contraceptives, oral
DOPA drugs (levodopa, methyldopa)
Gout meds: colchicine, allopurinol
Mood drugs: amitriptyline, amoxapine, desipramine, doxepin (Adapin, Sinequan), haloperidol (Haldol), imipramine, nortriptyline, protriptyline, trimipramine
Metals: gold, lithium (Eskalith, Lithane)
Nitrofurantoin (Furadantin, Macrodantin)
Probenecid (Benemid, Proban)
Pyridostigmine (Mestinon)
Retinoids (Etretinate, Tegison)
Thyroid drugs: carbimazole, thiouracils, iodine
Ulcer meds: cimetidine, famotidine, ranitidine
Valproic acid (Depakene, Depakote)

- Pregnancy (or oral contraceptives).
- Systemic illness, severe.
- Surgery, usually w a general anesthetic.
- Other:

Accidents
Acute blood loss
Acute psychiatric illness
Acute trauma
Crash dieting

Pathophys: Hair loss assoc w pregnancy follows delivery by 2–4 mo because large numbers of hair follicles that had been growing continuously during pregnancy and that had simultaneously entered the resting phase after delivery now are shed w renewal of anagen growth.

Sx: None.

Si: Diffuse but modest ↓ in scalp hair w/o scalp inflammation.

Crs: Onset often delayed 2–4 mo after the stress since telogen hair must be pushed out of its follicle by restart of anagen before hair is shed; reversible w normal thickness returning 6–12 mo after stress is removed; reversal may not occur in older persons who might have been in early stages of genetic balding anyway.

Lab: None useful; *hair-pull test*: hair gently pulled between 2 fingers should not bring out >2 hairs unless telogen loss is still in progress (if >2, repeat in 1–2 mo) (see DX.5).

Rx: Removal of inciting cause or recognition of what had been the cause 2–4 mo prior to hair loss; then reassurance that the hair will regrow.

12.1.B. TOXIC (ANAGEN) ALOPECIA

Cause: Hair follicles are esp vulnerable to damage during their anagen (growth) phase; meds: cancer chemotherapeutic agents, esp cyclophosphamide, dactinomycin, doxorubicin, paclitaxel, and vincristine, high dose of vitamin A, and synthetic retinoids (Soriatane, Accutane).

Pathophys: Hair growth disruption during anagen may be severe since 80% of scalp follicles are in anagen; the newly made hair shaft is weak and prone to breakage.

Sx: None.

Si: Hair loss may be extensive, leaving only those 20% of hairs not in anagen but these will be lost w later courses of chemotherapy; no scalp inflammation.

Crs: Starts 1–2 wk after chemotherapy; reversible; hair sometimes regrows w different texture.

Lab: Dx usually determined by hx; microscopic examination of hair shaft shows thinned portion at proximal end where hair growth was weakened (see DX.5).

Rx: None but reassurance that hair will regrow.

12.1.C. TRICHOTILLOMANIA

Arch Derm 1995;131:720, 723. Am J Psych 1991;148:365.

Cause: Self-induced plucking or cutting of scalp hair, sometimes of other hairy areas; DSM-IV classification: impulse-control disorder (312.39) rather than an obsessive-compulsive disorder.

Epidem: Children: boys = girls; adults: women >> men; 1%–2% of college students have hx.

Sx: Pt commonly denies hair pulling but this habit can be observed by family members; pts experience an increasing sense of tension before pulling and pleasure or relief when pulling (DSM-IV, American Psychiatric Assoc, 4th ed, 1994:618).

Si: Look for a nearly bald area on an otherwise normal, noninflamed scalp; hairs are shortened or a stubble in a round, irregular, or bizarre pattern; the area is not completely bald as seen in alopecia areata (see 12.3.a.); note that some shave, rather than pluck, hair; other common sites: eyebrows and eyelashes.

Crs: May be transient periods in childhood (benign or "habit") or chronic in adulthood w episodes over wks, mos, or yrs; continuous or episodic; sites may vary.

Lab: As hairs have no intrinsic defects, hair pluck shows roots to have a normal anagen-telogen ratio (80:20); distal ends may be frayed if broken off or neatly cut if snipped or shaved; bx, if performed, shows normal or traumatized follicles but no inflammation (see DX.5).

Rx: Tactfully confront pt w knowledge that you know the cause; this may be sufficient to stop the behavior, although denial of the deed is typical; refer recalcitrant cases to psychiatry/psychology (Nejm 1989;321:497).

12.1.D. HAIR SHAFT WEAKNESS, ACQUIRED

Cause: Usually excessive trauma from hair styling; may have underlying disorder, ie, **trichorrhexis nodosa**, which becomes evident only after sufficient trauma; endocrine, nutritional, and general medical disorders leading to hair loss: hypo- or hyperthyroidism, iron deficiency anemia (Clin Endocrinol 1992;36:421); alopecia is the most common skin effect of chemotherapy for cancer (J Am Acad Derm 1999;40:367).

Epidem: Usually confined to women who braid, dye, apply permanent waving solutions, or use excessive heat when drying hair.

Si: Hairs are short and broken, rather than reduced in numbers; may be numerous short hairs on pillow in morning.

Crs: Chronic but pts do not become bald.

Lab: Do hair pull and examine hairs microscopically (see DX.5.); look for frayed tips or nodes along the shaft, rather than square, barber-cut, distal ends; obtain thyroid function tests and serum ferritin level (should be >40 μg/L).

Rx: Depending on what is found in w/u, suggest change in hair styling and/or rx an underlying thyroid or iron deficiency condition.

DIFFUSE SCALP HAIR LOSS, GRADUAL (MANY MONTHS TO YEARS)

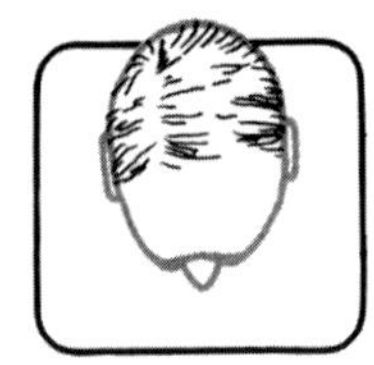

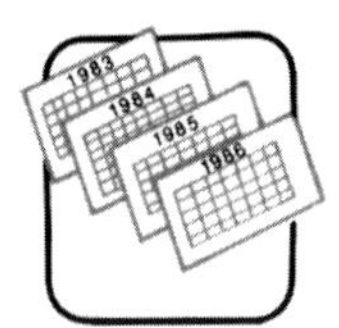

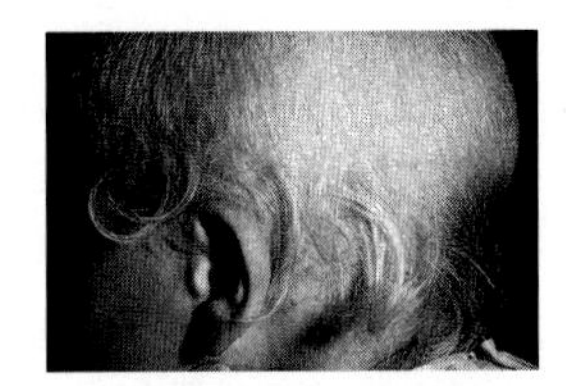

Congenital hair shaft weakness

12.2.A. HAIR SHAFT WEAKNESS, ACQUIRED

Summary: Hairs are short and broken, rather than reduced in numbers; may be numerous short hairs on pillow in morning (see 12.1.d.).

12.2.B. HAIR SHAFT WEAKNESS, CONGENITAL

Whiting DA, Hair shaft defects, in Olsen EA, ed, Disorders of hair growth, McGraw-Hill, New York, 1994:91.

Cause: Numerous conditions, all rare; many autosomal dominant, but may be other inheritance patterns or sporadic; includes **trichorrhexis nodosa** (bamboo hair), **monilethrix** (beaded hair), **pili torti** (ringed hair).

Si: Hair shaft breaks easily, usually short hairs, sometimes only a few cm in length; unruly hair rather than short in some conditions; hair may be normal in length, but sparse; **Netherton's syndrome**: short, broken hairs w a widespread skin eruption resembling atopic dermatitis.

Crs: Sparse, fine, or wiry hair since birth or early childhood; severity varies within same family and over time in the affected person; many diminish w age; dental and nail anomalies and mental retardation may be assoc w some of these syndromes.

Lab: Rare cases are assoc w disorders of copper or amino acid metabolism.

Rx: None available; all are so rare that the PCP generally seeks consultation w dermatology or pediatric dermatology.

12.2.C. TRICHOTILLOMANIA

Summary: Self-induced plucking or cutting of scalp hair, sometimes of other hairy areas; nearly bald area on an otherwise normal, noninflamed scalp; hairs are shortened or a stubble in a round, irregular, or bizarre pattern; may start suddenly or gradually and may be diffuse, although a single symmetric patch is more usual (see 12.1.c.).

PATCHY SCALP HAIR LOSS, SUDDEN (WEEKS)

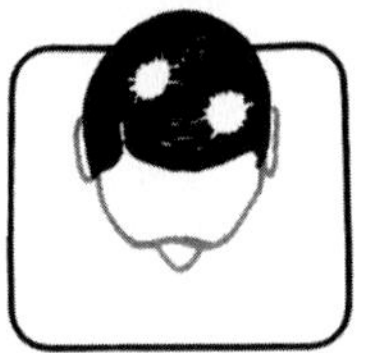

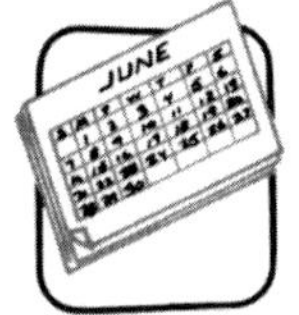

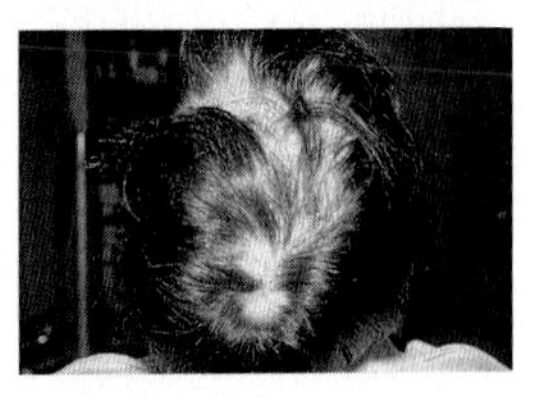

Alopecia areata

12.3.A. ALOPECIA AREATA

Jaad 2000;42:549; Derm Clin 1996;14:661.

Cause: Unknown; immunologic mechanism is suspected; role for emotional or physical trauma preceding hair loss is unproven recurring theme.

Epidem: Most <40 yo; men = women; 10% familial.

Sx: Usually none.

Si: Patches usually localized to sharply defined areas; hair loss in each patch is complete, leaving round or oval, hairless areas; almost no inflammation; may involve other hairy areas; pitting and striations of nails occur in 1/4 (see NAILS, 20.6.b.).

Crs: Appears abruptly, over days to wks; most get regrowth within a few mos; 1/4–1/2 experience recurrences, sometimes yrs later and often worse; rarely hair loss progresses to complete alopecia, of either scalp alone (**alopecia totalis**) or entire body (**alopecia universalis**); worse prognosis: 2nd or later episode, extensive hair loss, occipital region involvement, familial cases.

Lab: Activity of episode may be determined by gentle tugging on hairs at margins: >2 loose hairs w each pull indicates an active expanding process; ↑ frequency of thyroid and epithelial antibodies, pernicious anemia, and vitiligo.

Rx: Time will resolve most cases spontaneously, but topical CS soln (see RX.5.) bid for 1–2 mo may provide benefit; intradermal CS (see RX.7.) w triamcinolone acetonide (Kenalog 10 mg/mL) diluted to 4 mg/mL given at multiple sites about 1 cm apart using about

0.1 mL at each site generally leads to irregular patchy hair regrowth, often w a slight depression, usually reversible; systemic CS rarely used except for rapidly progressing, extensive loss; correction of underlying thyroid problem or anemia does not improve alopecia areata; dermatologists often use alternative therapies: PUVA, induction of irritation w topical irritants or allergens (Lancet 1997;349:222; J Am Acad Derm 1998;39:751).

Contact National Alopecia Areata Foundation (710 C Street, Suite 11, San Rafael, CA 94901; 415.456.4644; www.alopeciaareata.com) for assistance w pt education.

12.3.B. SYPHILIS, SECONDARY

Summary: Many patterns; most common: widespread, slightly scaly, tan, copper-colored, nonitchy patches, lesions on palms and/or soles; recent or healing genital ulcer; moist, wartlike genital growths (condylomata lata); painless oral erosions and mucous patches; "moth-eaten" scalp hair loss; mild or absent constitutional si and sx; LN↑, esp epitrochlear nodes; no blisters except in newborn; 2° lesions appear few wk after 1°; rash disappears.

For additional details, see BODY, 3.1.f.

12.3.C. TRICHOTILLOMANIA

Summary: Self-induced plucking or cutting of scalp hair, sometimes of other hairy areas; nearly bald area on an otherwise normal, noninflamed scalp; hairs are shortened or a stubble in a round, irregular, or bizarre pattern; may start suddenly or gradually and may be diffuse, although a single symmetric patch is more usual (see 12.1.c.).

12.3.D. FUNGAL INFECTION (TINEA CAPITIS)

Summary: Itchy areas or patches of thinned and broken scalp hairs; may be scaly w minimal inflammation, resembling seborrheic dermatitis, or crusted or pustular; most are in prepubertal children, often in minor epidemics.

For additional details and rx, see SCALP, 24.4.a.

PATCHY SCALP HAIR LOSS, GRADUAL (MANY MONTHS TO YEARS)

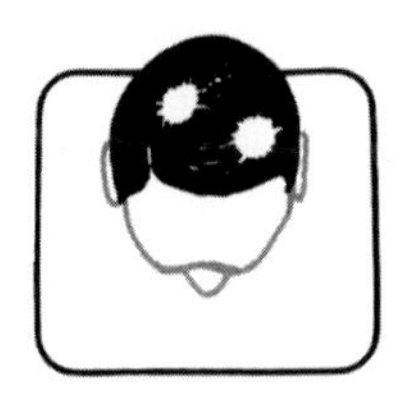

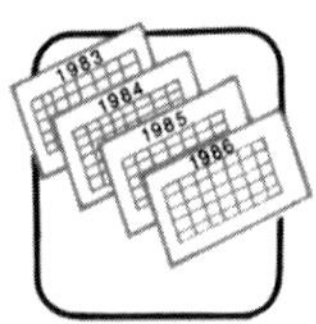

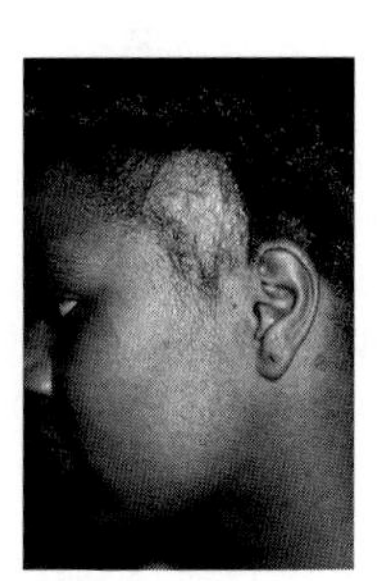

Traction alopecia

12.4.A. ANDROGENETIC ALOPECIA (COMMON OR PATTERN BALDING)

BMJ 1998;317:865. Am J Med 1995;98:95S.

Cause: Genetics determines onset and extent; time of onset and extent are not good measures of aging.

Epidem: Asians and American Indians < whites.

Pathophys: Each follicle has an intrinsic clock that initiates balding; only absence of androgens prior to puberty that trigger predetermined genetic patterns prevents the “clock” from being set, as in the case of males castrated before puberty and those w Klinefelter syndrome who never become bald; elevated androgen levels in masculinizing disorders of women produce baldness in a pattern similar to that seen in men; growing (anagen) phase shortens and number of resting (telogen) hairs ↑.

Si: Male: thinning usually starts in frontal hairline and vertex, first w development of sparse, fine hairs because of thinning, atrophic follicles; female: tends to be diffuse over top of scalp, while retaining the frontal hairline.

Crs: Slow, progressive, usually over decades.

Lab: Male: none necessary if pattern is typical; female: consider androgen excess w male pattern balding (see HAIR INCREASE, 13.2.).

Rx:

- Male: most reluctantly accept slow balding; if rx is desired: topical minoxidil (Rogaine ES 5% bid, OTC, $20/mo) (Jaad 1999;41:717) and/or finasteride (Propecia 1 mg qd, Rx, Merck, $$) (J Am Acad Derm 1998;39:578); finasteride's safety and efficacy have been shown only in men 18–41 yo and 4% experience reduced sexual interest or ability (compared to 2% on placebo) (Derm Clin 1998;16:341); surgical: hair transplants to move plugs of hair-bearing scalp from areas that usually retain hair, ie, fringe around back of head, to thinned frontal or crown areas; surgical scalp reduction to excise bald areas from crown, bringing hair-bearing areas closer together; a dermatologic surgeon or plastic surgeon can provide additional information and evaluation.
- Female: topical minoxidil may be beneficial; surgical techniques are not practical as hair loss is diffuse; finasteride is not safe or effective in women (Jaad 2000;43:768).

12.4.B. TRACTION (TRAUMATIC) ALOPECIA

Cause: Continuous or excessive pulling leads to thinning because of broken hair shafts and damage to the follicle; overtight hair curling, ie, cornrows, ponytails, sleeping w curlers, hot combs used to straighten hair.

Sx: None.

Si: Hair thinning is usually most noticeable at margins of scalp or between tightly braided hairs; scalp usually appears normal; most are black females (Derm Clin 1988;6:387).

Crs: Begins gradually and worsens as ever-tighter curls are attempted to conceal thinning; thinning may become permanent from scarring.

Rx: Suggest a change to a less traumatic form of hair care.

HAIR DECREASE

12.4.C. TRICHOTILLOMANIA

Summary: Self-induced plucking or cutting of scalp hair, sometimes of other hairy areas; nearly bald area on an otherwise normal, noninflamed scalp; hairs are shortened or a stubble in a round, irregular, or bizarre pattern; may start suddenly or gradually and may be diffuse, although a single symmetric patch is more usual (see 12.1.c.).

13 Hair Increase

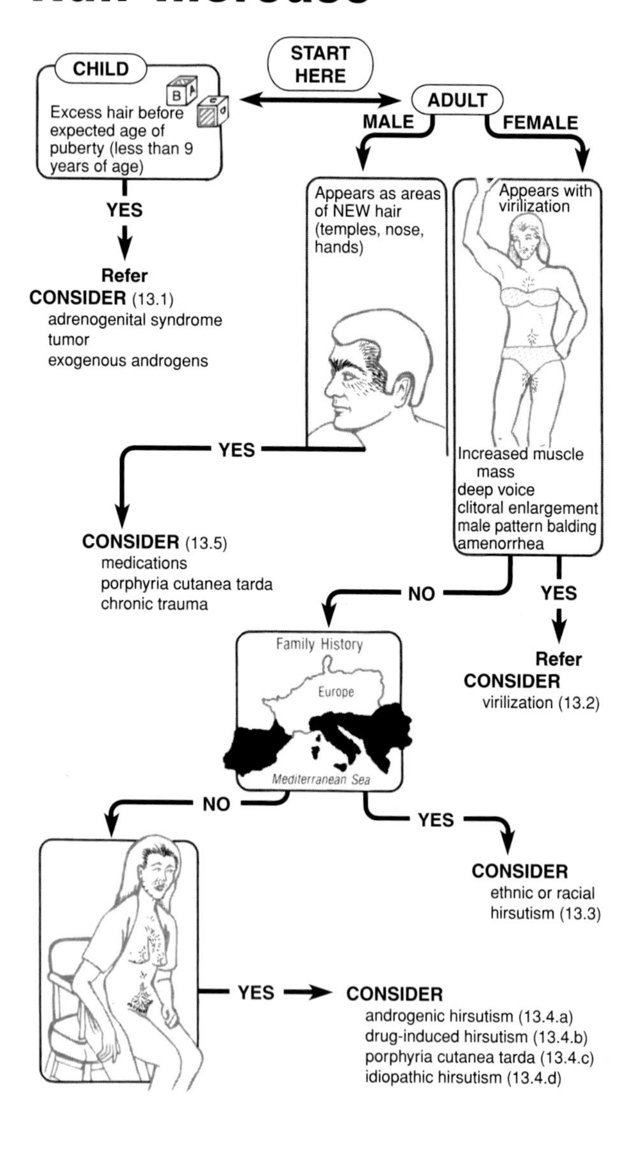

Written in collaboration with Marc R. Blackman, MD, Professor, Medicine, The Johns Hopkins Medical Institutions, Baltimore, Maryland.

Harman SM, Blackman MR, Common problems in reproductive endocrinology, in Barker LR, Burton J, Zieve PD, eds, Principles of ambulatory medicine, 5th ed, Williams & Wilkins, Baltimore, 1998:1168–1197. Cur Opin Ob Gyn 1995;3:344. J Am Acad Derm 1993;28:901.

CHILD

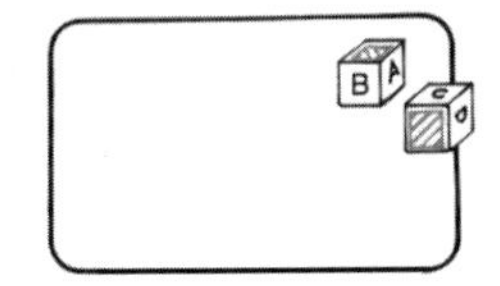

13.1. HIRSUTISM IN THE CHILD (PRECOCIOUS PUBERTY)

Cause: Excess androgens; hyperplasia or tumor of gonads, adrenals or pituitary gland (see 13.2.) or certain meds (see 13.4.b.).

Si: Hypertrichosis and/or 2° sexual hair w normal adult distribution; abn if appears <8 y age in female or <10 y age in male; early penile or clitoral development, ambiguity of external genitalia; other signs of endocrine disorder: obesity, hyperpigmentation, acne, striae, hypertension, hypokalemia.

Crs: Early growth spurt, but early epiphyseal closure and short stature.

Rx: Obtain prompt endocrinologic consultation.

ADULT, FEMALE, VIRILIZATION

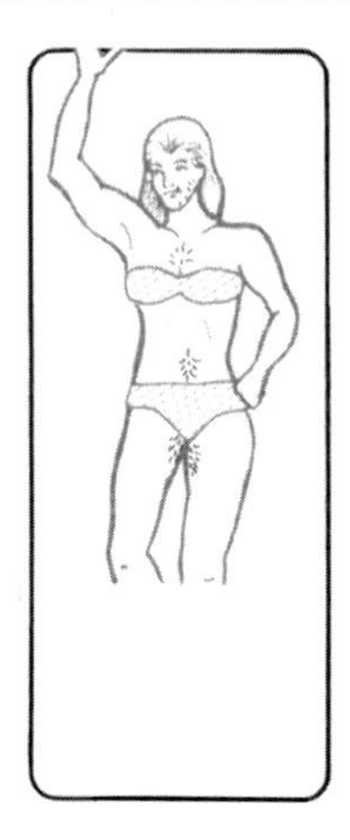

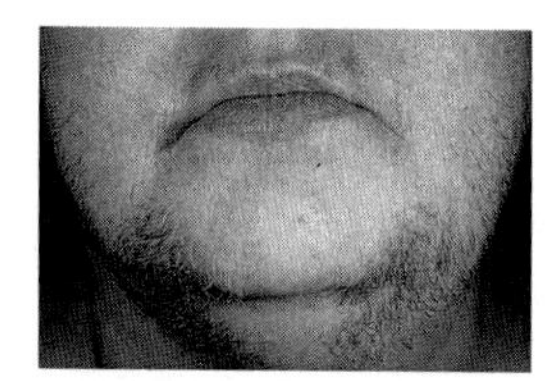

Hirsutism with virilization

13.2. VIRILIZATION

Cause: Use of exogenous androgens; ↑ androgen levels w adrenogenital syndrome, congenital adrenal hyperplasia, Cushing's syndrome, Stein-Leventhal syndrome, malignant adrenal or ovarian tumors (rare).

Epidem: Females only; males already maximally androgen stimulated and cannot become overvirilized.

Pathophys: ↑ androgen levels from exogenous androgens; or endogenous adrenal or ovarian source; most frequent cause of ↑ androgens: hyperplasia and benign tumors of ovaries or adrenal glands; hirsutism from this cause is usually not accompanied by virilization.

Si: Male pattern balding, acne, ↑ muscle mass, clitoral enlargement, deepening of voice, amenorrhea, hirsutism of male pattern w facial and body hair.

Crs: If rapid, more likely to be tumor, benign or malignant.

Lab:

1. Plasma total testosterone (normal <85 ng/dL) to r/o ovarian or, rarely, adrenal source; normal serum testosterone suggests idiopathic hirsutism and excludes major ovarian disorders; free testosterone level is not a screening test as most pts w ↑ free testosterone levels also have ↑ total testosterone levels; moreover, the test is expensive, however, if total testosterone is high normal and DHEA-S is normal, particularly if irregular menses are present, up to 20% have ↑ levels of free testosterone.
2. Serum DHEA-S level (normal <700 μg/dL) to r/o adrenal source of androgens; *note*: DHEA-S levels normally decrease after age 30, falling to $^1/_4$–$^1/_3$ by age 70.
3. **Cushing's syndrome**; screening tests:
   (a) *Dexamethasone suppression test*: 1 mg dexamethasone po at 11–12 PM, obtain serum plasma cortisol level at 7–8 AM the next morning; normal: <5 μg/dL (140 nmol/L), 5–10 μg/dL is borderline, and >10 μg/dL is abn; false-pos rate: 15%–20% due to obesity, depression, alcoholism.
   (b) *24-h urine free-cortisol*: >275 nmol/d (100 μg/d) is suggestive of Cushing's syndrome; false-pos rate of 5%–10%; false-pos rate for both (a) and (b): <1%–2%; less convenient for pts than (a) but obtain (b) if (a) is equivocal.

Rx: Refer all women w hirsutism and virilization, esp w ↑ levels of testosterone, DHEA-S, or plasma or urinary cortisol to endocrinologist or gynecologist.

ADULT, FEMALE, NO VIRILIZATION

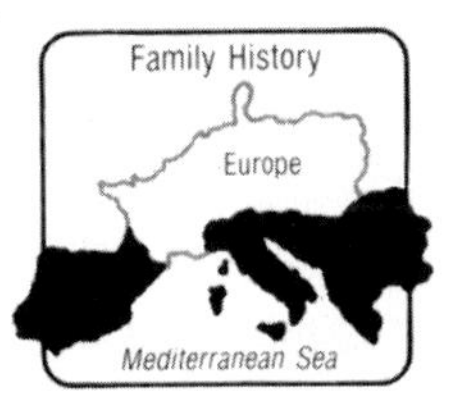

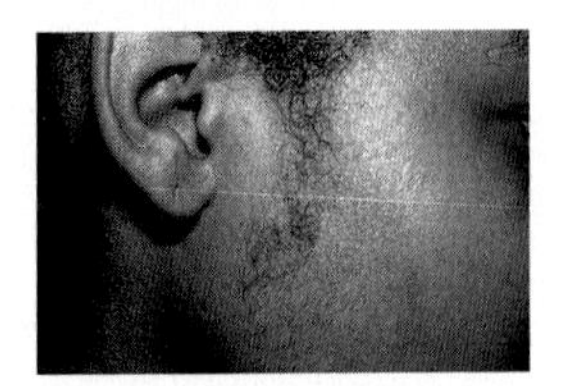

Ethnic hirsutism

13.3. ETHNIC OR RACIAL HIRSUTISM

Epidem: ↑ hair is normal in women from southern parts of Europe; Asians and American Indians have less body hair than do whites; blacks are in the intermediate range.

Si: ↑ sexual hair in male distribution; no menstrual irregularities or virilization.

Crs: Hair appears at puberty and persists w/o much change.

Lab: Not needed if hx is compatible; get lab tests (see 13.2.) if in doubt.

Rx: If mild: remove (pluck, hot wax, and depilatories) or bleach (Jolen, Fairfield, CT); electrolysis to permanently destroy hair follicles but requires repeated rx; removal does not cause hair to grow faster or thicker; laser techniques to remove hair have not been shown to be permanent and are costly (Jaad 1999;40:143); although not a hair removal product, eflornithine cr (Vaniqa 30 gm applied sparingly bid, not for use in pregnancy or breast feeding) reduces or prevents local hair regrowth so that plucking, waxing, or depilatory use may be decreased.

ADULT, FEMALE, NONETHNIC, NO VIRILIZATION

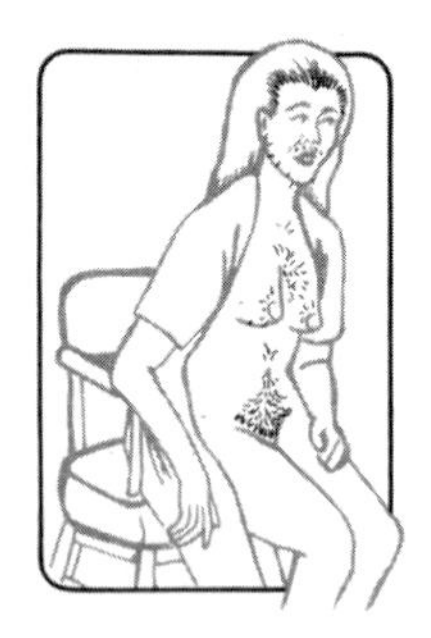

13.4.A. ANDROGENIC HIRSUTISM

Cause: About 2/3 of nonvirilized hirsute women have excess plasma or urinary ovarian and/or adrenal androgens, abn cortisol suppression test results, or alteration in normal diurnal androgen levels; adrenogenital syndrome causes 6%–12%.

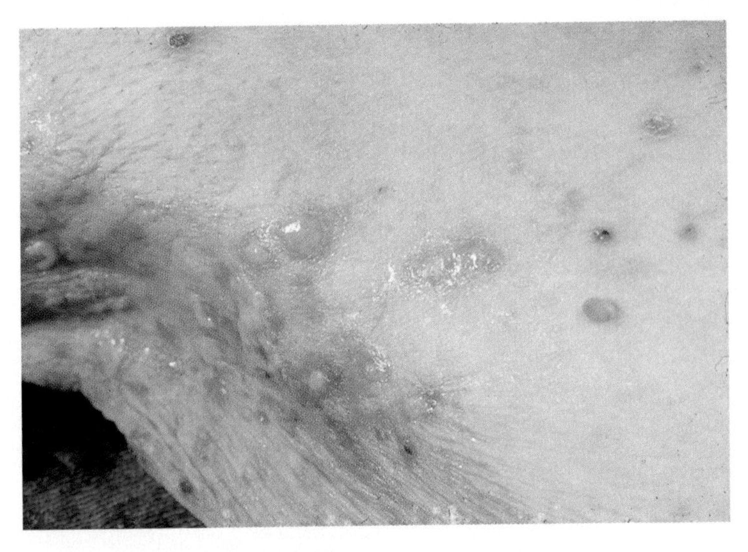

2.4.d.: Bullous pemphigoid

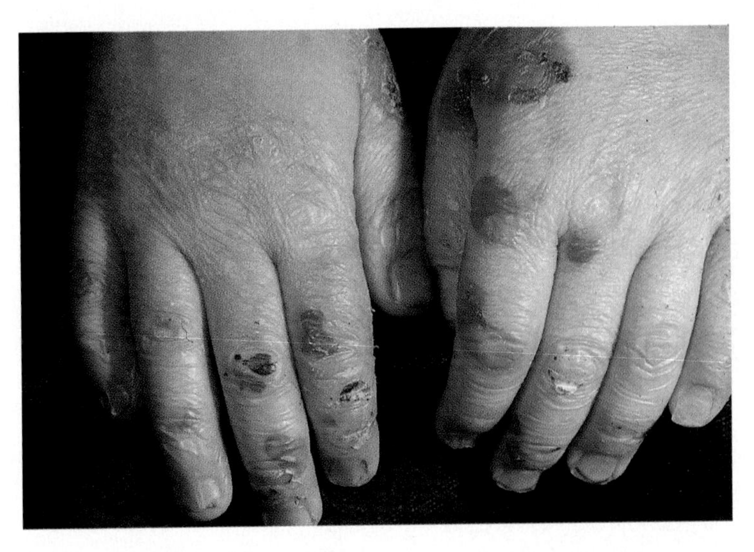

2.6.c.: Epidermolysis bullosa

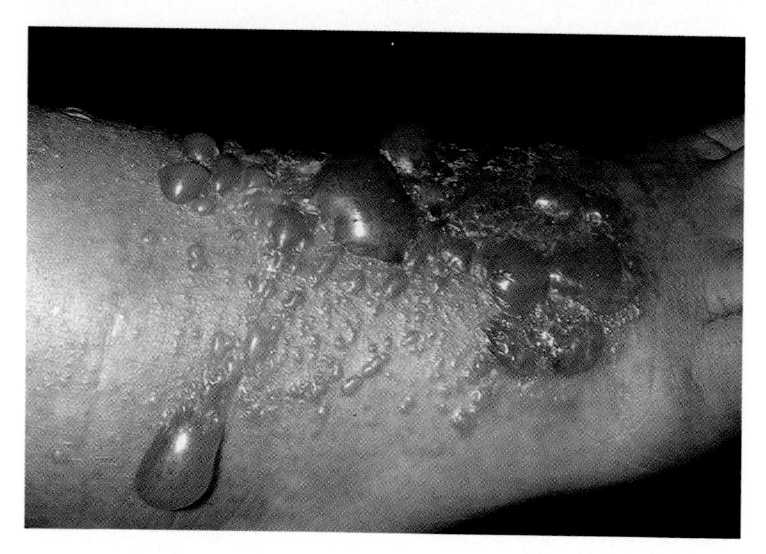

3.1.a.: Poison ivy dermatitis

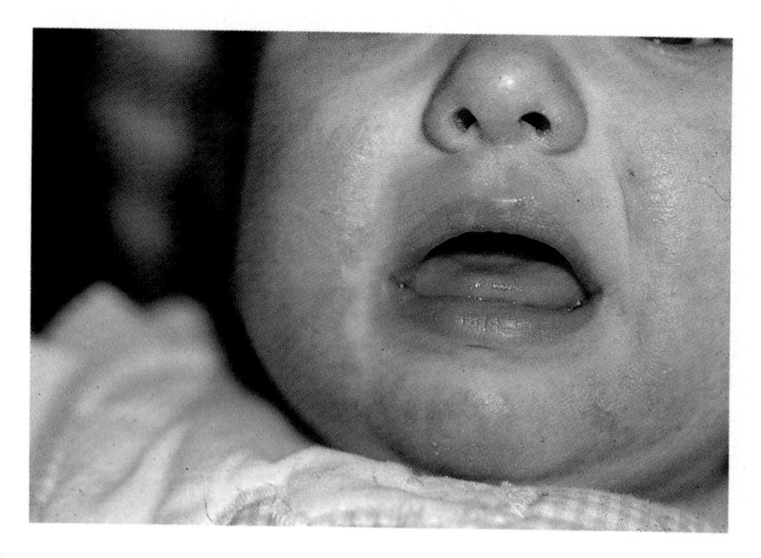

3.1.a.: Irritant dermatitis to acidic food

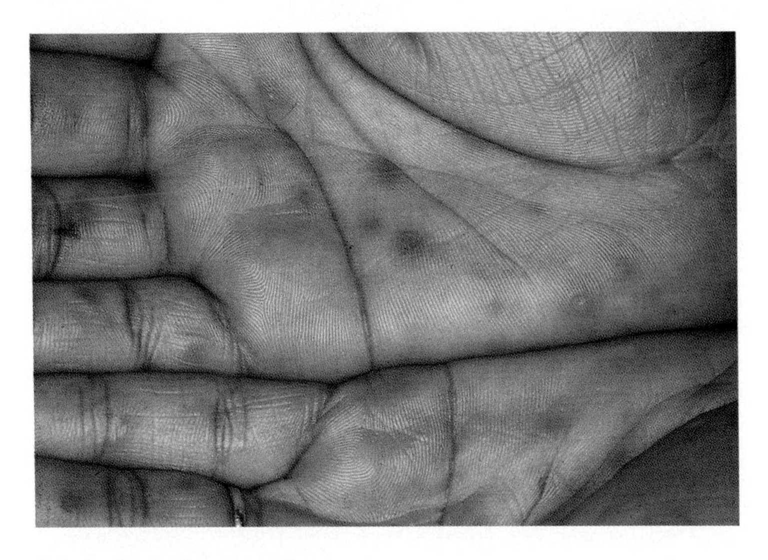

3.1.f.: Syphilis-secondary

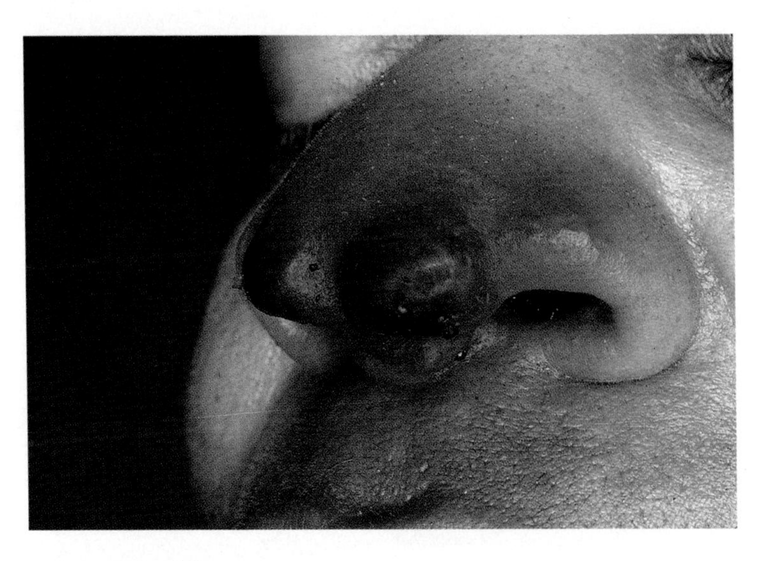

3.3.o.: Sarcoid

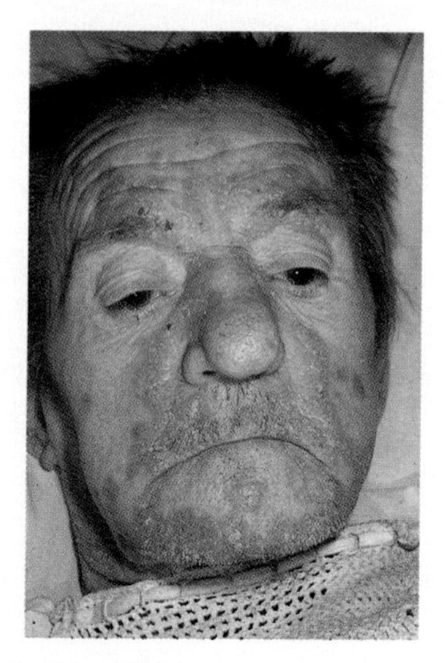

6.2.a.: Seborrheic dermatitis

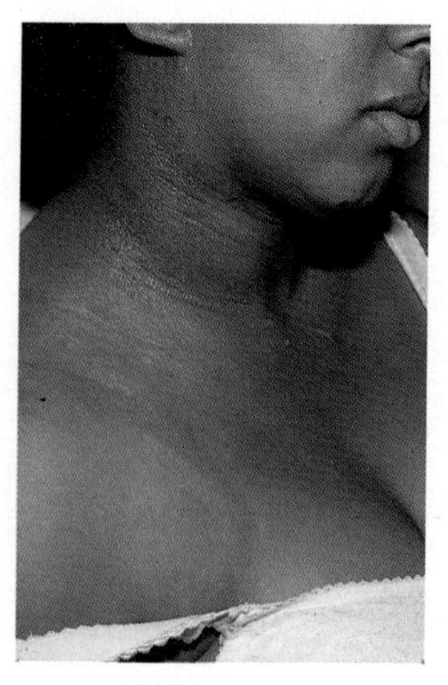

6.6.b.: Contact dermatitis to hair dye (note drip on chest)

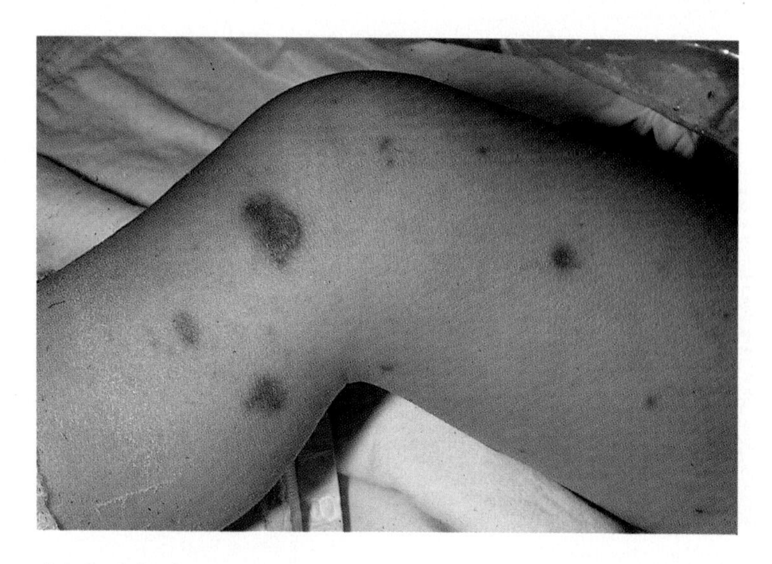

8.1.1.: Meningococcemia

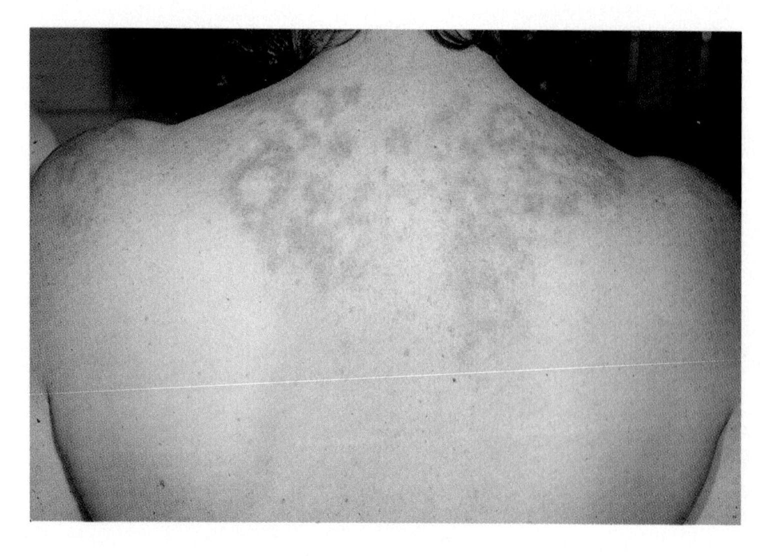

8.3.a.: Lupus erythematosus-systemic

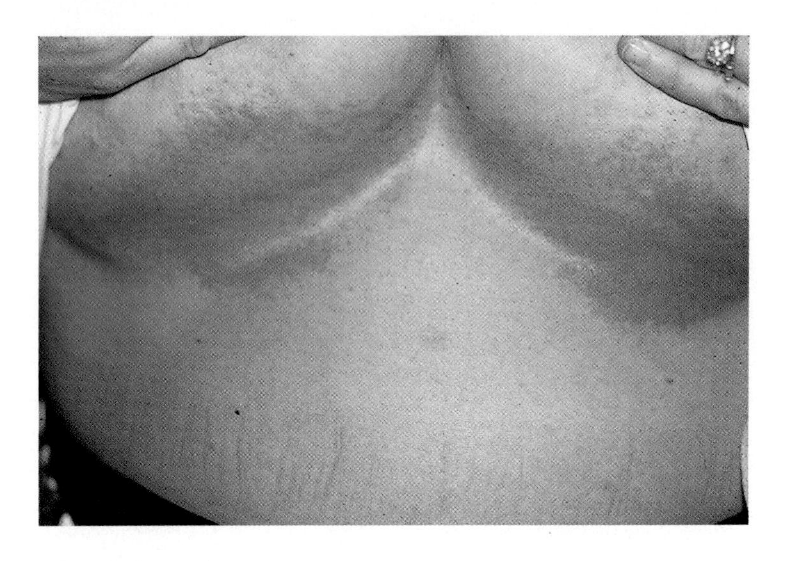

10.4.a.: Intertrigo

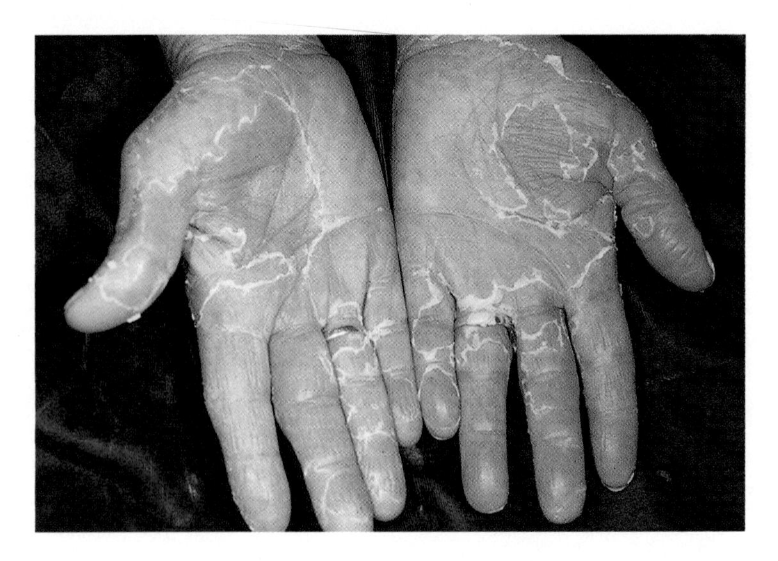

14.6.e.: Post-inflammatory desquamation after drug rxn

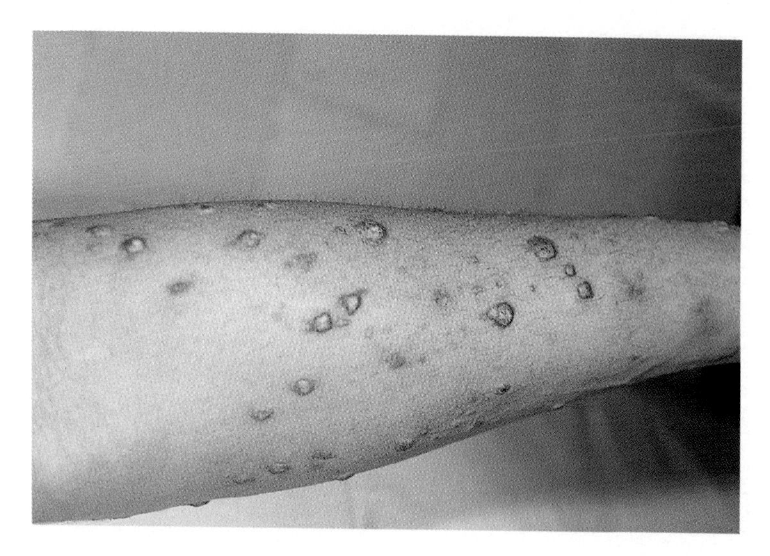

17.1.a.: Prurigo nodularis

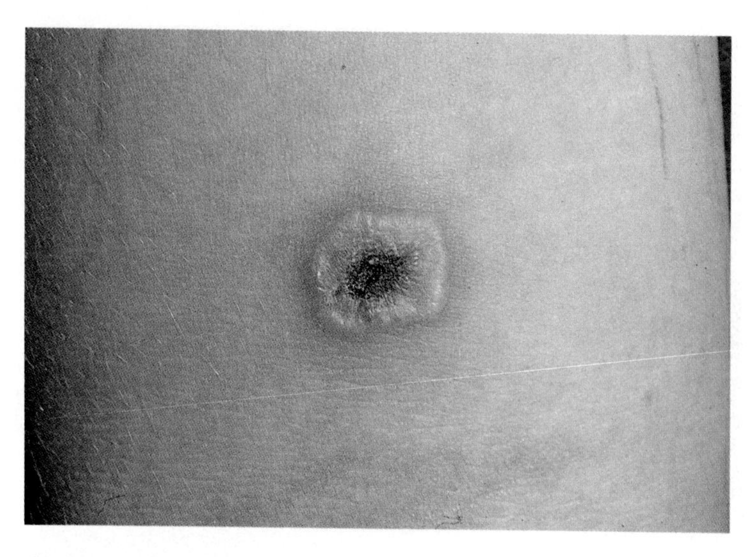

17.2.a.: Spider bite

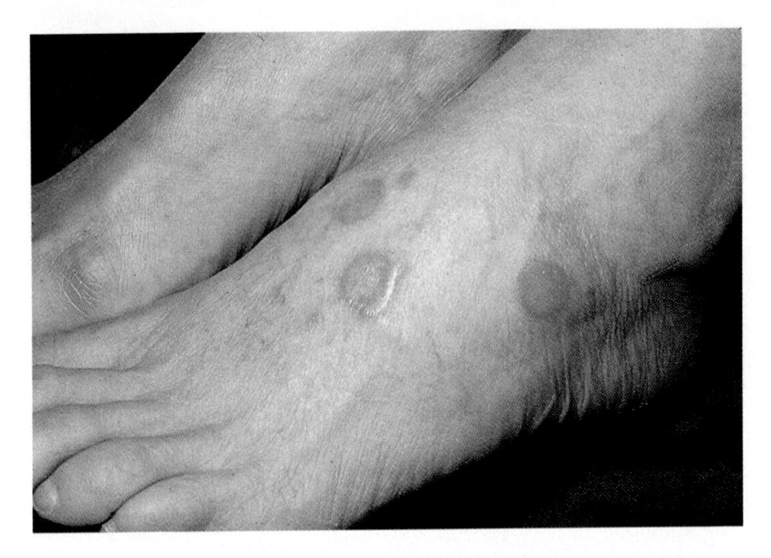

17.2.b.: Granuloma annulare

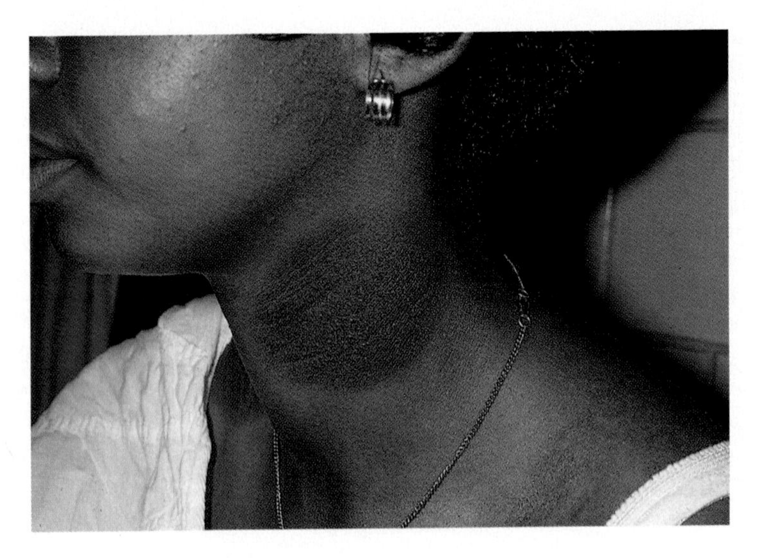

22.4.d.: Fixed drug eruption

Si: Male hair pattern w/o masculinization; menstrual periods often irregular.

Crs: Often occurs during pregnancy and after menopause.

Lab: Screen for *Cushing's syndrome* (see 13.2.); screen for *excess androgens* (see 13.2.); *high*: if total testosterone is >200 ng/dL, or plasma DHEA-S is >700 μg/dL r/o malignant neoplasia and refer to specialists; *moderate*: if total testosterone level 85–200 ng/dL and DHEA-S is <700 μg/dL, cause is usually benign ovarian or adrenal neoplasia or polycystic ovaries; normal DHEA-S makes an adrenal androgen cause unlikely (Nejm 1994;331:968); hirsutism w/o elevated total or free testosterone or DHEA-S is "idiopathic" hirsutism (see 13.4.d.): however, testosterone levels are normal in *congenital adrenal hyperplasia*: deficiency in enzyme in steroid synthesis; 21-hydroxylase deficiency most common; usually manifests as ambiguous genitalia, salt-retaining hypertension; may only become evident w hirsutism in early adulthood; if suspected, refer to endocrinologist (Nejm 1990;323:849).

Rx:

- *High*: refer to endocrinologist or gynecologist to r/o adrenal or ovarian tumors.
- *Moderate or normal*: consider a trial of androgen suppression w either spironolactone (up to 1 mg/lb) or cyclically administered estrogen-progestin combination or both (Jaad 2000;43:498; J Am Acad Derm 1999;41:64), esp if woman is fertile since the antiandrogen effect of spironolactone precludes its use during pregnancy; noticeable response takes mos and hair will return after withdrawal of rx; if no clinical response in 6 mo or repeat testosterone level at 6 mo shows an ↑, refer pt to an endocrinologist or gynecologist.
- Hair removal: if mild: remove (pluck, hot wax, and depilatories) or bleach (Jolen, Fairfield, CT); electrolysis or laser to permanently destroy hair follicles but requires repeated rx; hairs that were initiated during androgen excess do not disappear when androgen is reduced but new growth will be less; although not a hair removal product, eflornithine cr (Vaniqa 30 gm applied sparingly bid, not for use in pregnancy or breast feeding) reduces or prevents local hair regrowth so that plucking, waxing, or depilatory use may be decreased.

13.4.B. DRUG-INDUCED HIRSUTISM

Cause: *Androgen-effect drugs*: anabolic steroids, bcp's, systemic CS, tamoxifen; *non-androgen-effect drugs*: benoxaprofen, cyclosporine, diazoxide, minoxidil, penicillamine, phenytoin, psoralens, streptomycin, zidovudine (↑ eyelashes).

Si: Androgen-like drug causes sexual hair growth and only in women; nonhormonal drugs cause general hair growth in both men and women.

Rx: Eliminate or change med; new excess hair may not disappear and must be removed physically (see 13.3.).

13.4.C. PORPHYRIA CUTANEA TARDA (PCT)

Cause: Liver disease, DM, exogenous estrogens; pts w chronic renal insufficiency on hemodialysis; ↑ assoc w hepatitis C infection and hemochromatosis.

Si: ↑ hair on dorsum of hands and face of either men or women; also blisters, skin fragility, hyperpigmentation, dark wine-colored urine.

For additional details and rx, see LIGHT REACTIONS, 18.1.c.

13.4.D. IDIOPATHIC HIRSUTISM

Cause: Hirsutism and normal hormone levels; most ovulate regularly.

Lab: Neg lab results (see 13.4.a.).

Rx: Spironolactone (up to 1 mg/lb); cyclically administered estrogen-progestin combination; or both (see 13.4.a.); or finasteride (Fertil Steril 1996;66:734).

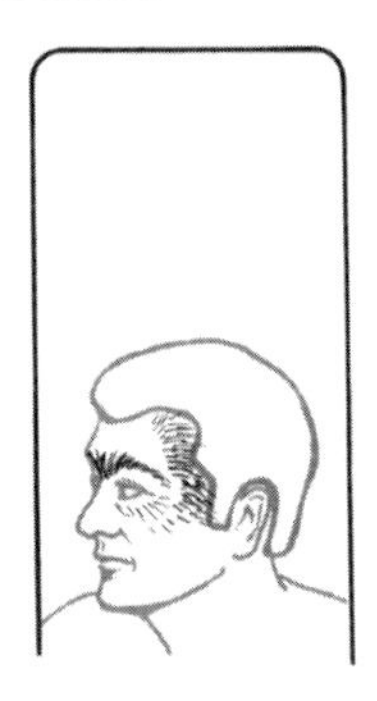

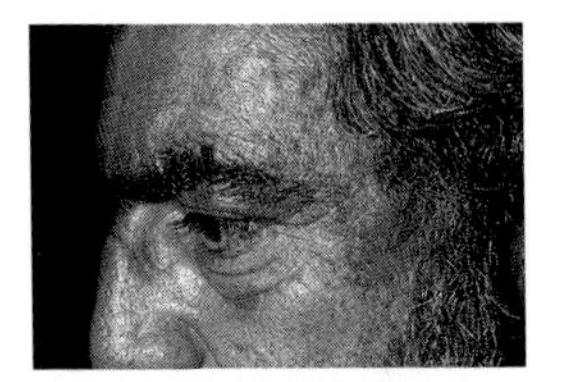

Porphyria cutanea tarda

13.5. HIRSUTISM IN ADULT MALE

Cause: Hair follicles in men already are maximally stimulated by androgens; only certain meds (see 13.4.b.), PCT (see 13.4.c.), and chronic trauma induce new hair growth in adult males.

14 Hands

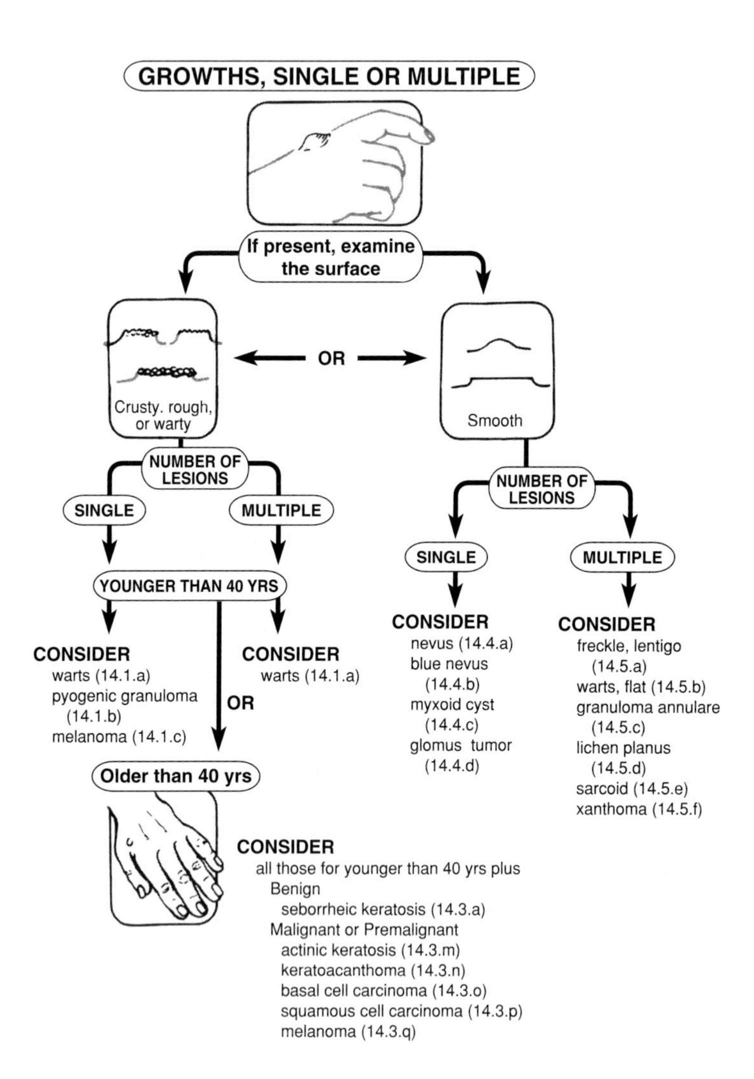

GROWTHS, SINGLE OR MULTIPLE
If present, examine the surface
Crusty. rough, or warty
OR
Smooth
NUMBER OF LESIONS
SINGLE
MULTIPLE
YOUNGER THAN 40 YRS
CONSIDER
warts (14.1.a)
pyogenic granuloma (14.1.b)
melanoma (14.1.c)
CONSIDER
warts (14.1.a)
OR
Older than 40 yrs
CONSIDER
all those for younger than 40 yrs plus
Benign
seborrheic keratosis (14.3.a)
Malignant or Premalignant
actinic keratosis (14.3.m)
keratoacanthoma (14.3.n)
basal cell carcinoma (14.3.o)
squamous cell carcinoma (14.3.p)
melanoma (14.3.q)
NUMBER OF LESIONS
SINGLE
MULTIPLE
CONSIDER
nevus (14.4.a)
blue nevus (14.4.b)
myxoid cyst (14.4.c)
glomus tumor (14.4.d)
CONSIDER
freckle, lentigo (14.5.a)
warts, flat (14.5.b)
granuloma annulare (14.5.c)
lichen planus (14.5.d)
sarcoid (14.5.e)
xanthoma (14.5.f)

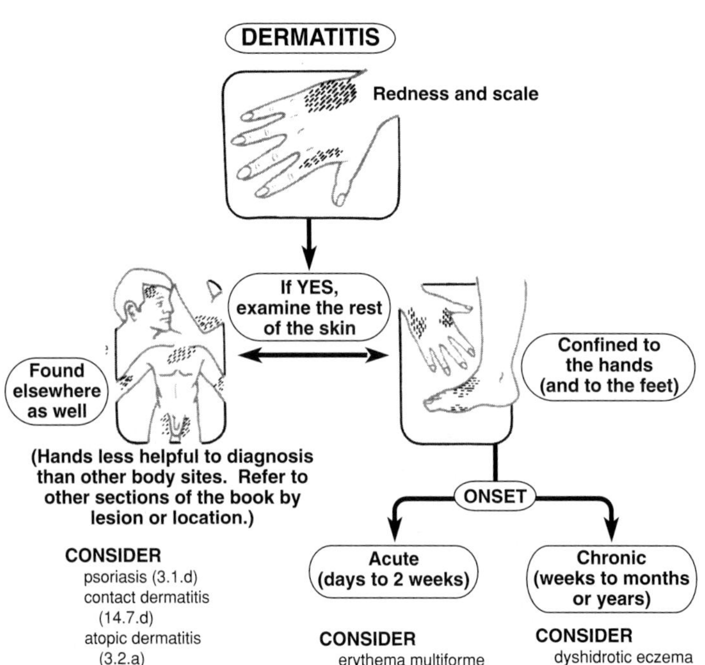

CONSIDER
- psoriasis (3.1.d)
- contact dermatitis (14.7.d)
- atopic dermatitis (3.2.a)
- syphilis, secondary (3.1.f)
- scabies (3.1.e)

Blisters on the palm

CONSIDER
- gonococcemia (8.1.l)
- dyshidrotic eczema (14.7.a)
- fungus infection (14.7.b)
- psoriasis (14.7.c)
- hand-foot-and-mouth disease (8.1.b)

Acute (days to 2 weeks)

CONSIDER
- erythema multiforme (14.6.a)
- vasculitis (14.6.b)
- Rocky Mountain spotted fever (14.6.c)
- syphilis, secondary (14.6.d)
- postinflammatory desquamation (14.6.e)
- paronychia, acute (14.6.f)
- anthrax (14.6.g)

Chronic (weeks to months or years)

CONSIDER
- dyshidrotic eczema (14.7.a)
- fungus infection (14.7.b)
- psoriasis (14.7.c)
- contact dermatitis (14.7.d)
- paronychia, chronic (14.7.e)

GROWTH, CRUSTY/ROUGH/WARTY, <40 YEARS OLD

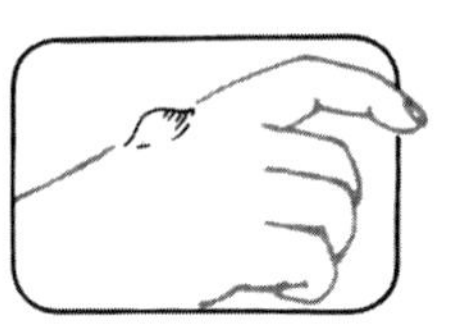

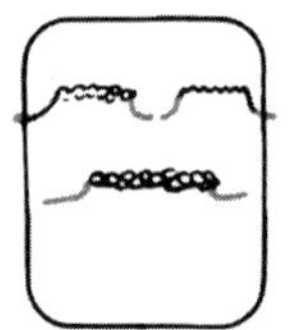

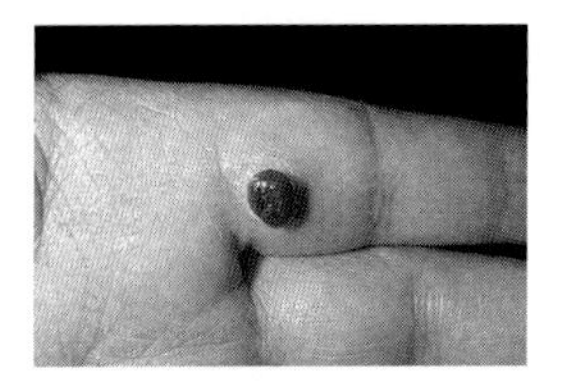

Pyogenic granuloma

14.1.A. VERRUCA VULGARIS (COMMON WARTS)

Cause: Papillomaviruses of several subtypes.

Epidem: Children > adults.

Sx: Painless unless traumatized.

Si: Raised, rough-surfaced, cauliflower-like growths; pinhead to marble sized.

Crs: Incubation: up to several mo; spread to other sites and to other persons; half involute spontaneously within 1 yr; resistant or extensive warts may be assoc w underlying immunodeficiency, lymphoma, DM, or systemic CS.

Ddx: Pare thick horny material that covers lesion: *wart*: cut surface has dark, speckled, or bleeding points; *corn*: cut surface is shiny and smooth.

Rx: If warts are not causing sx or rapidly spreading, observe for spontaneous resolution over mos; if rx is necessary (Review of Rx: Brit J Derm 2001;144:4):

- *Home rx*: salicylic acid–lactic acid combinations (Duofilm, Viranol, OTC, $): pt soaks wart in warm water for 5 min before bedtime; pt or parent pares hard surface material w single-edged razor blade or file; applies med just to wart; lets dry; leaves open or, if not responding in a few wk, covers w an occlusive tape and removes tape in morning; skips rx for day or so w excessive irritation; re-examine pt monthly.

- *Office rx*: LN2: painful during and after rx; therefore, difficult to do in small children; fast and convenient in older children and adults (see RX.18.); extensive or unresponsive warts may be treated by D&C (see RX.17.); other techniques available, generally performed by a dermatologist, include cantheridin, IL bleomycin ($$$), topical 5-FU (see RX.19), sensitization to antigens, such as squaric acid (Jaad 2000;42:803); imiquimod cr (Aldara, $$$); po cimetidine found not effective in controlled trials (J Am Acad Derm 1999;41:123).

14.1.B. PYOGENIC GRANULOMA

Summary: Single, bright red, raspberry-like growth; pea or bean sized; often friable and bleeds easily when traumatized; most are on exposed parts, esp face, arms, legs, hands, fingers; any age group.

For additional details and rx, see GROWTHS, 11.5.a.

14.1.C. MELANOMA

Summary: Black or brown, occasionally normal skin color; irregular in outline, may be itchy, bleed, or ulcerate; may have black, white, blue speckles; most common on back; also common on shins of women; whites >> blacks.

For additional details and rx, see GROWTHS, 11.4.b.

GROWTH, CRUSTY/ROUGH/WARTY, SINGLE OR MULTIPLE, >40 YEARS OLD

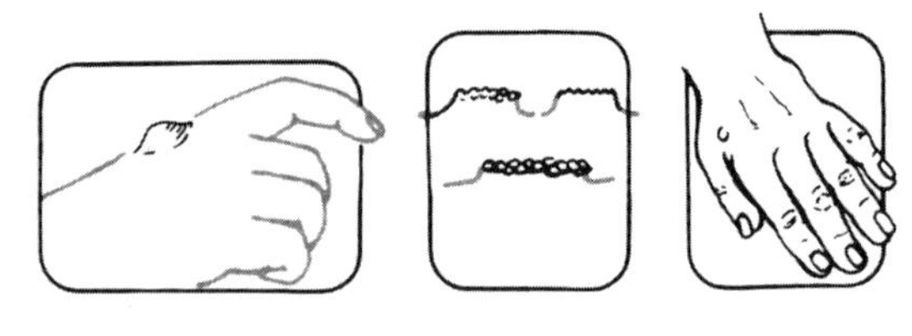

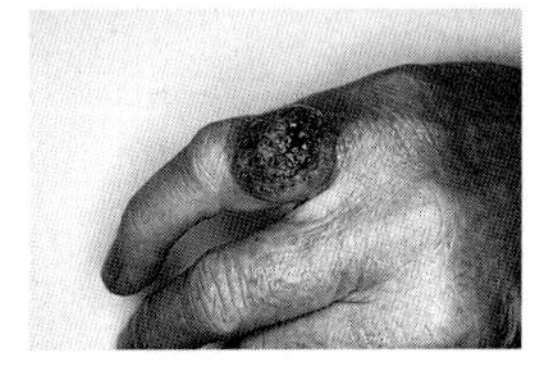

Keratoacanthoma

- The ddx is same as those <40 yo and, in addition, includes:

14.3.A. SEBORRHEIC KERATOSIS

Summary: Common benign growths, tan to dark brown, slightly roughened, waxy, crumbly; feels "stuck on" surface; usually fhx of similar lesions; most >40 yo.

For additional details and rx, see GROWTHS, 11.10.b.

14.3.M. ACTINIC KERATOSIS

Summary: Discrete; persistent; scaly, pink to red; esp in light-complexioned persons >40 yo; hx of excessive sun exposure; considered premalignant but few become SCC.

For additional details and rx, see GROWTHS, 11.11.a.

14.3.N. KERATOACANTHOMA

Summary: Single; pea to bean sized; umbilicated, hard, keratotic central plug; usually on sun-exposed areas; may appear and grow quickly over wks or mos; some, esp on face, can be quite aggressive; SCC resembles keratoacanthomas and is distinguished by bx.

For additional details and rx, see GROWTHS, 11.6.b.

14.3.O. BASAL CELL CARCINOMA (BCC)

Summary: Single or few; shiny or pearly colored; telangiectasias over surface; depressed center; slowly spreading; usually on light-exposed areas, esp face, neck, forearms; about 80% of skin cancers.

For additional details and rx, see GROWTHS, 11.6.c.

14.3.P. SQUAMOUS CELL CARCINOMA (SCC)

Summary: Usually single; painless; scaly, keratotic, bleeding, friable surface; most are on light-exposed areas, but appear on covered areas as well, sometimes adjacent to areas of trauma, ie, chronic leg ulcers, burn scars, or sites of radiation rx; lower lip is frequent location because of chronic sun exposure, as well as chronic tar and heat exposure in smokers.

For additional details and rx, see GROWTHS, 11.6.d.

14.3.Q. MELANOMA

Summary: Black or brown, occasionally normal skin color; irregular in outline, may be itchy, bleed, or ulcerate; may have black, white, blue speckles; most common on back; also common on shins of women; whites >> blacks.

For additional details and rx, see GROWTHS, 11.4.b.

GROWTH, SMOOTH, SINGLE

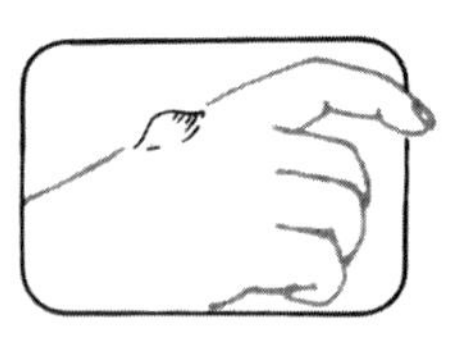

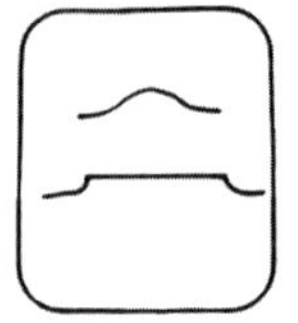

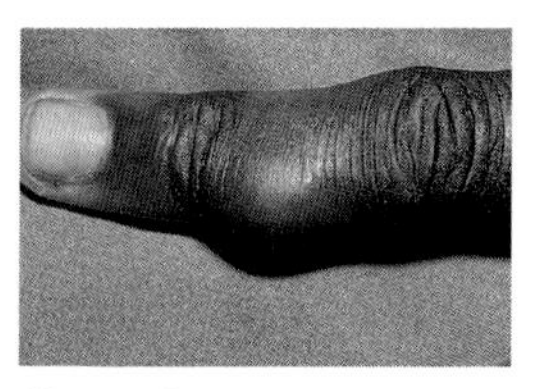

Giant cell tumor

14.4.A. NEVUS, MELANOCYTIC (MOLE—JUNCTIONAL, COMPOUND, AND INTRADERMAL)

Summary: Round; tan to dark brown; sharply outlined, present since young adulthood; average white adult has 20; prophylactic removal of all nevi is neither possible nor necessary; excise or bx a nevus that has changed, has bled, or is irregular or black.

For additional details and rx, see GROWTHS, 11.1.a.

14.4.B. BLUE NEVUS

Summary: Slightly raised; about size of split pea; mostly on extensor side of hand or forearm, or leg; blue-black; ddx: melanoma; normal skin markings are preserved while they are lost over melanoma; blue nevi persist but are not premalignant.

For additional details, see GROWTHS, 11.1.b.

14.4.C. MUCOID (MYXOID) CYST

Cause: Benign; mucin forming; extension of joint space, similar to ganglion.

Sx: Painless.

Si: Pea-sized swelling; skin colored to glistening in color; usually on dorsum of finger near tip or about nail; painless; if cyst impinges on nail plate, a depression or crease in nail may develop (Arch Derm 1996;132:225).

Crs: Persistent; prone to rupture but re-forms.

Ddx: *Epidermal inclusion cyst*: covered by normal-appearing skin; painless, unless ruptured; more likely on dorsum of hand rather than near fingertip; *benign tumor of tendon sheath*: on 1 finger; more proximal, deeper than mucoid cyst.

Rx: Repeated drainage may be sufficient; IL triamcinolone acetonide (10 mg/mL diluted to 5 mg/mL) (see RX.7); cryosurgery w LN2 (see RX.18) after drainage; excision; consider referral to dermatologist or surgeon.

14.4.D. GLOMUS TUMOR

Cause: Derived from smooth muscle cells; highly innervated.

Sx: Typically severe radiating pain; triggered by pressure or heat, or spontaneous.

Si: Solitary tumor; usual location is periungual skin, fingertip fat pad, nail bed; pinhead to a BB in size; blue to pink if visible (J Am Acad Derm 1997;37:887).

Crs: Usually clears spontaneously in wks.

Lab: None needed; multiple and visceral glomus tumors are rare; bone defect underlying a large glomus tumor may be visible by x-ray.

Rx: Reassure pt; protect finger from triggering trauma; persistent or extensive cases may require local excision.

HANDS

GROWTH, SMOOTH, MULTIPLE

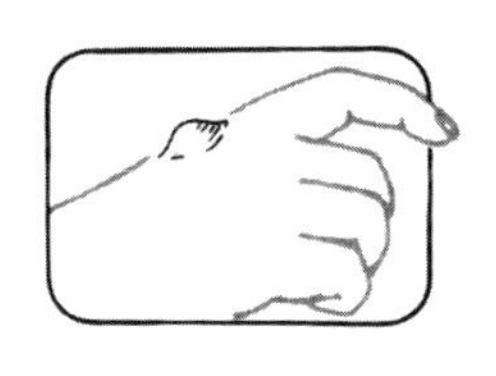

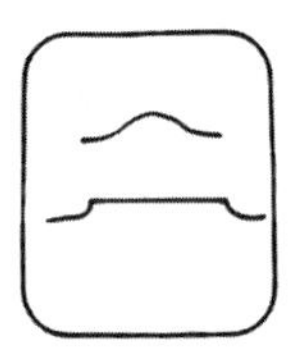

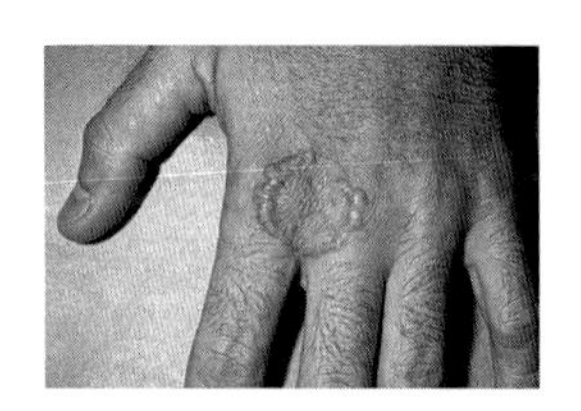

Granuloma annulare

14.5.A. FRECKLE/LENTIGO

Summary: *Freckle*: common; 1–3 mm; multiple; brown; flat; genetically determined on face; presence on trunk and arms indicates past intense sun exposure; not premalignant; rx not necessary or practical; *lentigo*: smaller and darker than freckle; fewer in number; not confined to sun-exposed areas; bx occasionally warranted to r/o melanoma.

For additional details and rx, see GROWTHS, 11.7.a.

14.5.B. WART, FLAT

Summary: Look like droplets of dried, skin-colored, rubber cement; multiple, smooth, round, slightly raised; common on face, neck, legs; asx.

For additional details and rx, see LEG RASH, 17.6.b.

14.5.C. GRANULOMA ANNULARE

Summary: Ring or plaque of pink BB-sized papules; not scaly; extensor surfaces, esp dorsum of hands, elbows, knees, ankles; usually itchy.

For additional details and rx, see LEG RASH, 17.2.b.

14.5.D. LICHEN PLANUS

Summary: Multiple pink to purple, flat-topped, itchy papules, often tightly grouped into plaques; look on wrists, lower legs, ankles, and for a lacy white patch on buccal mucosa.

For additional details and rx, see BODY, 3.3.n.

14.5.E. SARCOID

Summary: Mimics other eruptions; most are pink to yellow; firm papules or plaques; pinhead to pea sized or larger; usually nape, face, extensor surfaces; minimal itching; may develop within preexisting scars; sometimes severe and may distort facial features; may be deep; may ulcerate; may lead to local hair loss; blacks >> whites.

For additional details and rx, see BODY, 3.3.o.

14.5.F. XANTHOMA

Summary: Numerous variations; plasma lipid and lipoprotein abn are not specific to clinical appearance; however, certain clinical patterns exist: cutaneous xanthomas are yellow elevated lesions, except for deep tendon or tuberous xanthomas where skin is normal in color; xanthomas on palms: (a) rare type III hyperlipidemia, (b) pts w obstructive liver disease, (c) pts w paraproteinemia.

For additional details, see BODY, 3.3.p.

DERMATITIS, CONFINED TO HANDS (MAY INCLUDE FEET), ACUTE (DAYS TO 2 WEEKS)

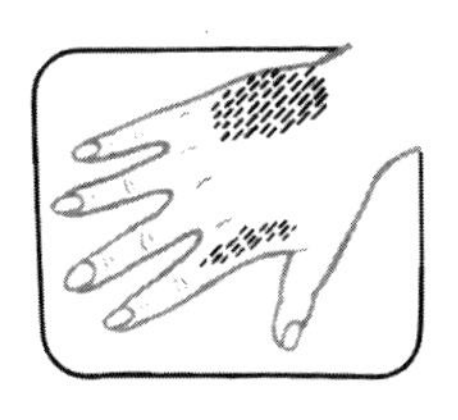

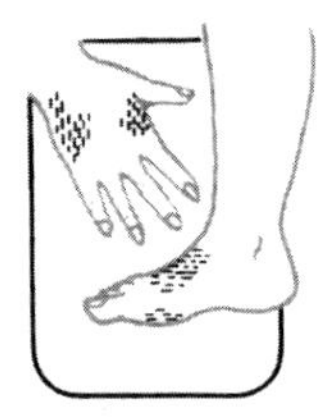

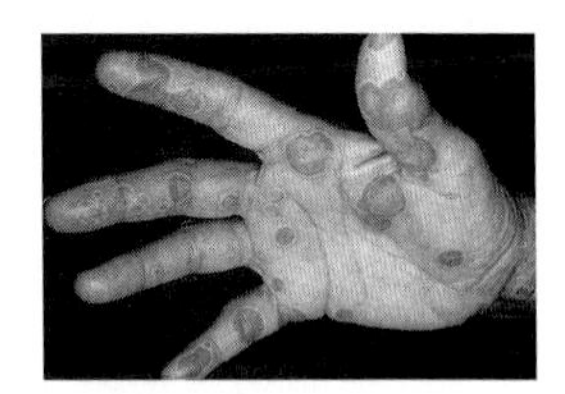

Erythema multiforme

14.6.A. ERYTHEMA MULTIFORME

Summary: Abrupt onset w flat, dusky lesions resembling dime- to quarter-sized hives; central part often is darker or blistering, like a bull's-eye or target; pain > itch; usually extensor surfaces; palmar and plantar lesions are tender; individual lesions persist longer than hives; severe cases may be hemorrhagic, peeling, or blistering; mucous membrane erosions are common and often disabling.

For additional details and rx, see BLISTERS, 2.1.b.

14.6.B. VASCULITIS

Summary: Palmar lesions are painful, palpable, purpuric; look for similar lesions elsewhere; ROS and w/u for fever, arthralgias, abdominal pain, or blood in urine or stool.

For additional details, see FEVER, 8.1.n.

14.6.C. ROCKY MOUNTAIN SPOTTED FEVER (RMSF)

Summary: Pt w fever and headache who develops a rash on hands and feet, often including palms and soles; eruption initially is light pink, but later becomes deeper red, even purpuric; may be accompanied by edema; spreads centrally.

For additional details and rx, see FEVER, 8.1.m.

14.6.D. SYPHILIS, SECONDARY

Summary: Many patterns; most common: widespread, slightly scaly, tan, copper-colored, nonitchy patches, lesions on palms and/or soles; recent or healing genital ulcer; moist, wartlike genital growths (condylomata lata); painless oral erosions and mucous patches; "moth-eaten" scalp hair loss; mild or absent constitutional si and sx; LN↑, esp epitrochlear nodes; no blisters except in newborn; 2° lesions appear few wk after 1° rash disappears.

For additional details, see BODY, 3.1.f.

14.6.E. POSTINFLAMMATORY DESQUAMATION

Summary: Peeling hands; sometimes peeling feet as well; no oozing, itch, inflammation suggestive of dermatitis; starts about 2 wk after any acute febrile illness; esp common and dramatic after streptococcal infection; typical for Kawasaki disease (see FEVER, 8.1.o.); no rx other than moisturizer.

See color plate section.

14.6.F. PARONYCHIA, ACUTE

Summary: Acute pain and swelling; single fingertip; pts may be febrile; may have tender LN↑; usually bacterial or herpetic infection.

For additional details and rx, see NAILS, 20.4.a.

14.6.G. ANTHRAX, CUTANEOUS

Nejm 1999;341:815; Jama 1999;281:1735

Cause: *Bacillus anthracis*, a few cases each yr normally occur from infected animal products, including hides, wool, and bones; now a terrorist weapon. Anthrax is not contagious from person-to-person.

Sx/Si: After 1–12 d incubation, a "malignant pustule"; painless but itchy papule (spider bites are painful) on an exposed area, i.e. hands, arms, head, or neck; lesion enlarges, develops blister, edema, and necrotic blackened center; pustules are not present and LN↑ is minimal.

Lab: Dx is established by culture of vesicle fluid, fluid under the eschar, punch bx from edge of central eschar or serum stored at –70°C for later analysis; contact local health department for additional instructions.

Rx: Ciprofloxacin 500 mg bid or doxycycline 100 mg bid or penicillin V 30 mg/kg in 4 equal portions q 6 hr until sensitivities are available; avoid doxycycline if under age 12 yr.

DERMATITIS, CONFINED TO HANDS (MAY INCLUDE FEET), CHRONIC (WEEKS TO MONTHS OR YEARS)

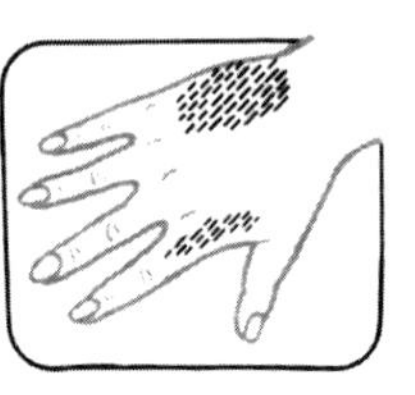

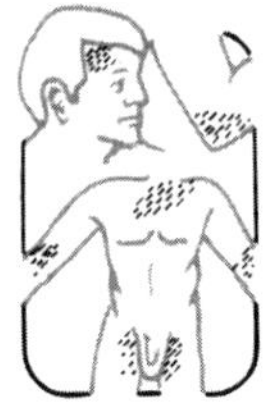

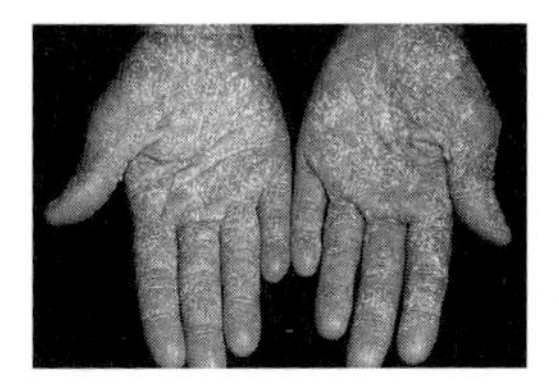

Psoriasis

14.7.A. DYSHIDROTIC ECZEMA (POMPHOLYX)

Summary: Intensely itchy; episodic; triggered by irritants; palms, sides of fingers may be studded w minute, sand grain–sized, deep blisters; acute inflammatory phase lasting 1–3 wk; followed by dry, cracking phase; assoc w hyperhidrosis.

For additional details and rx, see FEET, 7.1.b.

14.7.B. FUNGUS INFECTION (TINEA MANUS)

Summary: Usually chronic; asx; scaling on palmar surface; typically only 1 hand but both feet are involved "one hand–two foot" syndrome; fingernails and toenails frequently involved (see NAILS, 20.3.a.); KOH test result (see DX.3.) is pos; antifungal agents, either topical (see RX.10.) or systemic (see RX.11.), may be used.

14.7.C. PSORIASIS

Summary: Either scaly patches as part of widespread psoriasis or 1 or 2 pustular patches on palms; often involves soles as well; most pts w pustular form do not have psoriasis elsewhere; rx: try TCS (class I) oint, topical calcipotriene, or tazarotene (see BODY, 3.1.d.); PUVA often effective; refer recalcitrant cases to dermatologist.

For additional details on psoriasis, see BODY, 3.1.d.

14.7.D. CONTACT DERMATITIS

Cause: Restricted to hands: consider formalin (paper towels), latex (gloves), detergents, oil (auto repair, machine trades), perfume (hand cr), *Rhus* (plants), finger or wrists (nickel or chrome); occupational hand dermatitis: beauticians, dentists, florists, printers, bartenders, new mothers; consider photo-rxn, usually from meds.

Sx: Itch.

Si: Worse on back of hands than palmar surface; diffuse, pink to red; blistering to thickened and scaly; may be edematous depending on severity and duration.

Crs: Chronic until cause is identified and eliminated; latex allergy, esp from powdered gloves, has become a major source of disability in medical professions (J Am Acad Derm 1998;39:1; J Am Acad Derm 1998;39:98; J Am Acad Derm 1998;38:36).

Lab: Patch testing (see DX.6.) by dermatologist may be necessary, but hx and elimination of suspected antigens usually are sufficient.

Rx: Reduce excessive exposure to soap and water hand washing; protective gloves; antigen avoidance if recognized; TCS (class I–III); protective applied before exposure (Clear Hands, OTC, EnviroDerm, 800.991.3376; Kerodex 51 for dry or oily work and Kerodex for wet work, OTC, Medtech, 800.443.4908).

14.7.E. PARONYCHIA, CHRONIC

Summary: Boggy, red, crusty; around 1 or several fingernails; women >> men; present for many wks to mos; nail plate is distorted and ridged; purulent material sometimes can be expressed.

For additional details and rx, see NAILS, 20.5.a.

15 HIV

MUCOCUTANEOUS SIGNS SUGGESTIVE OF HIV INFECTION

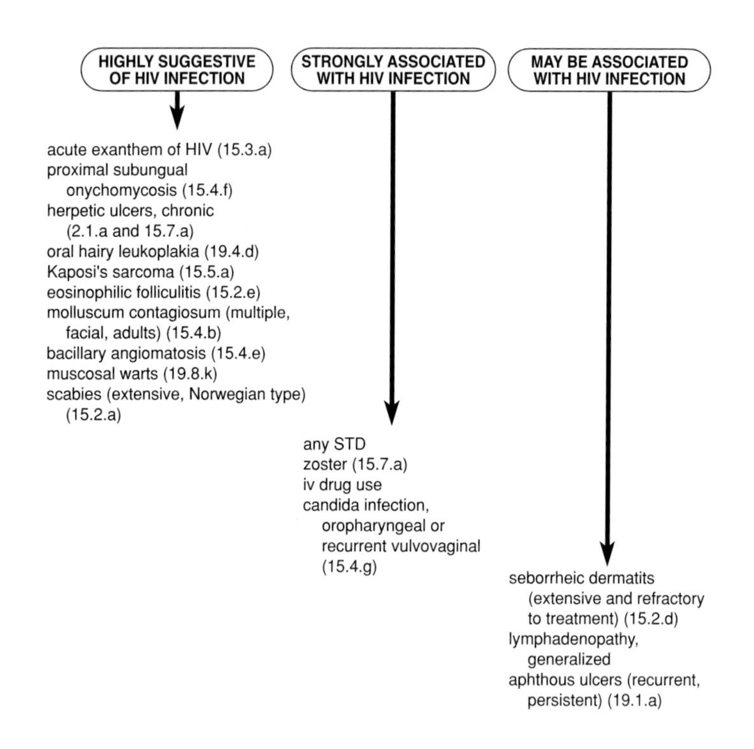

SKIN DISORDERS IN PERSONS WITH HIV

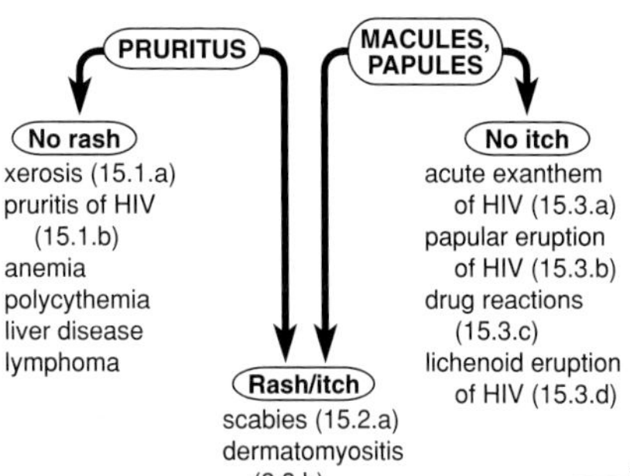

PRURITUS

No rash
- xerosis (15.1.a)
- pruritis of HIV (15.1.b)
- anemia
- polycythemia
- liver disease
- lymphoma

Rash/itch (PRURITUS; MACULES, PAPULES)
- scabies (15.2.a)
- dermatomyositis (8.3.b)
- atopic dermatitis (3.2.a)
- seborrheic dermatitis (15.2.d)
- folliculitis (15.2.e)
- ichthyosis (15.2.f)

MACULES, PAPULES

No itch
- acute exanthem of HIV (15.3.a)
- papular eruption of HIV (15.3.b)
- drug reactions (15.3.c)
- lichenoid eruption of HIV (15.3.d)

PAPULES, PLAQUES, NODULES

Infectious
- scabies (15.2.a)
- bacterial infections (15.4.a)
- folliculitis (15.2.e)
- molluscum contagiosum (15.4.b)
- verruca vulgaris (15.4.c)
- secondary syphilis (15.4.d)
- bacillary angiomatosis (15.4.e)
- fungal infection, superficial (15.4.f)
- candida infection (15.4.g)
- fungal infection, deep (15.4.h)
  - blastomycosis
  - coccidioidomycosis
  - cryptococcosis
  - sporotrichosis
- mycobacterial infection (15.4.i)
- pneumocystosis (15.4.j)

Neoplastic
- Kaposi's sarcoma (15.5.a)
- skin cancer (15.5.b)
- lymphoma (15.5.c)

Inflamed
- psoriasis (15.6.a)
- atopic dermatitis (3.2.a)
- nummular dermatitis (3.3.c)

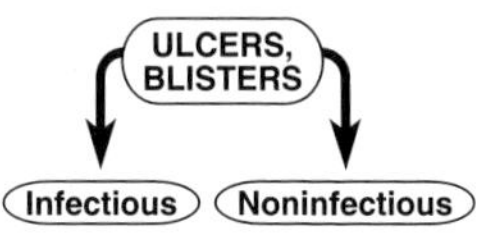

ULCERS, BLISTERS

Infectious
- viral (15.7.a)
  - CMV
  - HSV
  - HZ
- bacterial
  - syphilis
  - impetigo
- fungal
  - coccidioidomycosis
  - sporotrichosis
  - mycobacterial

Noninfectious
- Skin cancer
- porphyria cutanea tarda (15.8.a)
- erythema multiforme
- Stevens-Johnson syndrome

ORAL LESIONS
- HSV (2.1.a)
- warts (6.9.h)
- candida infection (19.1.f)
- oral hairy leukoplakia (19.4.d)
- Kaposi's sarcoma (19.2.g)
- oral cancer (19.2.h)

Written in collaboration with Jihad M. Alhariri, MD, Instructor, Dermatology, The Johns Hopkins Medical Institutions, Baltimore, Maryland.

Jaad 2000;43:409; Med Clin N Am 1998;82:1033. Arch Derm 1998;134:1208. J Am Acad Derm 1997;37:450. Br J Derm 1997;137:595. Ann IM 1996;125:485. Arch IM 1991;151:1295.

National CDC AIDS Hotline: 800.342.AIDS (2437); Spanish CDC AIDS Hotline: 800.344.7432; AIDS "Warm" Line (American Academy of Family Physicians): 800.933.3413; American Foundation for AIDS Research (newsletter and rx directory): 212.806.1600.

Internet sites: www.cdc.gov; www.actis.org; www.aidsnyc.org/network/; www.ama-assn.org/special/hiv/; hiv.medscape.com; hivinsite.ucsf.edu/.

In the course of HIV infection, 90% have HIV-assoc skin disease (Arch Derm 1991;127:714).

15.1.A. XEROSIS

Summary: Similar to xerosis ("dry" skin) in healthy, older pts (see ITCH, 16.1.a.); scratch marks; rx: emollients (see Bathing Instructions for Dry Skin, RX.3.).

HIV pointers: Common; r/o scabies.

15.1.B. PRURITUS OF HIV

Summary: Cause: unknown; may be severe w scratch marks; rx: UVB if emollients are not effective; may progress to *prurigo nodularis*: chronic nodular/papular form; multiple lesions; unremitting itch; resistant to rx.

HIV pointers: 20%–30% of pts w HIV infection develop severe itching.

15.2.A. SCABIES

Summary: Excoriated, red papules, some w a thin "burrow"; numerous scratch marks, lichenified patches; genital lesions include pea-sized lumps on penis and scrotum or vulva; look for excoriated lesions or scratch marks at finger webs, elbows, areolae, umbilicus, lower abdomen, wrists, antecubital fossae, and gluteal cleft; itching worse at night; conjugal partner is involved; for additional details and rx, see BODY, 3.1.e.

HIV pointers: 20% of HIV-pos pts; severe forms may develop: *Norwegian (crusted) scabies*, and palmoplantar hyperkeratosis resembling psoriasis; ivermectin (200 μg/kg, single dose, Rx, $$$) is effective (Nejm 1995;333:26).

15.2.D. SEBORRHEIC DERMATITIS

Summary: Usually diffuse but may be patchy; yellowish greasy scale; mild redness and itching; similar scale and itching often present in ear canals, retroauricular areas, eyebrows, nasolabial folds; for additional details and rx, see FACE, 6.2.a., and SCALP, 24.3.b.

HIV pointers: Most common skin condition (50%–85% incidence) assoc w HIV infection; difficult to control in HIV-pos pts; worsens w ↓ CD4 count.

15.2.E. FOLLICULITIS

Summary: Minute pustules centered at hair follicles; *bacterial*: *Staphylococcus aureus*; consider gram-neg folliculitis in pts on broad-spectrum antibiotics (see FACE, 6.1.d.); *fungal*: *Pityrosporum ovale*; *parasitic*: *Demodex folliculorum*; *perforating*: keratotic follicular papules extruding dermal components (J Am Acad Derm 1999;40:300); rx: direct at specific infectious agent, if known.

- **Eosinophilic pustular folliculitis**: itchy esp at night; pink; follicular papules and pustules are excoriated; few to hundreds; mostly upper body (above nipple line) and face; blacks = whites; rare except w HIV-pos pts; CD4 count usually 50–250/μL; bx

HIV

confirmatory but not usually necessary; r/o scabies; rx: UVB may help (Nejm 1988;318:1183); itraconazole 200 mg bid × 1–2 mo may help; isotretinoin 40 mg/d may help (review: Arch Derm 1992;127:206).

HIV pointers: More generalized if CD4 count <100/μL.

15.2.F. ICHTHYOSIS

Summary: Thick dirty scaling; worse on legs; may become generalized (J Am Acad Derm 1990;22:1270); rx: topical lactic acid (for details, see ITCH, 16.2.d.).

HIV pointers: If generalized, CD4 count usually <100/μL; may be assoc w concomitant HIV and HTLV II infection, esp in iv drug users (J Am Acad Derm 1993;29:701).

15.3.A. ACUTE EXANTHEM OF HIV (ACUTE SEROCONVERSION SYNDROME)

Summary: Pink red; roseola-like rash (40%–80%); morbilliform (Am Fam Phys 1999;60:535; J Am Acad Derm 1990;23:483); trunk and upper arms; 2–4 wk after infection; assoc w flulike syndrome, often severe w fever (80%–90%), fatigue (70%–90%), headache (30%–70%), LN↑ (40%–70%), ↓ wbc (40%), ↓ platelets (45%); antibodies may be evident; HIV-1 RNA level (viral load) by PCR becomes pos within 11 d of infection (Transf 1995;35:91); bx: not specific.

HIV pointers: Highly infectious during acute exanthem w high viral load > 50,000 copies/mL (Nejm 1998;339:33).

15.3.B. PRURITIC PAPULAR ERUPTION OF HIV

Summary: Cause: unknown; asx or mildly pruritic; rapid onset; skin-colored to erythematous papules; trunk, extremities (J Am Acad Derm 1991;24:231); rx: sx; responded to po pentoxifylline

(Trental) 400 mg tid in uncontrolled study (J Am Acad Derm 1998;38:955).

HIV pointers: Common; may be first sign of HIV infection; starts within wks to mos of HIV infection.

15.3.C. DRUG REACTIONS

Summary: Most common: trimethoprim-sulfamethoxazole (10%–40%), clindamycin (20%–30%), amoxicillin (20%–60%), tbc drugs (10%); widely distributed erythema; often edematous macules and patches; itching may be severe; drugs assoc w pruritus w/o rash: antimalarials, amphetamines, chlorpromazine, bcp's, hydralazine, isoniazid, opiates, reserpine, salicylates; serious rxns: erythema multiforme–like lesions; rarely, TEN.

HIV pointers: Occurs in >50%; ↑ incidence as immune function deteriorates (Nejm 1993;328:1670); drug rxns to trimethoprim-sulfamethoxazole do not preclude reuse as 50% of those w allergic rxn can be treated through adverse rxns w antihistamines (Arch IM 1994;154:2402).

- Protease inhibitors: induce skin and habitus changes **(peripheral lipodystrophy)**: cushingoid-like changes of buffalo hump, ↑ abdominal fat; sunken cheeks, thin extremities, breast hypertrophy, striae, ↑ lipids, insulin resistance; causes social distress as sunken cheeks proclaim the person is HIV infected on protease inhibitors; onset is more rapid and profound w ritonavir and sequinavir combination than w indinavir (Jaad 2000;42:129; Jaad 1999;41:467; Lancet 1998;352:1881).

15.3.D. LICHENOID ERUPTION OF HIV

Summary: Multiple; violaceous hyperpigmented; flat; papules and plaques w shiny surface; sometimes scaling and eczematous; most are on sun-exposed areas; may be caused by photosensitizing meds; blacks >> whites.

HIV pointers: CD4 count usually <50/μL.

15.4.A. BACTERIAL INFECTIONS

Summary: Lesions: folliculitis, abscesses, furuncles, impetigo, ecthyma gangrenosum; for details: see Index for specific infection or body area; get c + s early to properly direct rx; culture for all organisms, using appropriate media (bacterial, fungal, viral, anaerobic).

HIV pointers: Similar as in pts w/o HIV infection; *S. aureus* nasal carrier rate 2 × > normal (Lancet 1989;2:558); other organisms more common in HIV-pos pts: *Pseudomonas*; *Haemophilus influenzae* (Jama 1992:268:3350); recurrences are common (Semin Derm 1993;12:296).

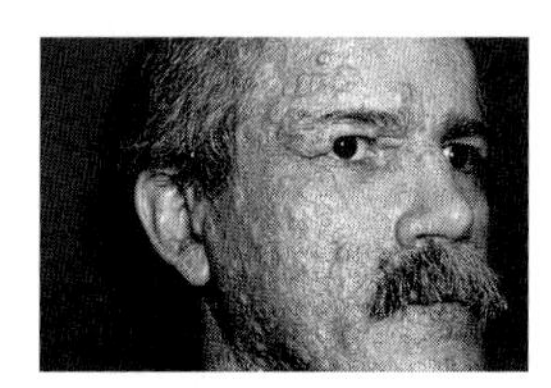

Molluscum contagiosum

15.4.B. MOLLUSCUM CONTAGIOSUM

Summary: Pale to pink, shiny, elevated bump or papule w light-colored dimple in center; look for lesions about genitals and lower abdomen, face; asx unless traumatized; DNA poxvirus; transmission is by close person-to-person contact; for additional details and rx, *see GENITAL, 9.7.b.*

HIV pointers: >20% of AIDS pts; CD4 usually <200/μL; giant molluscum lesions may appear; regress w protease inhibitors or cidofovir (Jaad 2000;43:409; Arch Derm 1997;133:987).

15.4.C. VERRUCA VULGARIS (COMMON WARTS)

Summary: Single to multiple; surface is raised, rough, cauliflower-like; pinhead to dime sized; most are on hands, feet, face; usually painless unless periungual or fingertip; condylomata acuminata in groin and perianal areas (see GENITALS, 9.7.a.); may be easily traumatized; may be extensive; resistant to rx; for details, see HANDS, 14.1.a., and LEG RASH, 17.6.a.

HIV pointers: >50% of homosexual men w AIDS; facial warts are early sign of HIV infection; rx is difficult (Arch Derm 1997;133:629).

15.4.D. SYPHILIS

Summary: Cutaneous: papulosquamous lesions; lues maligna; sclerodermiform lesions; extensive mouth ulcerations; keratoderma; widespread gummas; rx: higher doses and longer rx than for pts w/o HIV infection (Arch IM 1996;156:321), although this was denied in a large randomized trial (Nejm 1997;337:307) (1°, see GENITALS, 9.2.a.; 2°, see BODY, 3.1.f.; 3°, see ULCER—LEG, 25.2.d.).

HIV pointers: Obtain RPR or VDRL results for all HIV-pos pts at time of HIV dx; high incidence in HIV-pos pts (Arch IM 1990;159:1297); may rapidly progress w greater severity (Ann IM 1994;121:94), esp CNS disease (Nejm 1994;331:1469, 1516); r/o neurosyphilis in HIV-pos pts by looking for neurologic and/or cognitive dysfunction (Arch Neurol 1991;48:700; Review Jaad 2000;43:409).

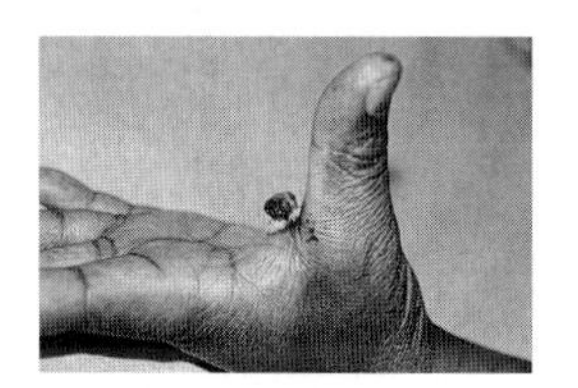

Bacterial angiomatosis

HIV

15.4.E. BACILLARY ANGIOMATOSIS (EPITHELIOID ANGIOMATOSIS)

Summary: Cutaneous: vascular lesions w pinpoint red to purple nodules are most common; sc nodules; crusted ulcerations; large exophytic masses (Br J Derm 1992;126:535; J Am Acad Derm 1990;22:501); any skin site; may resemble KS; underlying bone may be invaded;

viscera may be involved, esp liver; cause: *Bartonella henselae*, causes *cat-scratch disease* in immunocompetent pt (Nejm 1997;337:1916); *Bartonella quintana*, cause of *trench fever* (Nejm 1992;327:1625); dx: clinical; bx w Warthin Starry stains to show organism; culture; rx: erythromycin 2 gm/d or ciprofloxacin (1–1.5 gm/d), or doxycycline (200 mg/d) for 2 mo, but up to 6 mo may be needed (Med Clin N Am 1998;82:1033); also clears w HIV suppression by protease inhibitors.

HIV pointers: Rare; confined to HIV-pos pts (Arch IM 1994;154:524).

15.4.F. FUNGAL INFECTIONS, SUPERFICIAL

Summary:

- *Tinea versicolor*: darker than normal skin to lighter than normal skin; patches on upper trunk; does not differ from non-HIV-infected pts except more common; rx, see BODY, 3.1.h.
- *Tinea pedis*: common dermatophytosis in pts w HIV infection; typical interdigital maceration w scaling and diffuse hyperkeratosis of sole.
- *Tinea cruris*: more severe w HIV infection; usually extends beyond groin onto trunk.
- *Onychomycosis*: common w HIV infection; most common pattern: crumbly material under end and sides of toenails and fingernails; *Trichophyton rubrum*: most common (see NAILS, 20.3.a.); *Candida*: common; chronic paronychia; irregular nail surface but not crumbly under nail (see NAILS, 20.5.a.).

HIV pointers: Superficial fungal infections may show little inflammation if pt is severely immunosuppressed; consider obtaining scale for KOH/culture if in doubt; prevalence of dermatophyte infections not ↑ in HIV but pts have more difficulty in clearing infection, infection may invade deeper, and recurrences are common (J Am Acad Derm 1994;31S:S60); nail fungal infections may have white discoloration under nail starting at lunula and progressing distally (*proximal subungual onychomycosis*).

15.4.G. *CANDIDA* INFECTION

Summary:

- Pseudomembranes: most common; white elevated plaque w cottage cheese–like appearance; rx, see MOUTH, 19.1.f.
- Erythematous (atrophic): flat red patches; hard and soft palate, tongue; rx, see MOUTH, 19.4.b.
- Angular cheilitis: redness, cracking, fissuring of folds at corners of mouth; rx, see MOUTH, 19.8.e.

HIV pointers: Most common (eventually in 90%) fungal infection in HIV-infected pts; oral candidal infection common (up to 70%) initial manifestation of HIV infection.

15.4.H. FUNGAL INFECTIONS, DEEP

ASPERGILLOSIS

Summary: Clinical forms: Primary cutaneous aspergillosis: fluctuant papules, pustules, vesiculopustular plaques, non-healing ulcers; most commonly develop at site of IV catheters, traumatic inoculation or 2° colonization of burns and other wounds; Dx: biopsy, fungal stains and tissue culture; Rx: debride w wide surgical excision, may need lifelong Rx w itraconazole. Secondary cutaneous aspergillosis: develops from direct extension from chest wall or hematogenous dissemination; usually quickly fatal.

HIV pointers: Risk factors: occlusive dressings at site of catheters, ↓wbc, CD4 <50/μl. fatal without prompt Rx (Arch Derm 2000;136:365,412).

BLASTOMYCOSIS

Summary: Cutaneous: widespread verrucous papules; nodules; plaques; prevalent in North America; *Blastomyces dermatitidis*; dx: bx and fungal stains; rx: fluconazole, itraconazole, or amphotericin B.

HIV pointers: Skin lesions may be widespread, even fatal, if HIV pos.

COCCIDIOIDOMYCOSIS

Summary: Cutaneous: papules; pustules; sc abscesses; verrucous granulomas; hyperkeratotic plaques; cold abscesses; concomitant pulmonary disease; *Coccidioides immitis*; dx: bx and fungal stains; rx: fluconazole, itraconazole, or amphotericin B.

HIV pointers: Meningitis common (Clin Infect Dis 1995;21S:S111).

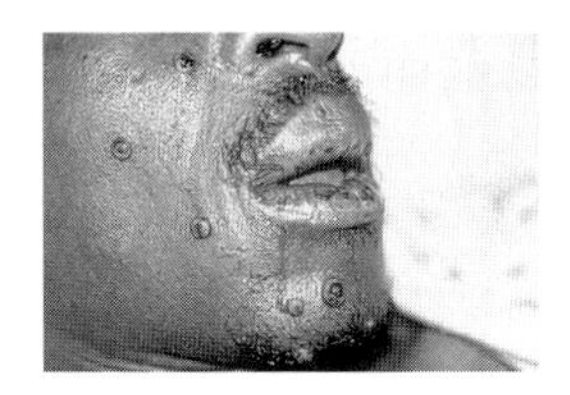

Cryptococcosis

CRYPTOCOCCOSIS

Summary: Skin lesions in 5%–10% of pts w disseminated disease; most common sites: face, neck, scalp; lesions are nonspecific: erythematous papules, pustules, umbilicated papules resembling molluscum contagiosum (Arch Derm 1996;132:545); dx: bx w Gomori methenamine silver stain shows budding yeast; culture.

HIV pointers: Leading cause of mortality and morbidity in pts w AIDS; meningitis common, do LP to exclude; rx: amphotericin 0.7 mg/kg qd w or w/o flucytosine 100 mg/kg po/d; consider prophylaxis, usually fluconazole 200 mg/d if CD4 count <50/μL and LP result is neg.

HISTOPLASMOSIS

Summary: Cutaneous lesions 10%–20% of pts w disseminated disease; erythematous papules; ulcerative plaques; eczematous or erythema multiforme–like lesions; *Histoplasma capsulatum*; dx: bx and fungal stains; rx: amphotericin B, itraconazole.

HIV pointers: Most common endemic mycosis in pts w AIDS; disseminated in 95% of pts w AIDS.

MUCORMYCOSIS (ZYGOMYCOSIS)

Summary: Large necrotic plaques and ulcers, mucous membrane involvement common, other involved sites: kidney, basal ganglia, respiratory tract; may be disseminated; Dx: skin bx, culture; Rx: surgical debridement and IV amphotericin B; mortality up to 40%.

HIV pointers: Usually in pts w advanced HIV disease w ↓ CD4 counts; active IV drug use, ↓ wbc; often rapid progression and fulminant course (Jaad 1994;30:904; Cutis 2000;66:15).

SPOROTRICHOSIS

Summary: Clinical forms: lymphocutaneous form, disseminated cutaneous form, systemic form; cutaneous: ulcers, papules, nodules, plaques, pustules; *Sporothrix schenckii*; dx: bx, culture, fungal stains; rx: fluconazole, itraconazole, or amphotericin B.

HIV pointers: Skin lesions may be widespread, even fatal.

15.4.I. MYCOBACTERIAL INFECTIONS

Summary: Cutaneous, varied: papules; nodules; hyperkeratosis; pustules; suppurative lymphadenitis; ulcerations (J Am Acad Derm 1995;33:433); *Mycobacterium avium-intracellulare*, *M. haemophilum*, others; rx: systemic multiple anti-tbc agents after suitable c + s testing.

HIV pointers: Skin lesions develop in 10% of HIV-pos pts who have systemic tbc (Clin Infect Dis 1995;21S:S66).

15.4.J. PNEUMOCYSTOSIS

Summary: Cutaneous: friable reddish papule or nodule in ear canal or nares (Am J Med 1991;127:250); dx: bx and special stains; rx: iv pentamidine.

HIV pointers: Rare; skin involved in pts using aerosolized pentamidine for prophylaxis of *Pneumocystis carinii* pneumonia.

15.5. NEOPLASTIC DISORDERS

Summary: See specific tumors in Index.

HIV pointers: AIDS-defining neoplasms: KS; non-Hodgkin's lymphoma: 2nd most common systemic malignancy after KS (Mayo Clin Proc 1995;70:665); 1° nervous system lymphoma; cervical carcinoma; general behavior; aggressive; higher-grade lesions, more advanced stage, and shortened survival compared to similar neoplasms in HIV-neg pts.

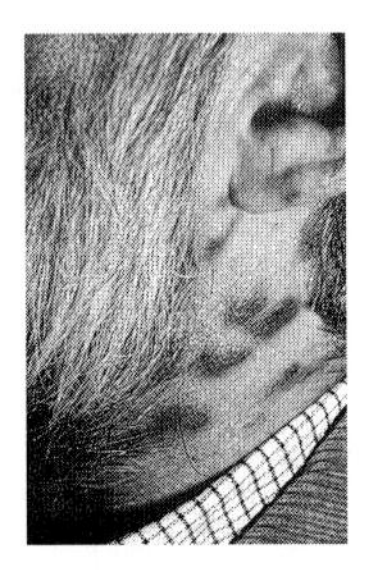

Kaposi's sarcoma

15.5.A. KAPOSI'S SARCOMA (KS, MULTIPLE IDIOPATHIC HEMORRHAGIC SARCOMA)

Summary: Cutaneous: pink to red to brown to purple; progresses from macules and patches to plaques, nodules, tumors; common sites: legs, feet, mucous membranes, scalp; internal: GI tract; cause: transmissible agent, probably human herpesvirus type 8; dx: confirmed by bx but bx not always necessary; for additional details and rx, see GROWTHS, 11.14.a.

HIV pointers: 15% of HIV-pos pts; most common HIV-assoc malignancy in homosexual and bisexual men; may need bx to r/o bacillary angiomatosis.

15.5.B. SKIN CANCERS

Summary: For appearance and general management, see GROWTHS, 11.

HIV pointers: BCE: ↑ incidence; can be aggressive; SCC: aggressive course w recurrence up to 20% after standard rx; eruptive dysplastic nevi and aggressive melanoma occur.

ANAL NEOPLASIA

Summary: Anal cancer and anal intraepithelial neoplasia; screen w anal PAP test; confirm by bx; rx: x-radiation, chemotherapy.

HIV pointers: Incidence: ↑ 40 × in homosexual men w AIDS, esp w receptor anal intercourse (Lancet 1994;343:636).

15.5.C. LYMPHOMA

Summary and HIV pointers: Most common AIDS-related lymphoma: high-grade B cell; 80%–90% are immunoblastic lymphoma or small noncleaved lymphoma; develops late in course of AIDS after various opportunistic infections; 80%–90% have systemic B cell lymphoma sx: fever, night sweats, ↓ weight; 60%–90% present w extranodal sites involved (compared to 40% non-HIV-pos pts); most common extranodal disease sites: CNS, GI, bone marrow, liver; other lymphomas: primary CNS lymphoma develops in 4% of pts w AIDS; Hodgkin's disease is assoc w drug use (Epstein-Barr virus?) (Nejm 2000;343:481) rather than AIDS (J Natl Cancer Inst 1993;85:1382).

15.6.A. PSORIASIS

Summary: Appearance similar to psoriasis in healthy pts (see BODY, 3.1.d.), but HIV may trigger or exacerbate severe psoriasis; spread rapidly; may become erythrodermic; rx, see BODY, 3.1.d.

HIV pointers: 5% of HIV-pos pts; arthritis is common; Reiter's syndrome may develop or worsen; avoid MTX as it worsens immune depression.

15.7.A. VIRAL INFECTIONS

CYTOMEGALOVIRUS (CMV)

Summary: Cutaneous skin lesions are uncommon, but include: ulcers; verrucous; palpable purpuric papules; blisters; perianal ulcerations 2° to chronic CMV colitis; retinitis leading to blindness; dx: viral culture and ↑ antibody titers; rx: ganciclovir; foscarnet; cidofovir (Arch IM 1998; 158:957; Nejm 1992;326:262).

HIV pointers: In up to 90% of AIDS pts; most appear when CD4 <50–100/μL; often dx when perianal ulceration does not improve after acyclovir rx.

HERPES SIMPLEX VIRUS (HSV)

Summary: Painful grouped vesicles on erythematous base; most heal in 2 wk; may develop chronic ulcers that last for mos; for additional details and rx, see BLISTERS, 2.1.a.

HIV pointers: Appears in 20%–50% of HIV-pos pts; rx: acyclovir: up to 800 mg po 5 ×/d or iv acyclovir 5–10 mg/kg q 8 h × 5–7 d; suppressive rx w famciclovir 500 mg bid is effective (Ann IM 1998;128:21); acyclovir resistance: foscarnet 40 mg iv q 8 h or 60 mg q 12 h.

HERPES ZOSTER (HZ)

Summary: Cutaneous: erythema; pain; hyperesthesia; blisters; dermatomal; for details and rx, see BODY, 2.3.d.

HIV pointers: CD4 usually 200–500/μL; 2nd episodes of HZ at same or different sites or multidermatomal may occur; varicella may occur sometimes assoc w fatal pulmonary infection (J Am Acad Derm 1989:20:637); other complications: PHN, scars, ulcers (Ann IM 1990;112:187); absorption of oral antiviral agents, except valacyclovir, may be ↓ due to atrophic gastritis; consider foscarnet 40 mg iv q 8 h or 60 mg q 12 h (Am J Med 1992:92:30S).

15.8.A. PORPHYRIA CUTANEA TARDA (PCT)

Summary: Fragile skin; blisters; hyperpigmentation; hands and other sun-exposed skin; ↑ facial hair; assoc w DM; alcoholism; (see LIGHT REACTIONS, 18.1.c.).

HIV pointers: ↑ incidence in HIV-pos pts; may be due to ↑ incidence of hepatitis C infection w ↓ liver function; rx: difficult as phlebotomy not useful if pt already is anemic; antimalarials (Arch Derm 1994;130:630); erythropoietin (Nejm 1990;322:315) has been used.

HIV

16 Itch

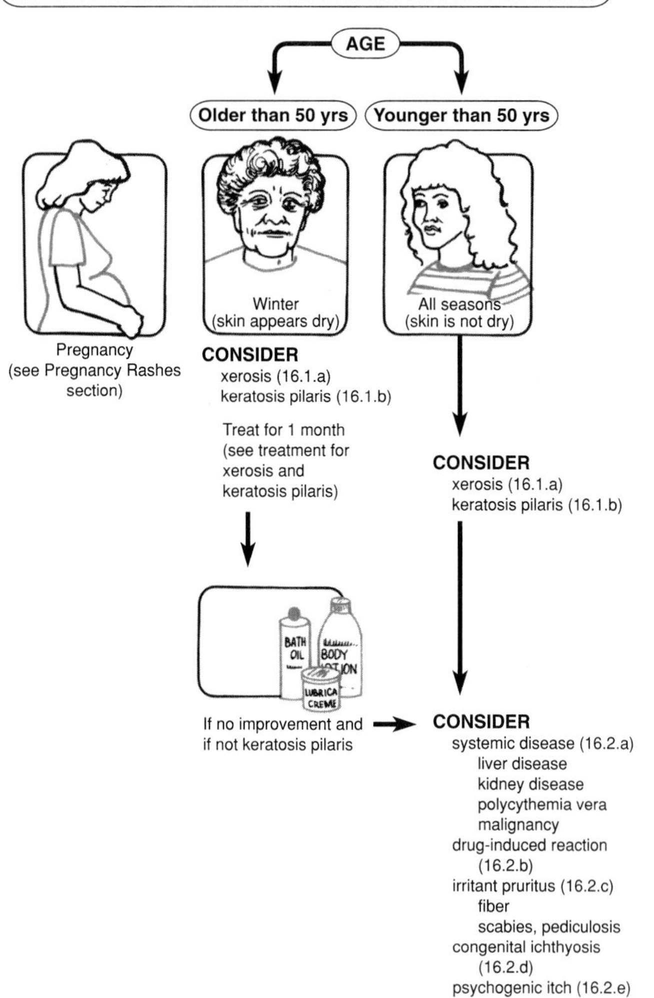

WITHOUT LESIONS EXCEPT SCALING AND/OR STRETCH MARKS
AGE
Older than 50 yrs
Younger than 50 yrs
Pregnancy
(see Pregnancy Rashes section)
Winter
(skin appears dry)
All seasons
(skin is not dry)
CONSIDER
xerosis (16.1.a)
keratosis pilaris (16.1.b)
Treat for 1 month
(see treatment for xerosis and keratosis pilaris)
CONSIDER
xerosis (16.1.a)
keratosis pilaris (16.1.b)
BATH OIL
BODY LOTION
LUBRICA CREME
If no improvement and
if not keratosis pilaris
CONSIDER
systemic disease (16.2.a)
liver disease
kidney disease
polycythemia vera
malignancy
drug-induced reaction (16.2.b)
irritant pruritus (16.2.c)
fiber
scabies, pediculosis
congenital ichthyosis (16.2.d)
psychogenic itch (16.2.e)

WITH WHEALS: HIVES, URTICARIA

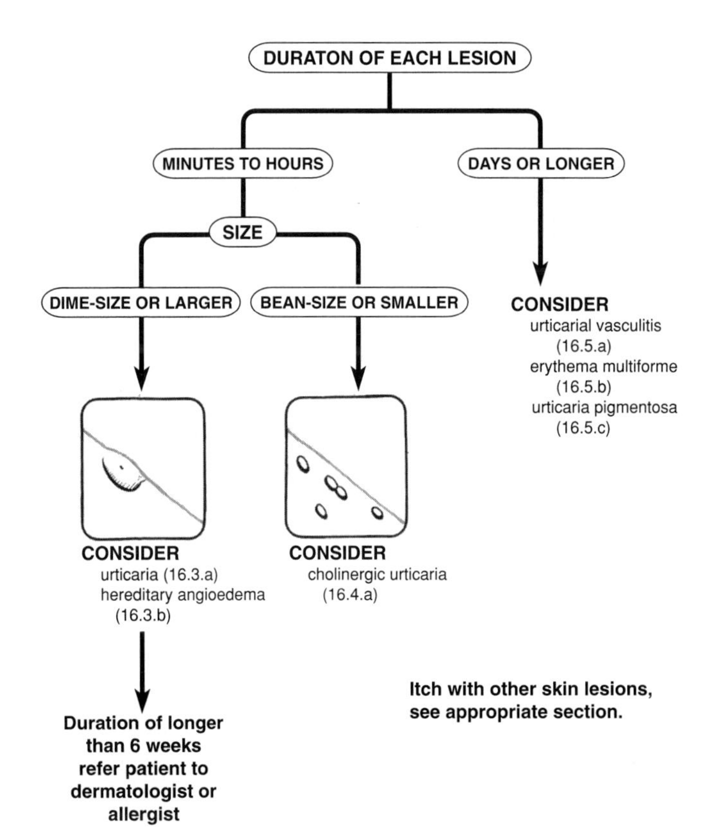

Itch with other skin lesions, see appropriate section.

NO LESIONS EXCEPT SCALING/SCRATCH MARKS, >50 YEARS OLD

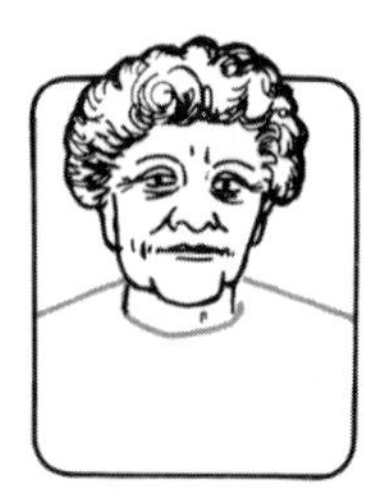

16.1.A. XEROSIS (ASTEATOSIS, DRY SKIN, WINTER ITCH)

Cause: Low humidity; dry, cold weather; excessive soap bathing; atopic tendency.

Pathophys: ↓ water-retaining lipids, esp common in aging.

Sx: Itching, worse on legs; may be generalized.

Si: Dry looking; scaly; even parchment like; scratch marks may not be present.

Crs: Recurs or worsens in winter; may not clear or improve in summer if pt lives/works in air-conditioned environment.

Lab: If not responsive to moisturizers and reduced bathing, consider evaluation for systemic disease (see 16.2.a.).

Rx: Older persons: reduce frequency to 2–3 ×/wk and length of bathing (see Bathing Instructions for Dry Skin, RX.2.); apply moisturizer while skin is still damp; advise installation of humidifier in house; avoid TCSs.

16.1.B. KERATOSIS PILARIS

Cause: Inherited; autosomal dominant; often assoc w atopic dermatitis.

Sx: Mild irritation.

Si: Discrete; pinhead sized; hard or horny, raised plugs, some pink; feels like sandpaper; most located on extensor surfaces of upper arms, thighs; may be generalized.

Crs: Most appear by age 10 yo; lesions are chronic but improve w age, most improve during summer (Br J Derm 1994;130:711).

Rx: Usually not necessary; if troublesome: try emollient cr w lactic acid or urea (OTC: AmLactin; Lacticare; UltraMide; rx: Lac-Hydrin); reduce soap use on area in winter.

NO LESIONS EXCEPT SCALING/SCRATCH MARKS, NOT RESPONDING TO DRY SKIN TREATMENT, NOT KERATOSIS PILARIS OR <50 YEARS OLD

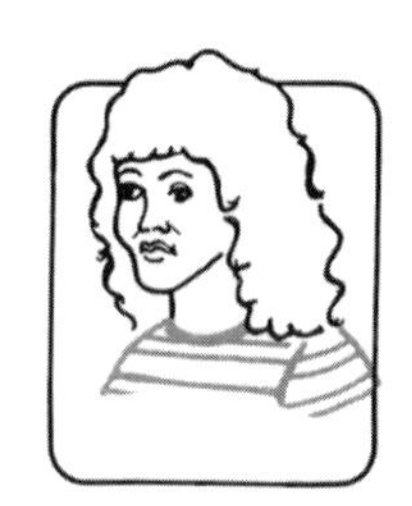

16.2.A. SYSTEMIC DISEASE

Cause: R/o renal insufficiency; hepatitis or obstructive liver disease; polycythemia vera; DM; endocrine disorders, esp thyroid and parathyroid disease; some malignancies, esp lymphomas, mycosis fungoides, Sézary syndrome (J Am Acad Derm 1990;22:19); HIV infection; psychogenic; if pt is pregnant (see PREGNANCY, 23.).

Sx: Pruritus is a sx, not a disease; more significant if it interferes w work or sleep or has started in last few wks or mos.

Crs: Depends on underlying cause; itch may clear even as disease progresses.

Lab:

- If onset is recent, esp if pt <50 yo: CBC, LFTs and RFTs, FBS; consider thyroid function tests, calcium, phosphorus, stool exam for ova and parasites; if lab values are WNL and there are no skin lesions, consider xerosis (see 16.1.a.), scabies (see GENITAL, 9.1.g.), an irritant cause (see 16.2.c.), psychogenic itch (see 16.2.d.),

malignancy, however, extensive screening for malignancy is not justified (J Am Acad Derm 1987;16:1179).
- If chronic, esp if pt >50 yo: defer lab tests; instruct pt in bathing and lubricating techniques (see 16.1.a.).

Rx: Pruritus may be improved by local or systemic measures even if underlying disorder cannot be corrected; modify bathing habits and advise lubrication (see 16.1.a. and RX.1.); avoid topical anesthetics or antihistamines as they are sensitizing; doxepin may be helpful, but avoid w liver disease; consider oral cholestyramine, 8–12 gm/d for liver pruritus; UVB helpful esp w renal (Jaad 2000;43:975) and HIV pruritus.

16.2.B. DRUG-INDUCED REACTION

Summary: Consider even in absence of eruption; drugs assoc w pruritus: antimalarials, amphetamines, chlorpromazine, bcp's, hydralazine, isoniazid, opiates, reserpine, salicylates.

16.2.C. IRRITANT PRURITUS

Summary: Wool clothing, esp in pts w atopy; antistatic dryer sheets (ie, Bounce); fiberglass-containing materials (ie, insulation, some draperies); scabies and pediculosis pubis w/o rash may be seen in persons who bathe frequently ("clean" scabies).

16.2.D. ICHTHYOSIS

Summary: Inherited disorders of keratinization of several subtypes:
- *Ichthyosis vulgaris*: most common; autosomal dominant; improves in summer; worse on extremities, palms, and soles and spares flexural regions; responds to lubrication (see 16.1.a.) or lactic acid or urea compounds (Lac-Hydrin and many similar OTC products).

- *X-linked recessive ichthyosis*: sons of asx female carriers; rare; large polygonal scale; may involve flexural areas; other physical abn present; steroid sulfatase deficiency.
- *Others*: rare; severe; esp if autosomal recessive.

Refer pts w suspected congenital ichthyosis to dermatology.

Contact F.I.R.S.T.—Foundation for Ichthyosis and Related Skin Types (POB 669, Ardmore, PA 19003-0669; 800.545.3286 or 610.789.3995; www.libertynet.org/~ichthyos) for pt education materials.

16.2.E. PSYCHOGENIC ITCH

Summary:

- **Neurotic excoriations**: no 1° lesions, just scratch marks, lichenification, healed and fresh erosions; most itchy when pt is not otherwise occupied, ie, reading or watching TV, esp in evening; itch does not wake pt from sleep; pt has been able to function well at work; responds to behavioral modification and/or nortriptyline (10–100 mg/d) or doxepin (10–100 mg/d); **prurigo nodularis**: chronic nodular/papular form; multiple lesions; unremitting itch; resistant to rx.
- **Delusions of parasitosis**: claims to find "bugs" or other particles in skin; probably a form of obsessive-compulsive disorder; may injure skin in attempt to remove foreign material; skin heals w stellate-shaped scars; pt often emotionally disturbed; not able to function well at work; generally resists psychiatric help; refer to dermatologist and/or psychiatrist.

HIVES, DURATION MINUTES TO HOURS, > DIME SIZED

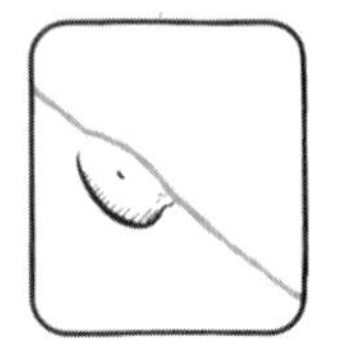

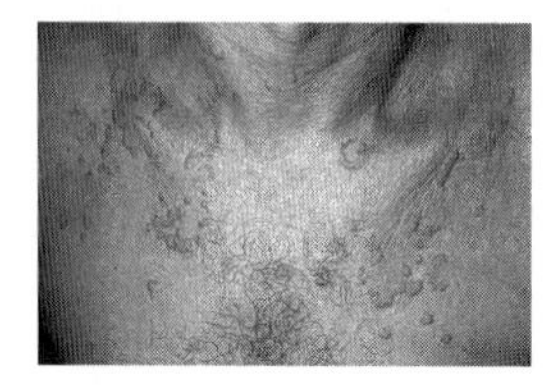

Urticaria

16.3.A. URTICARIA (HIVES)

Cause: Histamine release induced in mast cells by either direct, nonallergic mechanisms or rxn to an allergen; mediated by IgE (type I hypersensitivity) and probably by other tissue and serum factors as well; *direct histamine releasers*: ROH, ASA, various opiates, hydralazine, some foods, esp nuts, shellfish, eggs, cheese, milk, berries, or those containing benzoic acid, a common preservative; *allergen histamine releaser*: (1) physical injury: light, cold, heat, pressure; **dermatographism**: hive localized to site of pressure, common, usually not due to underlying allergy, rx not needed; (2) systemic allergen: topical agents (soaps, cosmetics, etc) are unlikely causes.

- The most common causes of hives are the 6 "I's":
  - *Ingestants*: esp meds: ROH, ASA, laxatives, foods, food additives.
  - *Injections*: vaccinations, dental work
  - *Infections*: viral, esp infectious mononucleosis, hepatitis; fungal, ie, tinea, *Candida* infection
  - *Inhalants*: pollens, aerosols
  - *Infestations*: insect bites, systemic parasites
  - *Internal disease*: malignancies, DM, autoimmune disorders, ie, SLE, RA, polymyositis, vasculitis

Sx: Intensely pruritic.

Si: Abrupt appearance of raised edematous wheal; flat-topped, doughnut, quarter-moon shaped; dime to a saucer in size; sharp edge; pinker than normal skin; any region; **angioedema**: deep tissue swelling.

Crs: Individual lesions are transient; min to few h; disappear w/o a trace; if individual hive lasts >d, consider urticarial vasculitis (see 16.5.a.); episodes of urticaria last days to wks w daily or so reappearances; an episode >6 wk defines *chronic urticaria*; perhaps 20% of pts w chronic urticaria continue to have intermittent problems for yrs.

Lab: Recent onset: identify cause from hx of recent change of drugs, foods, or other exposures; as duration of episode lengthens, identification of the inciting cause becomes more difficult; chronic urticaria: may require extensive evaluation, including blood and urine screening, x-rays of suspected loci of infection or tumor, allergy skin or radioallergosorbent test, skin bx, isolation of pt from home and work environment, elimination diets; refer pts w chronic urticaria to dermatologist or allergist; cause is not identified in 3/4 of cases.

Rx:

- *Mild*: relieve itching w topical calamine or Burow's shake lotion w 0.25% menthol (see RX.3.); systemic antihistamines: hydroxyzine, 10–25 mg qid (see RX.12.); doxepin (Adapin, Sinequan, Rx), 10–25 mg hs to qid (do not use w MAO inhibitors, ROH, or in children or pregnant women); TCSs do not help; *chronic urticaria*: avoid systemic CSs when possible.
- *Acute and extensive*: may require systemic CS (20–40 mg prednisone daily in divided doses for up to 2 wk) as a temporary measure, but CSs have a limited role as they delay identification of underlying cause, may hide underlying infection, and generate side effects (see RX.8.); angioneurotic edema or laryngeal edema requires urgent care: aqueous epinephrine 1:1000 (0.1% or 1 mg/mL), 0.3–0.5 mL sc or im (children: 0.01 mL/kg but <0.3 mL/dose) immediately and up to q 15–20 min × 2; also: diphenhydramine 50 mg (children: 1 mg/kg) po or im q 4–6 h; elevate legs; maintain airway; oxygen.

16.3.B. HEREDITARY ANGIOEDEMA

Summary: Rare; autosomal dominant; recurrent urticaria; angioedema; intestinal colic; life-threatening laryngeal edema; cause: defect in esterase that inhibits a component of C′.

HIVES, DURATION MINUTES TO HOURS, < DIME SIZED

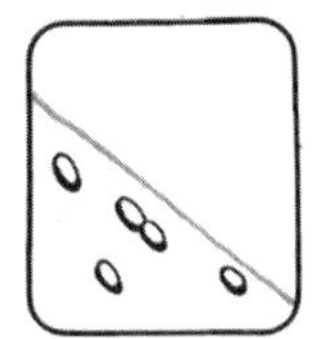

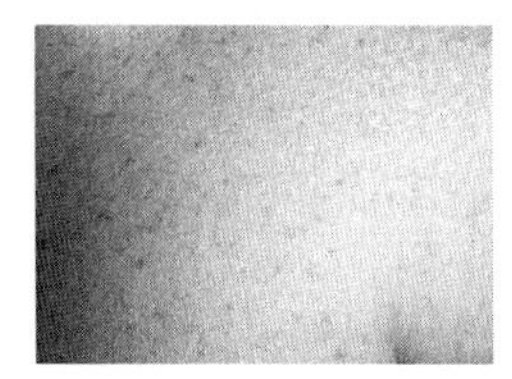

Cholinergic urticaria

16.4.A. CHOLINERGIC URTICARIA (HEAT-INDUCED URTICARIA)

Summary: Evanescent wheals; multiple; bean size or smaller; itchy; induced by heat or exercise; disappears shortly after cooling off; pts almost never have lesions at time of office visit; course lasts mos or yrs; antihistamines, esp hydroxyzine or cyproheptadine, often suppress sx, but large doses may be needed (see RX.12.).

HIVES, DURATION DAYS OR MORE

16.5.A. URTICARIAL VASCULITIS

Summary: Appears similar to urticaria but wheals persist longer, 1–3 d; may be assoc w mild purpura, arthralgias, abdominal pain, glomerulonephritis; may accompany hepatitis B infections, infectious mononucleosis, drug eruptions, anaphylactoid purpura, SLE; lab: ESR usually ↑; bx: venulitis and leukocytoclasis; obtain tests for hepatitis B antigen, heterophile agglutinin, ANA, cryoglobulins, RF (J Am Acad Derm 1998;38:899; Arch Derm 1998;134:88).

16.5.B. ERYTHEMA MULTIFORME

Summary: Abrupt onset; flat, dusky lesions resembling hives; individual lesions persist longer than hives; central part often darker or blistering, like a bull's-eye or target; pain > itch; usually extensor surfaces; palmar and plantar lesions are tender; severe cases: may be hemorrhagic; peeling; blistering; mucous membrane erosions are common and often disabling.

For additional details and rx, see BLISTERS, 2.1.b.

16.5.C. URTICARIA PIGMENTOSA (MASTOCYTOSIS)

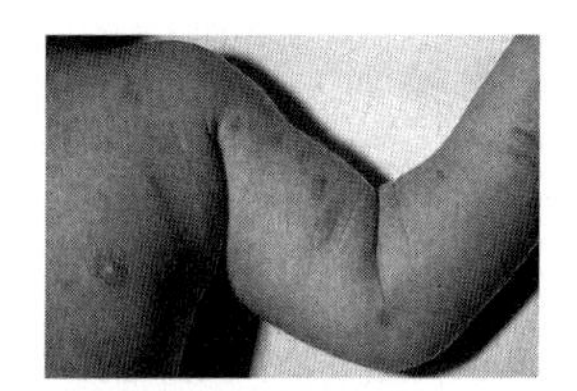

Urticaria pigmentosa

Brit J Derm 2001;144:682; Arch IM 1999;159:401. Am Fam Phys 1999;59:3047. J Am Acad Derm 1996;32:545.

Cause: ↑ numbers of mast cells; limited to skin or systemic; occas malignant.

Sx: 2° to release of histamine and other chemical mediators from mast cells; *skin lesions*: itchy, esp if rubbed or after hot shower; *systemic*: flushing, palpitations, headache, tachycardia, syncope, hypotension, GI complaints, ie, abdominal pain, diarrhea.

Si: Pencil eraser size; tan; flat to slightly raised; multiple; densest on trunk; urticate, becoming raised, reddened, and itchy after a hot shower or when rubbed (*Darier's sign*); if bone marrow involved: pain, anemia, fractures.

Crs: *Benign, skin only*: onset before puberty; lesions lighten or disappear in yrs (urticaria pigmentosa); *benign, systemic*: onset adulthood; skin lesions in 85% and persist (J Invest Derm 1991;96:5S); bone marrow is 2nd most common organ involved; *mast cell leukemia* may develop; most frequent in elderly symptomatic pt w/o skin lesions (J Invest Derm 1995;104:885).

Lab: Skin bx (see DX.7.): special stains for mast cell granules; preserve granules in suspected cases by infiltrating around, not under, lesion and use local anesthetic w/o epinephrine; further w/u not needed in children or unless ROS suggests systemic involvement; labs if systemic mastocytosis suspected: ↓ cholesterol, ↑ eos, ↑ LFTs, ↑ plasma tryptase, bone x-rays and scans, endoscopy w upper GI sx; bone marrow bx when onset in adulthood (Ann Allergy 1994;73:197).

Rx: If asx, do not treat; ↓ factors that trigger histamine release: extremes of heat, cold, exercise; drugs: ASA, NSAIDs, ROH, narcotics, quinine, reserpine, iodine-containing x-ray contrast media; use histamine H1 antagonists, ie, hydroxyzine, doxepin, chlorpheniramine (see RX.12.), or combination w an H2 antagonist, ie, cimetidine; cromolyn sodium (Gastrocrom, Rx, $$$), 200 mg qid, to ↓ diarrhea and abdominal pain; PUVA provides help for some (Am J Med Sci 1995;309:328) (see RX.15.); advise pts w systemic mastocytosis to wear a medical alert bracelet and carry an adrenaline syringe.

17 Leg Rash

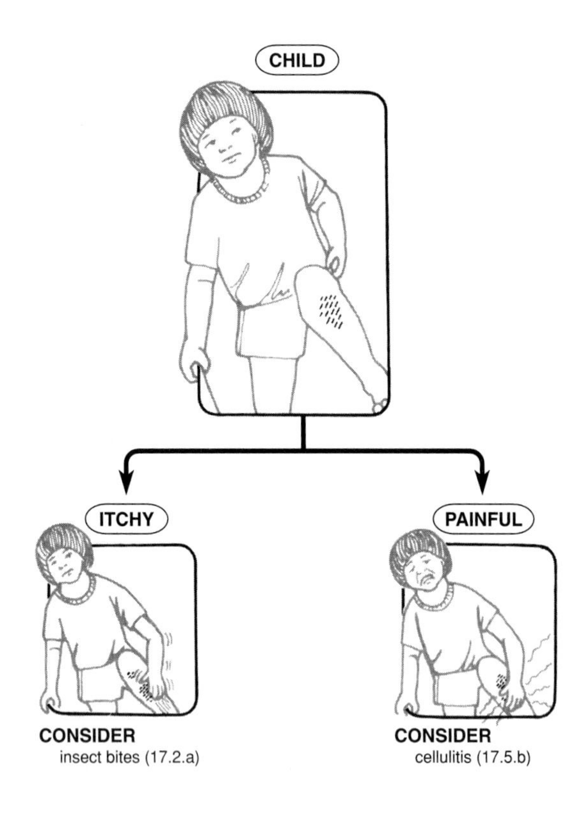
BUMPS OR NODULES
(KNEES TO ANKLES OR SEE FEET)
CHILD
ITCHY
PAINFUL
CONSIDER
insect bites (17.2.a)
CONSIDER
cellulitis (17.5.b)

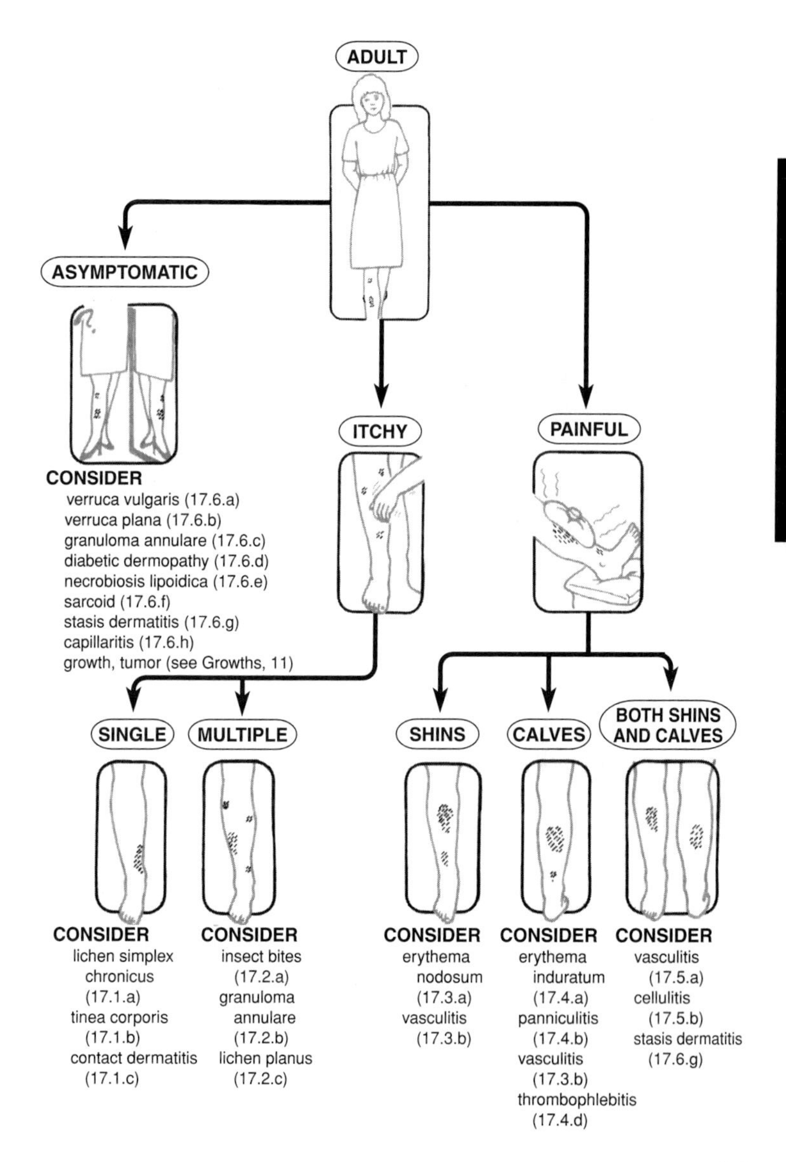
ADULT
ASYMPTOMATIC
CONSIDER
verruca vulgaris (17.6.a)
verruca plana (17.6.b)
granuloma annulare (17.6.c)
diabetic dermopathy (17.6.d)
necrobiosis lipoidica (17.6.e)
sarcoid (17.6.f)
stasis dermatitis (17.6.g)
capillaritis (17.6.h)
growth, tumor (see Growths, 11)
ITCHY
PAINFUL
SINGLE
MULTIPLE
SHINS
CALVES
BOTH SHINS AND CALVES
CONSIDER
lichen simplex chronicus (17.1.a)
tinea corporis (17.1.b)
contact dermatitis (17.1.c)
CONSIDER
insect bites (17.2.a)
granuloma annulare (17.2.b)
lichen planus (17.2.c)
CONSIDER
erythema nodosum (17.3.a)
vasculitis (17.3.b)
CONSIDER
erythema induratum (17.4.a)
panniculitis (17.4.b)
vasculitis (17.3.b)
thrombophlebitis (17.4.d)
CONSIDER
vasculitis (17.5.a)
cellulitis (17.5.b)
stasis dermatitis (17.6.g)

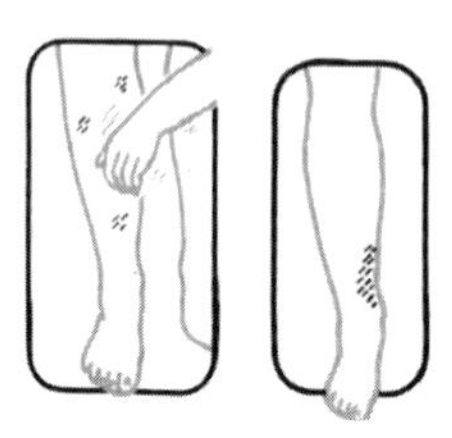

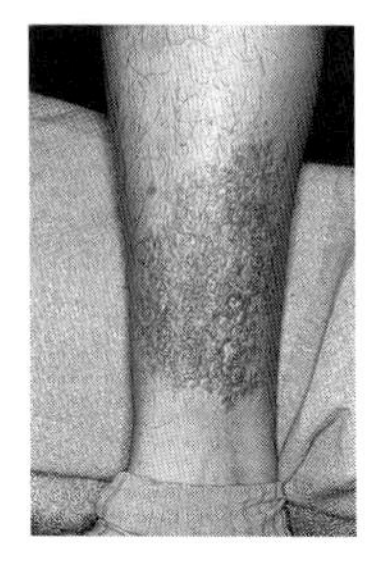

Lichen simplex chronicus

See color plate section.

17.1.A. LICHEN SIMPLEX CHRONICUS (LOCALIZED NEURODERMATITIS)

Cause: Self induced; most pts appear "high strung" and intense but not emotionally disabled; role of psychogenic factors or local abn cutaneous nerve endings is unclear.

Sx: Consuming paroxysmal itch, typically worse during unoccupied evening hrs or at times of emotional stress.

Si: Scaly, thickened patch; usually single; location: lower leg or ankle, nape, hand; **prurigo nodularis**: chronic nodular/papular form; multiple lesions; unremitting itch.

Crs: Usually has been present for many mos to yrs; waxes and wanes.

Lab: Bx not diagnostic, but may be necessary to r/o tumor, psoriasis.

Rx: Protect site from scratching and reduce itch w TCS (class I–III) cr under occlusive waterproof tape, ie, Blenderm (3M) (see RX.6.) or tape w CS in its adhesive (Cordran tape, 60/200 cm, Rx, $$), apply either for 36 h, then uncover for 12 h to prevent maceration; alternative: IL triamcinolone acetonide (Kenalog, 10 mg/mL) diluted to 2.5–4 mg/mL w saline (see RX.7.); consider nortriptyline (10–100 mg at dinner) or a serotonin-uptake inhibitor.

17.1.B. TINEA CORPORIS (FUNGUS INFECTION)

Summary: 2 forms:

- 1 or more patches of scaly, inflamed dermatitis; resembles tinea, or "ringworm," infections elsewhere.
- Pinhead-sized pustular, crusty, itchy eruption about hair follicles; only in women who shave their legs; caused by *Trichophyton rubrum* that penetrates hair follicles after repeated shaving trauma.

Confirm dx by KOH exam (see DX.3.) or culture of scale or plucked hairs.

For additional details and rx, see BODY, 3.1.g.

17.1.C. CONTACT DERMATITIS

Summary: Allergic or irritant rxn to ingredient of socks, shoes, foot med, etc; worse or restricted to dorsum, tops, or tips of toes and ankles; distribution often corresponds to outline of contactant, ie, a shoe tongue, at toe-grip of leather sandals or shower shoes; itchy.

For additional details and rx, see FEET, 7.3.a., and BODY, 3.1.a.

ADULT, ITCHY, MULTIPLE

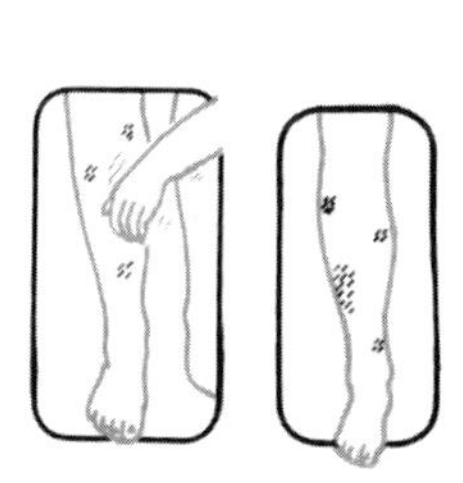

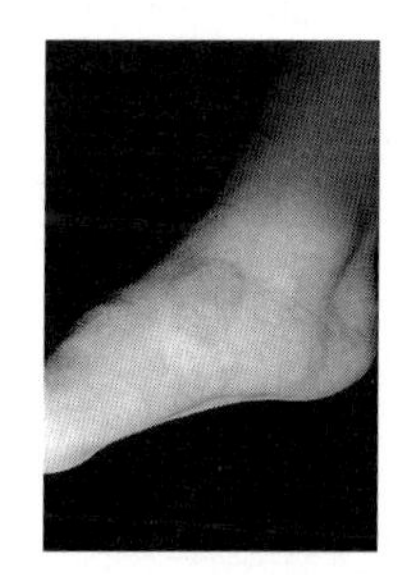

Granuloma annulare

17.2.A. INSECT BITES

J Am Acad Derm 1997;35:243. Arch Derm 1987;123:98.
See color plate section.

Cause: *Fleas:* worse when pet, the preferred host, is removed from household; may live 2 mo off host; *spiders*: most common in Americas: *Loxosceles* (brown recluse) has violin-shaped spot on top of brown body; not aggressive but moves into houses in fall and bites if caught in clothing pressed against skin (Derm Clin 1997;15:307); *bees and wasps* (Hymenoptera): most cases of insect bite hypersensitivity; 40 deaths/yr in U.S.

Sx: Itchy except spider bites: painful, often delayed a few h after the bite.

Si: *Fleas*: isolated itchy lesions below knees; lesions in rows are from stinging insects that crawl; *chiggers (trombiculid or harvest mites)*: most often at edges of shorts or underwear as they bite when meeting an obstruction; *mites*: intensely itchy eruption; may be widespread; follows exposure to paper, grain, flour, birds (Semin Derm 1993;12:46); scabies: see BODY, 3.1.e.; *spiders*: toxin is cytotoxic w necrosis or neurotoxic; systemic si/sx of fever, arthralgias, abdominal pain, headache, rare fatalities; *ticks*: see FEVER, 8.1.d.; *bees and wasps*: pain followed by localized erythema; edema; *allergic local rxn*: swelling, warmth, itch; not cellulitis, and antibiotics are generally not indicated; lasts up to 5 d; *systemic rxn*: start in min to 2 h or so; generalized urticaria, itch, erythema, angioedema, laryngoedema, asthma, abdominal cramps, ↓ BP, shock.

Crs: *Itchy bites*: depends on sensitization and kind of insect; clearing may take wks to mos; **papular urticaria**: an initial bite followed by similarly appearing, itchy, urticarial papules that may recur in large numbers after later bites (Ped Derm 1996;13:246); *painful bites*: usually spider, mild: resolve in few d; more severe: central blister, eschar, ulcer; prolonged healing; often leaves depressed scar; occas becomes systemic (Jaad 2001;44:561).

Cmplc: Infection; spider bites may lead to necrotic ulcers and to intravascular hemolysis, renal failure (Am J Clin Path 1995;104:463).

Rx:

- *Itchy bites*: partial relief may be provided by a shake lotion, ie, calamine w menthol (see RX.3.) or TCS (class II–IIII); infected lesions may require antibiotics; eradicate source: for temporary prevention: apply insect repellents to lower legs and socks; exterminate indoor fleas w readily available house aerosol insecticide "bombs" that kill both fleas and eggs; treat pets; most effective repellents contain DEET (diethyltoluamide) (Ann IM 1998;128:931; J Am Acad Derm 1997;35:243).

- *Painful bites*: rest, ice compresses, elevation (RICE therapy); analgesics (1 aspirin/d); dapsone use is controversial (Jama 1983;250:648) but may be helpful in moderate to severe lesions (50 mg/d and determination of G-6-PD status, if normal (pos) inc to 50 mg bid); avoid surgical debridement; heparin has been used to prevent DIC (Jama 1984;251:889); systemic CS not helpful; antivenin to *Loxosceles* not yet available.
- *Systemic rxn*: aqueous epinephrine 1:1000 (0.1% or 1 mg/mL), 0.3–0.5 mL sc or im (children: 0.01 mL/kg but <0.3 mL/dose) immediately and up to q 15–20 min × 2; also: diphenhydramine 50 mg (children: 1 mg/kg) po or IM q 4–6 h; elevate legs; maintain airway; oxygen; discuss venom immunotherapy or refer to allergist; systemic CSs do not alter lesion size or progression and should not be routinely used (Jaad 2001;44:561).

17.2.B. GRANULOMA ANNULARE

Cause: Unknown but probably immunologic; generalized form assoc w DM (Br J Derm 1984;111:325), thyroid disease, AIDS (Cutis 1995;55:158).

Sx: Mildly itchy.

Si: Pink papules or a ring of BB-sized papules or larger nodules; not scaly; most common over joints, esp elbows, ankles, hands; may be sc (Peds 1997;100:965).

See color plate section.

Crs: Episodes develop over several wk; typically form ring w raised border and flat center; most clear by 2 yr; 1/2 recur.

Lab: Bx (see DX.7.) confirms dx, but bx often unnecessary if si are typical.

Rx: If itchy or unsightly: TCS (class I–III); *not responding*: consider TCS w occlusion (see RX.6.) or TCS incorporated in tape adhesive (Cordran tape, 60/200 cm, $$); IL triamcinolone acetonide (Kenalog, 10 mg/mL) diluted to 2.5–4 mg/mL (see RX.7.); *extensive*: consider PUVA (see RX.15.) (Arch Derm 1997;133:1605).

17.2.C. LICHEN PLANUS

Summary: Multiple pink to purple, flat-topped, itchy papules, often tightly grouped into plaques; look on wrists, lower legs, ankles and for a lacy white patch on buccal mucosa; hypertrophic type: less common; mostly on legs of blacks; thickened, itchy, chronic.

For additional details and rx, see BODY, 3.3.n.

ADULT, PAINFUL, SHINS

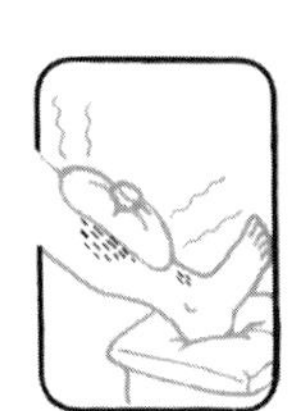

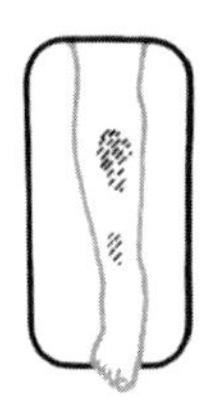

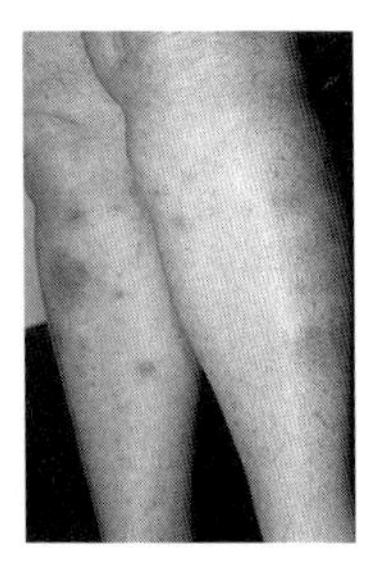

Erythema nodosum

17.3.A. ERYTHEMA NODOSUM

Clin Infect Dis 1995;20:1010. Curr Opin Rheum 1990;2:66.

Cause: Immunologic; antigens assoc; infections: streptococcal, tbc, deep fungal, viral, chlamydia, psittacosis, lymphogranuloma venereum, cat-scratch disease, HIV (J Am Acad Derm 1991;25:113); also, sarcoidosis (Arch Derm 1997;133:882), lymphoma (J Rheum 1990;17:383), colitis, drugs: bcp's, sulfonamides, aspartame, iodides, gold.

Epidem: Most are adults, 20–40 yo; occas children (Ped Derm 1996;13:447); women >>> men.

Sx: Painful, not itchy.

Si: Red to purple; deep nodules; most are only on shins but occas arms; bilateral; multiple.

Crs: Prodrome: malaise, arthralgias; episodes often last 1–3 mo; individual lesions resolve in 2–4 wk; resolve like deep bruises w dusky-greenish yellow; heal w/o ulceration or scarring; up to 1/3 recur.

Cmplc: Leg edema often develops; arthropathy may be severe w pain, swelling, residual stiffness.

Ddx: Resemble cellulitis or abscesses of shins, but do not ulcerate.

Lab: Bx: septal panniculitis; supports dx but not essential if case is typical; may have ↑ wbc w slight left shift; if cause (see above) is not obvious, get chest x-ray, PPD, throat culture, CBC, ESR; cause cannot be identified in half (Med Clin N Am 1998;82:1359).

Rx: Acute episode: sx relief w bed rest, leg elevation, support stocking, analgesia w salicylates or acetaminophen; only consider systemic CS (prednisone 20 mg/d) if systemic infection has been r/o and lesions are disabling; alternatives: SSKI (J Am Acad Derm 1983;9:77) or hydroxychloroquine; confirmation of dx and choice of rx may require dermatology referral.

LEG RASH

17.3.B. VASCULITIS

Summary: Typical lesions: discrete palpable purpuric or petechial; esp legs and buttocks; palmar lesions are painful; ROS and w/u for fever, arthralgias, abdominal pain, or blood in urine or stool.

For additional details, see FEVER, 8.1.n.

ADULT, PAINFUL, CALVES

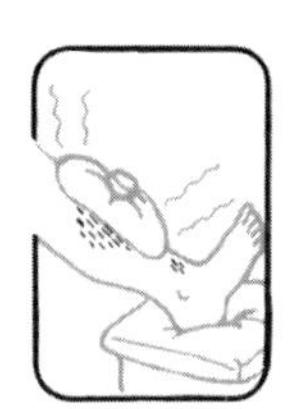

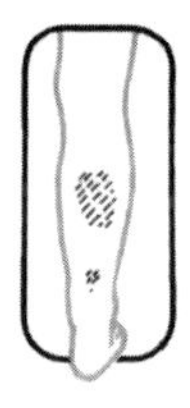

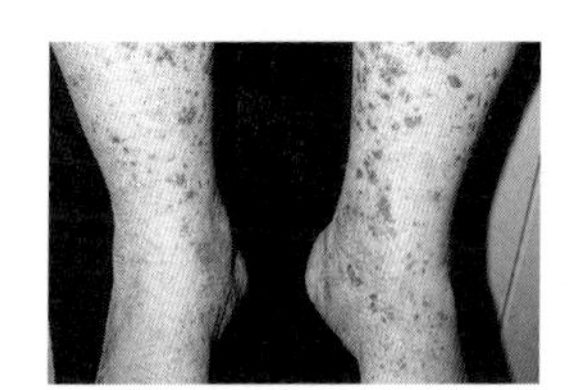

Vasculitis

17.4.A. ERYTHEMA INDURATUM

Summary: Chronic, deep, painful plaques/nodules; lower legs, esp calves; often ulcerate and scar; rare; women >>> men; pathophysiology resembles tbc; search for active tbc elsewhere (J Am Acad Derm 1994;31:288); mycobacteria in lesions have been found by PCR (Am J Dermatopath 1997;19:323; J Am Acad Derm 1997;36:99); rx is anti-tbc therapy; refer to a dermatologist for confirmation of dx and rx.

17.4.B. PANNICULITIS

Summary: General term for inflammation of sc fat; tender firm nodules; various forms: some indolent; some assoc w fever, suppuration, scarring, vasculitis; r/o local trauma; bacterial, fungal, mycobacterial, spirochetal, HIV infections; collagen vascular disease; lymphoma; paraproteinemia; a_1-antitrypsin deficiency; pancreatitis; **fasciitis-panniculitis syndrome**: inflammation, induration, eos fasciitis; dx may require bx, cultures; often difficult to classify; refer to dermatology and rheumatology.

17.4.D. THROMBOPHLEBITIS

Summary: Thrombus formation and inflammation of blood vessel wall; predisposed by surgery, trauma, immobilization, pregnancy, hypercoagulable state, estrogens, neoplasms; most develop in veins, esp varicose veins, but some in arteries; local tenderness; palpable or visible tender "cord"; may ulcerate; $\uparrow$wbc and $\uparrow$ESR; almost no risk of pulmonary embolus from superficial phlebitis; deep vein phlebitis may show as leg edema and pain but often is asx, esp if pt is confined to bed because of surgery or illness; pain during dorsiflexion of foot (Homans' sign) is not a reliable si.

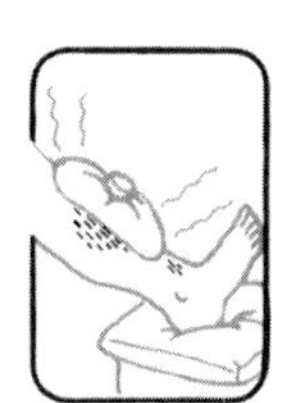
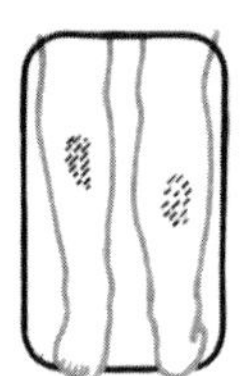
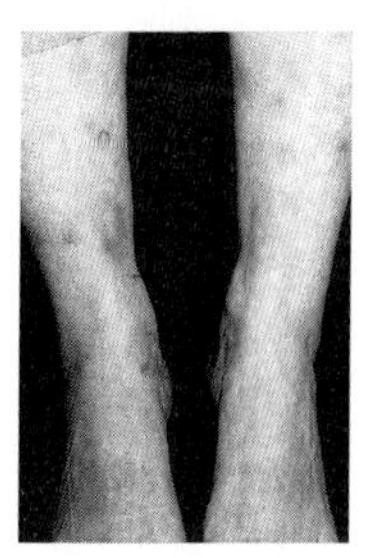

Panniculitis

17.5.A. VASCULITIS

Summary: Typical lesions: discrete palpable purpuric or petechial; esp legs and buttocks; palmar lesions are painful; ROS and w/u for fever, arthralgias, abdominal pain, or blood in urine or stool.

For additional details, see FEVER, 8.1.n.

17.5.B. CELLULITIS, BACTERIAL

Nejm 1996;334:240.

Cause: Usually assoc w chronic stasis; trauma, inc cat/dog bites; chronic lymphedema; underlying disease, esp DM; chronic dermatitis allowing entry of infection, esp tinea pedis; usual bacteria are pathogenic *Staphylococcus aureus, S. pyogenes*, or streptococci, but gram-neg and anaerobic infections also are found.

Sx: Tenderness and pain.

Si: Edema; red; *coin-sized, isolated or few*: furuncles, or abscesses; *larger, deep, and expanding*: cellulitis; ascending lymphangitis: about 20% w cellulitis; unilateral LN↑ in 80%; may be systemic infection: chills, fever, ↑ wbc.

Crs: Begins abruptly; single episodes clear w rx; recurrences are common if predisposing factors persist.

Cmplc: Recurrence may lead to chronic lymphedema and fibrosis.
Ddx: Distinguish from **varicose eczema**: patchy and itchy dermatitis w/o fever or pain; common in winter in older persons; assoc w varicose veins; Rx w support stockings and TCS (BMJ 1999;318:1672); **Group A Streptoccal Necrotizing Fasciitis** "flesh-eating disease": rare, but highly destructive and potentially lethal; assoc w severe, unrelenting pain unresponsive to NSAIDs, fever, tachycardia, GI sx, myalgias, ↓ BP; confirm w blood culture, MRI; surgical debridement and clindamycin + penicillin may be effective (Infect Med 2001;18:198).
Lab: C + s not necessary for single or isolated furuncles but may be appropriate if lesions are draining or are multiple, recurrent, or appeared while pt was hospitalized, esp if pt is immunocompromised (often gram-neg); culture of deep lesions may require punch bx; culture attempts using a small syringe and flushing deep tissue w sterile saline free of preservatives and antibacterial agents may be tried but is usually not productive (pos <20%) (Arch Derm 1991;127:493).
Rx: Depends on organism; antibiotics, po or iv: dicloxacillin, erythromycin, nafcillin, cephalexin, or cefazolin; *animal bites*: ampicillin-clavulanate, ampicillin-sulbactam, cefoxitin; recurrent episodes are cellulitis and lymphangitis: consider prophylactic monthly im benzathine penicillin or qd po erythromycin.

ADULT, ASYMPTOMATIC

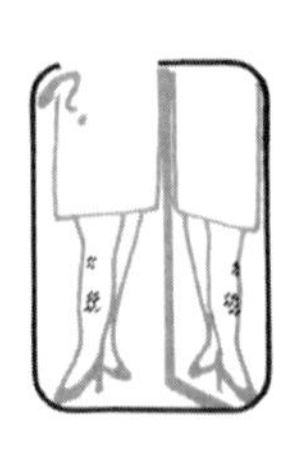

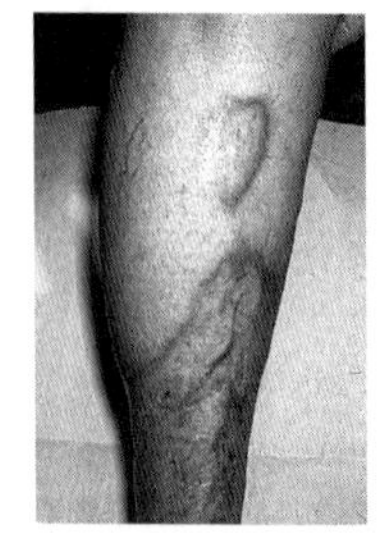

Necrobiosis lipoidica

17.6.A. VERRUCA VULGARIS (COMMON WARTS)

Summary: Single to multiple; surface is raised, rough, cauliflower like; pinhead to dime sized; most are on hands, feet, face; usually painless unless periungual or fingertip; may be easily traumatized.

For additional details and rx, see HANDS, 14.1.a.

17.6.B. VERRUCA PLANA (FLAT WARTS)

Cause: Transmissible HPV; antigenic type distinct from other warts.

Epidem: Both children and adults are susceptible.

Sx: Asx.

Si: Few to hundreds; smooth, round, slightly raised; 1 to few mm; like droplets of dried, skin-colored rubber cement; mostly on face, backs of hands, shins.

Crs: Steadily ↑ in number; spread by autoinoculation; tend to disappear spontaneously in children but are more persistent in adults.

Ddx: Lichen planus, esp in children.

Lab: None, but bx occasionally needed to confirm dx (see DX.7.).

Rx: *If few*: thin coat of salicylic acid/lactic acid in flexible collodion (Duofilm, Salactic Film, or Viranol, OTC) hs; defer when irritation develops, then restart; *if numerous or unresponsive*: tretinoin cr (Retin-A, 15/45 gm, Rx, $$) hs–bid, aim for mild irritation of warts w/o inducing uncomfortable irritation of normal skin, clearing may take mos; *large lesions*: may require light D&C or LN2 cryotherapy; avoid more aggressive surgical procedures that might cause scarring; use of electric razor or depilatory, rather than blade shaving, to ↓ nicking and autoinoculation; refer pts w large numbers of warts or those resistant to rx to dermatology.

17.6.C. GRANULOMA ANNULARE

Summary: Typically, lesions appear in ring of pink BB-sized papules; w/o scaling; most common on extensor surfaces, ie, elbows, shins, and hands; may be itchy; papules usually spread out over several wk w raised border and flat center; 1/2–3/4 of cases spontaneously remit by 2 yr; nearly 1/2 of pts have recurrences.

For additional details and rx, see 17.2.b.

17.6.D. DIABETIC DERMOPATHY

Int J Derm 1998; 37:113.

Summary: Multiple; red to brown; <1 cm; scaly patches and depressed, atrophic depressions, like healed trauma; shins; asx; assoc w DM; microangiopathy; rx not available.

17.6.E. NECROBIOSIS LIPOIDICA

J Am Acad Derm 1994;30:519. J Am Acad Derm 1991;25:735. J Am Acad Derm 1988;18:530.

Cause: Unknown; strongly assoc w DM: 2/3 have DM; 1/2 of rest have pre-DM by GTT (Jama 1966;195:433); more recent studies show lower (25%) assoc w DM (Br J Derm 1999;140:283); angiopathy w granuloma formation that progresses to atrophy.

Epidem: Uncommon; <0.5% of DM; most are insulin-dependent DM rather than those controlled by diet; women >> men; children: assoc w DM complications (Ped Derm 1995;12:220).

Sx: Asx unless painful ulcerations develop.

Si: Plaques; yellowish-pink tint; fine surface telangiectasias; slightly depressed, sometimes raised; 1 or 2 or several; shins and occas arms and elsewhere.

Crs: Chronic and progressive; progression is not affected by tight control of blood sugar.

Lab: Bx not necessary if appearance is typical as healing of bx may be slow or bx may ulcerate.

Rx: None usually, as rx is not effective and lesions are asx; improve glucose control; if active inflammation, consider TCS and occas IL CS but further atrophy and ulceration are a risk; skin grafts may be needed if ulcerated; consider dermatology consultation.

17.6.F. SARCOID

Summary: Mimics other eruptions; most are pink to yellow; firm papules or plaques; pinhead to pea sized or larger; usually nape, face, extensor surfaces; may be scaly when on legs; minimal itching; may develop within preexisting scars; sometimes severe and may distort facial features; may be deep; may ulcerate; may lead to local hair loss; blacks >> whites; may 1st manifest as erythema nodosum: infiltrated, painful plaques over shins (see 17.3.a.).

For additional details and rx, see BODY, 3.3.o.

17.6.G. STASIS DERMATITIS

Summary: Painful but not so severe as to interfere w sleep; pain of arterial insufficiency is worsened by elevation; that from venous insufficiency is worsened by dependency; leg edema; brown, speckled pigmentation from hemosiderin; dry scaling and itching precede ulcer, if present (for leg ulcer, see ULCER—LEG, 25.2.a.(1).); palpable pedal pulses suggest venous rather than arterial cause; varicosities nearly always present; support stockings provide compression of superficial veins, as well as protection from minor injury; the best are labeled as supplying 20–40 mm of pressure but are expensive ($70 and not covered by most insurers) and difficult to put on, but an acceptable alternative can be purchased in local pharmacies for about $20 (Jobst and Sigvaris); **varicose eczema**: patchy and itchy dermatitis w/o fever or pain; common in winter in older persons; assoc w varicose veins; Rx w support stockings and TCS (BMJ 1999;318:1672).

For additional details and rx, see ULCER—LEG, 25.2.a.1.

17.6.H. CAPILLARITIS (SCHAMBERG'S DISEASE, PROGRESSIVE PIGMENTARY DERMATOSIS)

Cause: Unknown; not assoc w cardiac or vascular disease; noninflammatory leakage of small capillaries.

Epidem: men>>women; often assoc w varicose veins.

Sx: Asx; sometimes slight itching.

Si: Fine, pinhead sized, cayenne pepper colored, puncta due to hemosiderin; diffuse, usually confined to lower shins and ankles, occasionally more widespread.

17.6.h. Capillaritis (Schamberg's disease, progressive pigmentary dermatosis), continued

Crs: Sudden onset which causes pt concern; slowly resolves over months as the iron from leaked rbcs is cleared; often recurs, even years later.

Cmplc: None.

DiffDx: Hyperglobulemic purpura; drug rxn: arsenic, atropine, bismuth, barbiturates, carbromal, chloramphenicol, chlorothiazide, chlorpromazine, diethyl stilbestrol, gold, hair dye, isoniazid, iodides, menthol, meprobamate, paraaminosalicylic acid, piperazine, quinidine, quinine, reserpine, snake venoms, sodium salicylate, sulfonamides, tartrazine and other food additives, thiouracil, tolbutamide and glyceryl trinitrate (Arch Derm 1974;109:49).

Lab: Bx or coagulation studies not necessary.

Rx: None; reassurance; support stockings may help.

18 Light Reactions

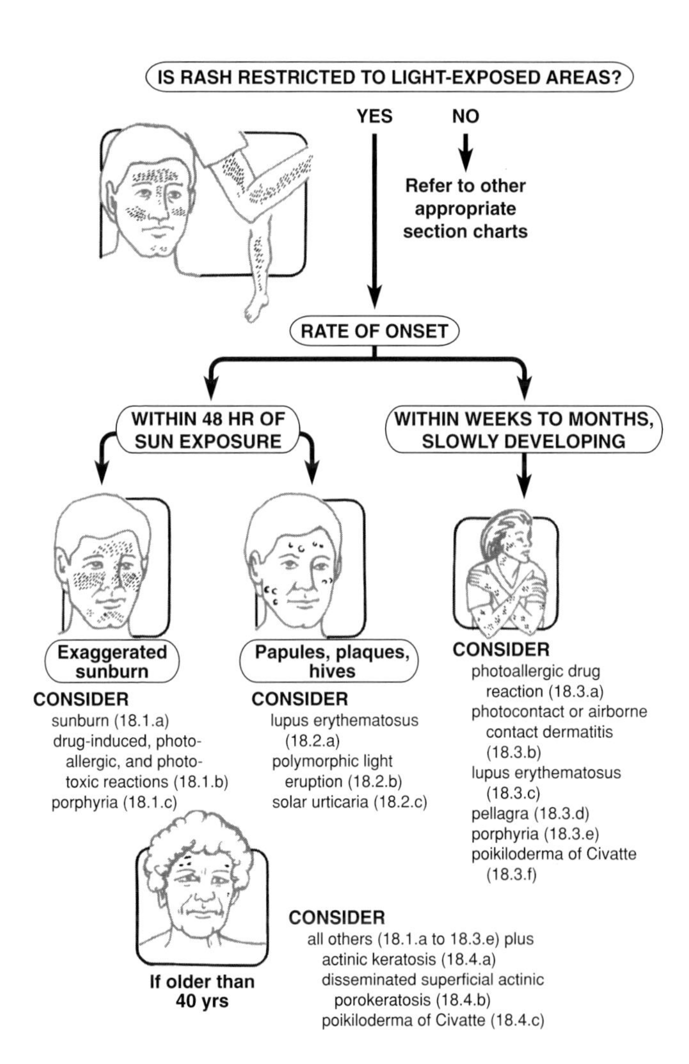

UV light is destructive radiation; there is no "safe" level of UV light exposure; tanning is a response to injury rather than nature's gift to beauty; melanin is skin's major protection against UV light, as is shown by ↑ frequency of skin cancers in albinos and ↓ wrinkling and ↓ frequency of skin cancers in blacks.

- *UVB*: short wave (290–320 nm); 10% of sun's energy that reaches earth, but about 1000 × > UVA to cause sunburn; leads to burning; acute and chronic damage, esp burns, wrinkling, and most BCEs and SCCs; also induces vitamin D synthesis, now only an incidental benefit because of fortified foods.
- *UVA*: long wave (320–400 nm); most of energy in UV light; leads to tanning; interferes w immune tumor suppression (J Natl Cancer Inst 1990;82:1392).

(Review: Dx of photosensitivity Arch Derm 2000;136:1152).

ONSET WITHIN 48 HOURS OF EXPOSURE, EXAGGERATED SUNBURN

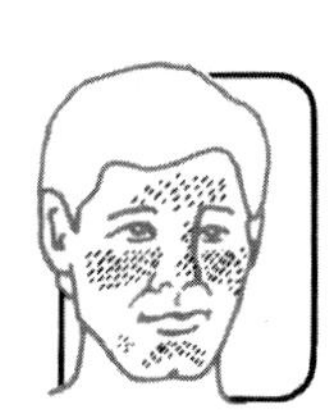

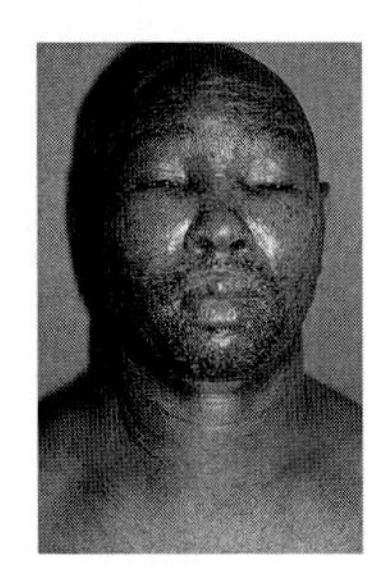

Photoallergy to tetracycline

18.1.A. SUNBURN

Summary: UVB plus external or systemic photosensitizer; pain, tenderness; red; maximal in 12–24 h; if severe: skin may blister or peel 1 d to several d later; heals w/o scarring unless 2° infection occurs; exaggerated response w an unexpected "burn": suspect concomitant photosensitizer (see 18.1.b.); tx: ASA or ibuprofen to ↓ pain and ↓ inflammatory rxn; soothe extensive burns w a 20-min colloidal oatmeal bath, made by adding 1/2 cup of Aveeno oatmeal (450 gm, OTC) to lukewarm or cool bath water; try to leave blister roofs intact as a pain-reducing biologic dressing; TCSs or systemic CSs provide no benefit; for sun protection, see RX.16.

18.1.B. DRUG-INDUCED, PHOTOALLERGIC, AND PHOTOTOXIC REACTIONS

J Am Acad Derm 1996;35:871. J Am Acad Derm 1995;33:551.

Cause: Aberrant responses to sunlight: either an exaggerated sunburn rxn or dermatitis, ie, hives, plaques, patches, or scaling; most common is PMLE (see 18.2.b.), but also solar urticaria (see 18.2.c.), porphyria (see 18.1.c.), LE (see 18.2.a.).

Sx: Pain if sunburn, or itching if dermatitis.

Si: Sun-exposed areas only; upper eyelids, neck under chin tend to be clear; if drug related: *exaggerated sunburn*: phototoxic; *dermatitis*: photoallergic.

Lab: Testing to discriminate between phototoxic and photoallergic rxns not often necessary as hx and appearance usually suffice; further evaluation requires referral to dermatologist.

Rx: Identify photo-inducing agent:

- Systemic drugs assoc w phototoxicity (Levine JI, Medications that increase sensitivity to light, Food and Drug Administration, Publication 91-8280, 1990).

Antibiotics

Ciprofloxacin
Griseofulvin
Sulfa drugs
Tetracyclines

Anticancer Drugs

Actinomycin
Dacarbazine
Doxorubicin
5-FU
Hydroxyurea
MTX
Procarbazine
Vinblastine

Antidepressants/Antipsychotics

"Amines"
Amoxapine
Doxepin
Isocarboxazid
Tricyclic antidepressants
Triptylines

Antihistamines

Brompheniramine
Carbinoxamine
Cetirizine
Chlorpheniramine
Cyproheptadine
Diphenhydramine
Loratadine
Terfenadine

Cardiovascular

Amiodarone
Beta-blockers
Bumetanide
Captopril
Diltiazem
Disopyramide
Enalapril
Methyldopa
Nifedipine
Verapamil

Diuretics

Amiloride
Chlorthalidone
Furosemide
Metolazone
Quinethazone
Thiazides

Hormones

Estrogens
Progestogens

Hypoglycemics

Acetohexamide
Chlorpropamide
Glipizide
Glyburide
Tolazamide
Tolbutamide

Lipid lowering agents

Clofibrate
Fenofibrate
Simvastatin

NSAIDs

Diclofenac
Indomethacin
Naproxen
Phenylbutazone
Profens
Piroxicam
Sulindac

18.1.C. PORPHYRIA

Summary: Eruption is sharply limited to sun-exposed areas; 2 major forms affect skin as well as a very rare congenital erythropoietic type.

18.1.C.(1). PORPHYRIA CUTANEA TARDA (PCT)

Br J Derm 1999;140:573. Clin Derm 1998;16:251,295. Lancet 1997;349:1613. Derm Clin 1993;11:583.

Cause: Defect: ↓ hepatic uroporphyrinogen decarboxylase; usually assoc w acquired liver insufficiency and liver cirrhosis; *men*: chronic alcoholism; *women*: alcoholism, estrogen med; provoked by iron overload, hepatitis; ↑ assoc w hepatitis C infection (J Am Acad Derm 1999;41:31; Arch Derm 1996;132:1503); ↑ assoc w hemochromatosis; hepatoma; DM; end-stage renal disease on hemodialysis (J Am Acad Derm 1993;29:499); HIV (J Am Acad Derm 1992;26:857); autosomal dominant enzyme deficiency underlies some cases.

Epidem: Most common porphyria (1:70,000).

Si: *Acute*: blisters, edema, restricted to sun-exposed skin; skin is fragile and shears or bruises easily from mild trauma; thin scars at sites of previously healed blisters; *later*: ↑ pigmentation, milia, thickening, ↑ hair in chronically light-exposed parts, esp glabella, temples, pinna, leading to "werewolf" appearance; urine may appear dark, like red wine, esp w flares.

Crs: Episodes start several to 24 h after exposure; pattern develops slowly over many mo.

Ddx: Photosensitivity, indistinguishable from PCT, develops in some pts w chronic renal failure on hemodialysis (Jaad 2000;43:975).

Lab: Submit screening test for urine porphyrins to commercial lab; urinary porphyrins may be WNL during clinical remission and only fecal porphyrins will be abn; quantitative tests: both uroporphyrins and coproporphyrins are ↑; uroporphyrins > coproporphyrins; further evaluation: LFTs; serum iron; TIBC; consider CT of liver and liver bx; generally consult w dermatology, hematology, GI specialties.

Rx: Can remit w/o specific rx if alcoholism or DM is controlled or if a causal med is dc'd; reduce excess iron stores w phlebotomy; iron chelators and chloroquine have been used but have risks; rx of PCT usually is undertaken at medical centers or in consultation w appropriate specialists.

Contact American Porphyria Foundation (POB 22712, Houston, TX 77227; 713.266.9617; www.enterprise.net/apf) for pt support information.

18.1.C.(2). ERYTHROPOIETIC PROTOPORPHYRIA (EPP)

Summary: Rare; autosomal dominant deficiency in activity of bone marrow heme synthetase; itching, burning, redness; immediately after sun exposure; fragile skin w/o blisters; pebbly scars develop; childhood onset; ↑ protoporphyrins in rbc's, feces, but not in urine; exposure of internal organs to OR lights during surgery has led to internal burns and severe complications; as condition is dramatic, most cases would be dx and followed at medical centers w special interest (Br J Derm 1999;140:573).

ONSET WITHIN 48 HOURS OF EXPOSURE, PAPULES/PLAQUES/HIVES

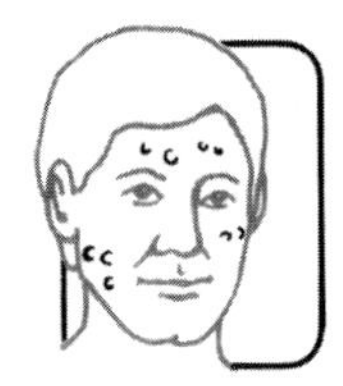

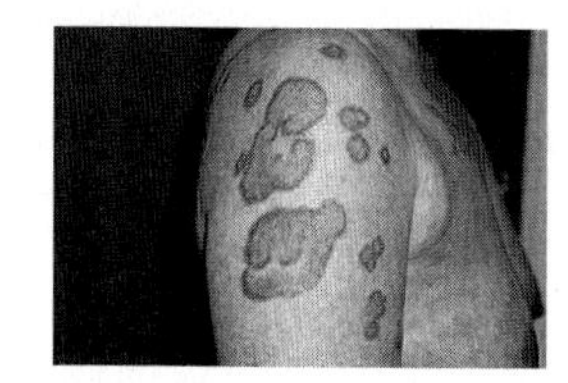

Subacute cutaneous lupus erythematosus

18.2.A. LUPUS ERYTHEMATOSUS (LE)

Summary: May flare after sunlight exposure; mostly involve light-exposed areas.

- *DLE*: pink to red; slightly scaly; often have areas of atrophy, esp in center, that are shiny, depressed, depigmented, hairless (see FACE, 6.2.c.).
- *SLE*: 60%–75% are photosensitive, most to UVB (J Am Acad Derm 1990;22:181); face or hands; pink, scaly, edematous; subset of pts w SLE (Ro pos) are highly sensitive to sunlight, but have ↓ likelihood to develop systemic, vascular, renal complications (see FEVER, 8.3.a); dx is confirmed by bx and ANA testing; also consider dermatomyositis (see FEVER, 8.3.b.).

For additional w/u and rx, see FACE, 6.2.c., and FEVER, 8.3.a.

18.2.B. POLYMORPHIC LIGHT ERUPTION (PMLE)

Semin Derm 1990;9:32. J Am Acad Derm 1980;3:329.

Cause: "Allergic" rxn to light; some evoked by UVA, some by UVB, some by visible light (400–800 nm).

Epidem: 10% of normal persons; most evident in whites; rare in children.

Si: Several forms: elevated papules, nodules, urticaria, scaly dermatitis; restricted to light-exposed areas: face, nape, V of neck, back of hands, shins in women; atrophy does not develop.

Crs: Appears w 1st intense sun exposure of season: spring or during a winter vacation in tropics; most improve and even clear completely w continued exposure over summer; some persist or worsen; recurrences each spring and summer are typical; tendency may persist for life.

Lab: Not necessary; hx confirms dx; occas skin bx to r/o LE; ask about potentially photoreactive drugs; specialized irradiation instruments are available at some dermatology offices and medical centers to determine inducing wavelengths, necessary to set up prevention plans.

Rx: If *UVB induced*: sunscreens are useful; if *UVA or visible light induced*: sunscreens less useful; tell pt to seek broad-spectrum products; dc photosensitizing meds (see 18.1.b.).

- Prior to winter vacation in tropics: pt may benefit from induction of tolerance by tanning or a short course of antimalarial hydroxychloroquine (Plaquenil, 200 mg) bid for 3 d before and during trip (J Am Acad Derm 1981;4:650); TCSs help during flares; systemic CS (prednisone, 40–60 mg/d) may be necessary.

18.2.C. SOLAR URTICARIA

Summary: Itching and burning followed by hives; within min of light exposure; hives last h or so; inciting wavelengths differ between pts; relative resistance to repeated irradiation for few d after severe rxn; rare; most in young adults; pts suspected of having this disorder need specialized phototesting and specialty care (J Am Acad Derm 1989;21:237).

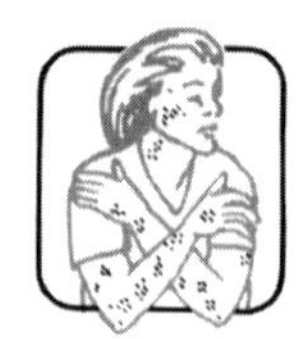

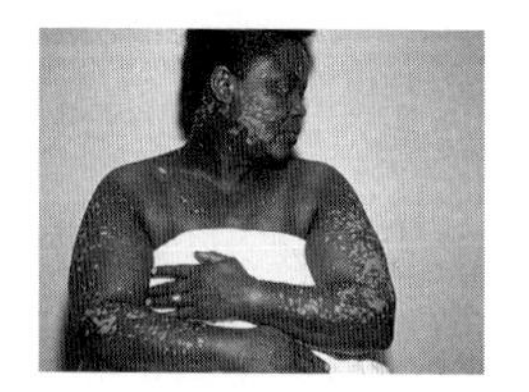

Photosensitivity to cyclamate

18.3.A. PHOTOALLERGIC DRUG REACTION

Summary: Non-sunburn rxn: papules, plaques, hives, or dermatitis; onset is delayed until drug sensitivity develops plus seasonal exposure to sunlight; therefore, pt often is not aware of the association (see 18.1.b.).

18.3.B. PHOTOCONTACT OR AIRBORNE CONTACT DERMATITIS

Summary: Limited to exposed skin: arms, face, neck; often chronic; rash usually itchy w scaling, hyperpigmentation, lichenification; cause is often airborne allergen, ie, ragweed; distribution similar to photodermatitis; ddx: regions protected from light, ie, skin below nose and chin and in eye sockets, are involved w airborne contactants but not photo-rxns; airborne contact rxns may also involve covered parts to which antigen was spread, ie, genitalia, which remain clear in photo-rxns; determination of cause requires patch testing and photo testing; refer pts to dermatologist or allergist.

18.3.C. LUPUS ERYTHEMATOSUS (LE)

Summary: DLE: slow to exacerbate after sun exposure, taking wks or mos (see FACE, 6.2.c.); SLE or photosensitive Ro-pos LE: acute flares may develop within hrs or days of exposure (see FEVER, 8.3.a.).

18.3.D. PELLAGRA

Summary: Deficiency of nicotinic acid, niacin, or its precursor, tryptophan; rare except in assoc w poor diet, esp w alcoholism or tea-and-toast diet of elderly; GI malabsorption; anti-tbc rx w isoniazid, which competes w nicotinic acid; some pts w carcinoid syndrome because tryptophan is diverted to serotonin production; scaly dermatitis and dusky brown pigmentation on sun-exposed parts, esp face, neck, backs of hands; diarrhea; dementia; oral fissures and ulcers; redness and swelling of tongue; muscle weakness; depression; fatal if not treated; if nutritional, reverses rapidly on normal diet (Semin Derm 1991;10:282).

18.3.E. PORPHYRIA

Summary: Although sunlight-induced reactivity may be present for mos or more, pts may not seek medical help until 2° changes, ie, scarring, hyperpigmentation, hirsutism, develop (see 18.1.c.).

18.3.F. POIKILODERMA OF CIVATTE

Cause: Chronic sun exposure.

Epidem: Fair skinned persons; women > men.

Sx: None.

Si: Reticulated hyperpigmentation on the sides of the neck w telangiectasias and light and dark areas, resembling post X-radiation; the area under the chin, shaded from the sun, is notably more normal in appearance.

Crs: Persists.
Lab:
Rx: None available although laser is being tried at some centers.

PATIENT >40 YEARS OLD

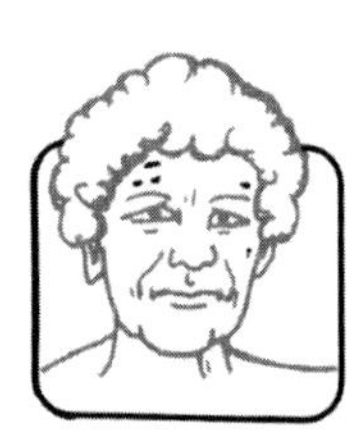

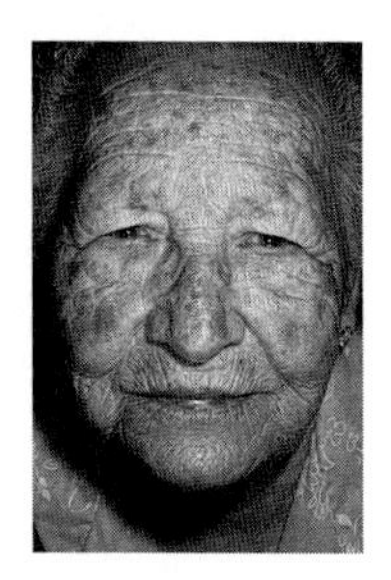

Actinic keratosis

18.4.A. ACTINIC KERATOSIS

Summary: Discrete; persistent; scaly, pink to red; esp in light-complexioned persons >40 yo; hx of excessive sun exposure; considered premalignant but few become SCC.

For additional details and rx, see GROWTHS, 11.11.a.

18.4.B. DISSEMINATED SUPERFICIAL ACTINIC POROKERATOSIS (DSAP)

Summary: Autosomal dominant; triggered by chronic light exposure; numerous scaly patches; brownish red; thread-like raised edge; up to a dime in size; most on arms and legs of light-complexioned, middle-aged women; appears or flares during summer; ↑ w age; dx confirmed by bx; LN2 sometimes effective (J Am Acad Derm 1989;20:1015).

18.4.C. POIKILODERMA OF CIVATTE

Summary: Reticulated hyperpigmentation on the sides of the neck w telangiectasias and light and dark areas, resembling post X-radiation; the area under the chin, shaded from the sun, is notably more normal in appearance; most evident >40 yo, but may appear earlier (see above, 18.3.f.).

19 Mouth

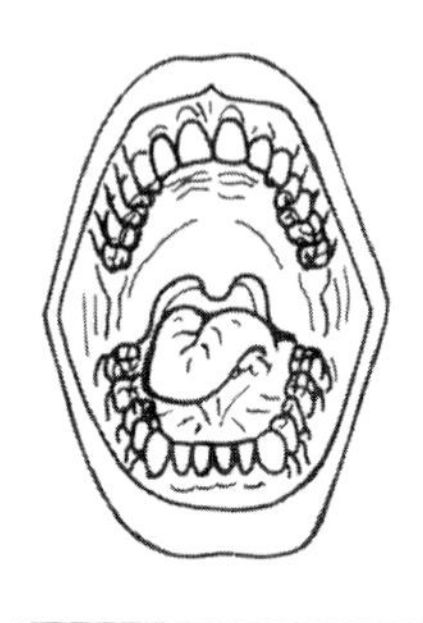

LESSIONS TO CONSIDER IN ALL LOCATIONS

Painful

Erosion, ulcer

CONSIDER

COMMON

aphthous stomatitis (19.1.a)
herpangina (19.1.b)
herpetic gingivostomatitis, primary (19.1.c)
erythema multiforme (19.1.d)
chemical burns (19.1.e)
candida infection (19.1.f)

UNCOMMON

pemphigus, pemphigoid (19.1.g)
Behçet's syndrome (19.1.h)
lichen planus (19.1.i)
lupus erythematosus (19.1.j)
syphilis (19.1.k)

Painless

Growth

CONSIDER

fibroma (19.2.a)
hemangioma (19.2.b)
pyogenic granuloma (19.2.c)
syphilis (19.1.k)
leukoplakia (19.2.e)
erythroplakia (19.2.f)
Kaposi's sarcoma (19.2.g)
cancer (19.2.h)

Burning, dryness

CONSIDER

xerostomia (19.3)
Sjögren's syndrome (19.3)

LESIONS TO CONSIDER IN SPECIFIC LOCATION

TONGUE

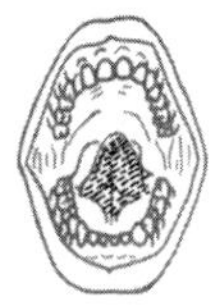

Burning, dryness
vitamin B deficiency (19.4.a)

Color change (and fuzzy)
candida infection (19.4.b)
hairy tongue (19.4.c)
hairy leukoplakia (19.4.d)

Deformed (chronic)
median rhomboid glossitis (19.4.e)
fissured tongue (19.4.f)
geographic tongue (19.4.g)

CHEEKS AND SOFT PALATE

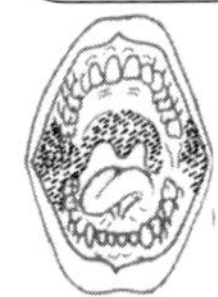

Dark ← Color Change → Light

Dark:
Addison's disease (19.5.a)
racial pigmentation (19.5.b)
hemangioma (19.5.c)
nevus, melanocytic (19.5.d)
metals, pigmentation (19.5.e)

Light:
Fordyce spots (19.5.f)
candida infection (19.4.b)
linea alba (19.5.h)
lichen planus (19.1.i)
white sponge nevus (19.5.j)

Painless growths
epulis (19.5.k)

GINGIVA AND HARD PALATE

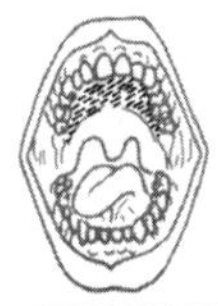

Inflammation
ANUG (19.6.a)

Dark ← Color Change → Light

Dark:
see misc (19.6.b)

Light:
candida infection (19.4.b)

Painless growths
torus palatinus (19.6.d)
parulis (19.6.e)

FLOOR OF MOUTH

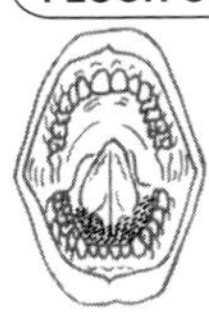

Painless growths
torus mandibularis (19.7.a)

LIPS

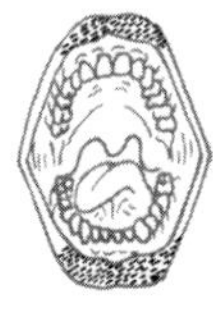

Inflammation
herpes labialis (19.8.a)
candida infection (19.4.b)
vitamin deficiency (19.4.a)
ill-fitting dentures

Burning, dryness
angular cheilitis (19.8.e)
cheilitis (19.8.f)

Light spots
Fordyce spots (19.8.g)
vitiligo (21.2.a)

Painless growths
mucocele (19.8.i)
vascular lesions (19.8.j)
verruca vulgaris (19.8.k)

Written in collaboration with Marc W. Heft, DMD, PhD, Professor, and James G. Green, MD, DDS, Associate Professor, Department of Oral and Maxillofacial Surgery and Diagnostic Services, University of Florida, Gainesville, Florida.

PAINFUL EROSIONS OR ULCERS, ANY LOCATION

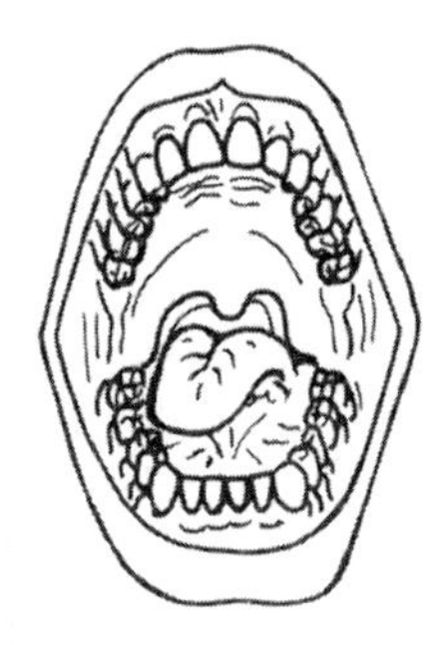

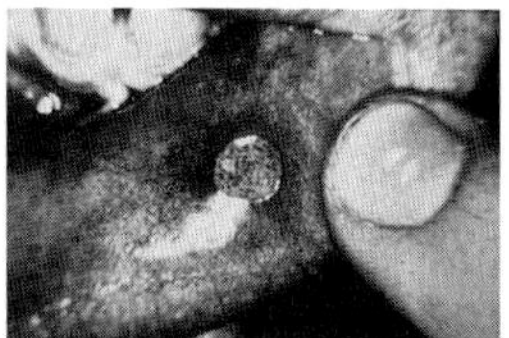

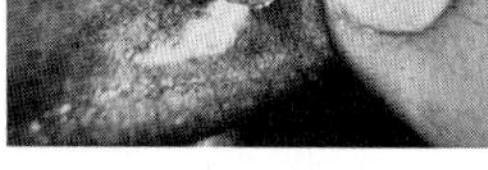

Aphthous stomatitis

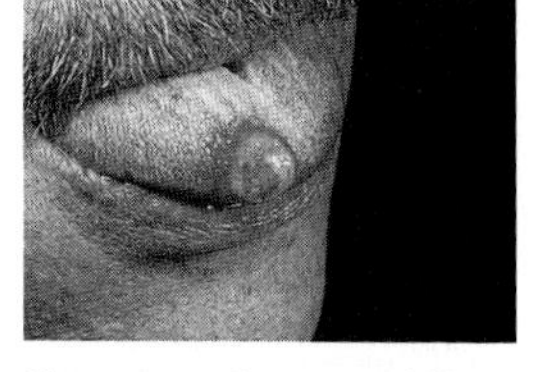

Chancre—primary syphilis

19.1.A. APHTHOUS STOMATITIS (CANKER SORES)

J Oral Path Med 1991;20:395. Curr Probl Derm 1991;3:107.

Cause: Unknown; may search for underlying disease; nutritional deficiency, Behçet's syndrome (see 19.1.h.) if genital ulcers and uveitis are present; Crohn's disease; celiac disease; ↑ numbers and depth in HIV-pos pts (Ann IM 1988;109:388).

Sx: Painful, often out of proportion to size of lesion.

Si: Crateriform fibrinous ulcerations w red halo on nonkeratinized portions of mouth (cheeks, tongue, floor of mouth, soft palate) but not gingiva or hard palate; *minor form*: 1–5 small ulcers <1 cm or clusters; *major form*: 1–10 lesions, larger, 1–5 cm.

Crs: Chronic, recurrent; *minor form*: clears 7–14 d w/o scarring; *major form*: may persist >6 wk and heal w scarring.

Lab: None.

Rx: TCS (dexamethasone 0.01% elixir, fluocinonide oint 0.05%); sx relief: topical local anesthetics (viscous lidocaine (Xylocaine), dyclonine); thalidomide has been used in HIV-pos pts (Nejm 1997;336:1487); refer pts w large or persistent ulcers to oral specialist.

19.1.B. HERPANGINA

J Peds 178;93:492.

Cause: Coxsackieviruses (A, B, echoviruses).

Epidem: Mostly infants or young children.

Sx: Fever, sore throat, headache, anorexia, myalgia, vomiting, malaise.

Si: 10–12 red macules that quickly form 2–4-mm blisters on tonsils, soft palate, pharynx; quickly rupture to leave painful gray ulcers w red halo.

Crs: Blisters appear 2 d after onset of sx; rupture in 1–2 d and heal in 7–10 d.

Lab: Culture and specific antibody titer are available; sometimes obtained by oral specialist in questionable cases.

Rx: None needed; maintain fluids.

19.1.C. HERPETIC GINGIVOSTOMATITIS, PRIMARY

Oral Surg Omop 1989;68:701.

Summary: *Herpesvirus hominis*, type 1 (usually) or 2; mostly infants and children, occasionally adults; vesicles, blisters, crusts; fever, malaise, irritability, sore throat; children: oral cavity; adults: pharyngotonsillitis; cervical LN↑.

For additional details and rx, see BLISTERS, 2.1.a.

19.1.D. ERYTHEMA MULTIFORME

Summary: Red, blistering, eroded lesions on lips, tongue, palate, cheeks; mouth may be bloody, crusted, swollen; look for multiple, target-shaped lesions on body as well.

For additional details and rx, see BLISTERS, 2.1.b.

19.1.E. CHEMICAL BURNS

Jama 1989;119:279. J Oral Ther 1965;2:101.

Summary: Tender reddening at site of trauma, turning to white film; trigger usually is obvious, includes local rx for toothache or chemical rxn to chemical in recent dental procedure; rx w topical protective coating, ie, Orabase Plain or benzocaine.

19.1.F. *CANDIDA* INFECTION (MONILIASIS, THRUSH, PERLÈCHE)

BMJ 2000;321:225; Jada 1992;123:77. Oral Surg Omop 1992;74:41.

Cause: *Candida albicans*; more severe in immunosuppressed, ie, DM, cancer, HIV pos, CS, broad-spectrum antibiotics.

Si: Forms: *acute pseudomembranous*: curdlike white patches that scrape off leaving a red, bleeding base; *acute atrophic*: multiple red lesions w loss of filiform papillae; *chronic atrophic*: usually confined to denture areas, esp palate; *angular cheilitis (perlèche)*: moist, split, commissures of mouth, esp in older pts.

Rx: *Topical*: nystatin oral suspension 1 tsp swished in mouth and swallowed qid for 7 d (100 000 units/mL, 60 mL, Rx, $); clotrimazole lozenges (clotrimazole, Mycelex Troche, 70 tab, pregnancy category B) dissolved slowly in mouth 5/d × 2 wk; systemic: ketoconazole (Sporanox, Rx, $$) bid × 2 wk or fluconazole (Diflucan, Rx, $$) qd–bid × 2 wk (see RX.11); *denture note*: add nystatin oral suspension to water overnight while soaking.

For additional details, see GROIN RASH, 10.2.a.

19.1.G. PEMPHIGUS VULGARIS, BULLOUS PEMPHIGOID, BENIGN MUCOUS MEMBRANE (CICATRICIAL) PEMPHIGOID

Oral Surg Omop 1993;76:453. J Oral Path Med 1990;19:16.

Summary: Group of immunologic disorders presenting w blisters, ulcers, painful erosions; individual or clusters; on oral mucosa, gingiva, may involve conjunctivae, larynx, other mucosal surfaces; skin lesions usually coexist; obtain oral surgical, ophthalmologic, and/or dermatologic consultation.

For additional details, see BLISTERS, 2.4.d.

19.1.H. BEHÇET'S SYNDROME

Jaad 1999;41:540; J Am Acad Derm 1999;40:1. Lancet 1990;335:1078. J Am Acad Derm 1988;19:767.

Cause: Unknown; probably immunologic.

Epidem: Most common in Middle East; genetics or environment may be important.

Sx: Painful oral, genital ulcers.

Si: Oral, genital ulcers; 0.5–3 cm; also uveitis; cutaneous vasculitis; erythema nodosum (Jaad 1999;41:540); migratory thrombophlebitis; arthritis (50%); GI w pain, diarrhea, bloating (40%); cardiac; renal; variety of neurologic changes and peripheral neuropathy; sterile pustule at site of minor trauma, ie, following blood drawing.

Crs: Chronic w episodic flare-ups; si vary over time; usually benign but may be fatal; high morbidity from ulcerations and ocular disease that may lead to blindness.

Lab: None diagnostic; skin bx: vasculitis and thrombosis; dx is clinical, difficult, often delayed.

Rx: Pts need multiple specialty referrals; rx may include systemic CS, colchicine, dapsone, MTX, thalidomide.

19.1.I. LICHEN PLANUS

BMJ 2000;321:225; Oral Surg Omop 1991;2:665. J Oral Path 1988;7:213.

Cause: Unknown; some from systemic meds.

Sx: Asx usually; bullous, atrophic, and erosive forms are painful.

Si: Network of interlacing or spidery, fine, white or bluish-white lines or streaks on buccal mucosa and/or tongue; erosive, plaque, atrophic, bullous forms exist; usually typical lichen planus on skin.

Crs: Persistent or sometimes episodic; may change form w time.

Cmplc: Erosive oral lichen planus has possible assoc w SCC.

Lab: Bx by oral surgeon.

Rx: Most cases are referred to dermatology and/or dentistry for confirmation of dx and rx.

For lichen planus involving skin, see BODY, 3.3.n.

19.1.J. LUPUS ERYTHEMATOSUS (LE)

Summary: Oral lesions of LE most commonly on buccal mucosa, lips, tongue; lesions show central reddening, depression, or atrophic areas, surrounded by a 2–4-mm, white, elevated border; interlacing white striae may extend beyond white border, resembling lichen planus; persistent.

For additional details and rx, see FACE, 6.2.c., and FEVER, 8.3.a.

19.1.K. SYPHILIS

Dentistry 1986;6:7. Oral Surg Omop 1967;23:45.

Summary:

- 1°: 3 wk after infection; intraoral, esp lips, tongue, gums, pharynx; painless or painful; lymphadenitis common.
- 2°: 6 wk after 1°; multiple, painless, grayish white, eroded "mucous patches."
- 3°: gumma; painless nodule that grows w destruction; 3–10 yr after 1°; midline of tongue, palate; palate perforation (other causes are

injury, cancer, chrome toxicity); 3° is most common syphilitic lesion seen in mouth; refer for bx to confirm dx and r/o cancer.

For additional details and rx, see BODY, 3.1.f., and GENITAL, 9.2.a.

GROWTHS, PAINLESS, ANY LOCATION

19.2.A. FIBROMA

Cause: Chronic irritation.

Si: Smooth, pink, firm, sessile, or pedunculated mass on tongue, cheek, palate, gums; usually <1.5 cm; most common benign soft-tissue growth in oral cavity.

Crs: Persistent, slowly growing.

Rx: Excision, usually by an oral surgeon, to eliminate irritation or establish dx.

19.2.B. HEMANGIOMA

Summary: Blue to red vascular lesions that are present from birth or shortly afterward; some assoc w neurologic complications; lesions that appear in adulthood usually follow trauma.

For additional details and rx, see GROWTHS, 11.2.a.

19.2.C. PYOGENIC GRANULOMA

Summary: Single, bright red, raspberry-like growth; pea or bean sized; often friable and bleeds easily when traumatized; surface often ulcerated; most common on gingiva, lips, tongue, other oral soft tissues; any age group; refer to dentist or oral surgeon to confirm dx and rx.

For additional details and rx, see GROWTHS, 11.5.a.

19.2.E. LEUKOPLAKIA (SNUFF DIPPER'S POUCH, WHITE PATCH)

BMJ 2000;321:225; Cancer 1989;64:1527. Cancer 1984;53:563.

Cause: Chronic irritation: smoking, snuff, alcohol, chronic sun exposure.

Si: White to yellowish white, usually single, leathery thickening of mucosa w/o adjacent reddening; most frequent sites: line of teeth closure, lower lip, tongue, palate, floor of mouth; cannot be scraped off.

Crs: Persistent or progressive unless cause is eliminated; mostly in older ages.

Cmplc: 20% are dysplastic at time of bx; 4% develop SCC.

Rx: Refer to oral surgeon or ENT for bx to r/o SCC and rx.

19.2.F. ERYTHROPLAKIA (RED PATCH)

Cause: Chronic irritation, smoking, alcohol.

Sx: None.

Si: Red, velvety lesion; most common sites: tongue, floor of mouth, soft palate; does not blanch w pressure; often has very distinct borders between normal and affected tissue; older persons; males > females.

Crs: Persistent.

Cmplc: 90% show severe dysplasia, carcinoma in situ, or SCC at time of bx.

Rx: Refer to oral surgeon or ENT for bx to r/o SCC and rx (BMJ 2000;321:225).

19.2.G. KAPOSI'S SARCOMA (KS)

Summary: Red to blue to purple; gingival or hard palate; starts flat; becomes nodular plaque; may become multiple and massive; may interfere w eating; assoc w pain and bleeding.

For additional details, see GROWTHS, 11.14.a., and HIV, 15.5.a.

19.2.H. CANCER

J Oral Max Surg 1991;49:1152. Cancer 1988;62:1796.

Summary: Refer any pt w a slowly growing, painless, persistent mass in mouth to a dentist, oral surgeon, or ENT; inciting causes: tobacco, smoked or chewed; most common sites: floor of mouth (45%), soft palate (30%), tongue (15%); most are SCCs; at dx 40%–50% have metastasized to LNs; 5-yr survival is 60%–70%.

DRYNESS AND/OR BURNING, ANY LOCATION

Oral Surg Omop 1992;74:158. Dent Clin N Am 1991;35:171.

19.3. XEROSTOMIA (DRY MOUTH)

Cause: Meds: tricyclic antidepressants, antiparkinsonian drugs, antihypertensives, GI antispasmodics; diseases: mumps, sarcoidosis, HIV infection, posttherapeutic x-ray; idiopathic; **Sjögren's syndrome**: chronic autoimmune disease, lymphocytic infiltration of glands, dry mouth and eyes; women >>> men; mostly middle-aged; Ro/SS-A often pos; ↑ ESR; arthritis; some develop lymphoma or Waldenström's macroglobulinemia (Arthritis Rheum 1993;36:340).

Sx: Sore mouth.

Si: Red, dry mouth; often rampant dental caries, periodontal disease, ↓ taste sensitivity.

Crs: Persistent or episodic.

Cmplc: Tooth loss; osteoradionecrosis if assoc w x-ray; poor diet from dysphagia.

Rx: If underlying cause is not evident, refer to dentist or oral surgeon who will rx to preserve teeth and may use topical fluorides and artificial saliva; Sjögren's syndrome: sx relief only, as disorder is not curable; observe for lymphoma.

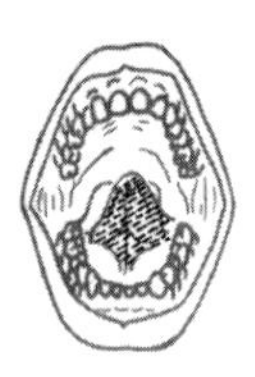

TONGUE, BURNING AND/OR DRYNESS

19.4.A. VITAMIN B DEFICIENCY

Summary: Elderly; mostly women; w sore or burning mouth or tongue; red, shiny tongue w/o papillae; consider deficiency of thiamine (B_1), niacin, riboflavin (B_2), B_{12}; obtain dietary hx; r/o pernicious anemia; if no cause found, try 1 tsp aqueous 0.5% diphenhydramine hydrochloride or viscous lidocaine retained in mouth for a few min before spitting out; refer to dentist or oral surgeon.

TONGUE, COLOR CHANGE AND FUZZY

19.4.B. *CANDIDA* INFECTION

Summary: Discrete white spots on mucosa; recent onset; easily wiped off (see 19.1.f.).

19.4.C. HAIRY TONGUE

J Oral Med 1977;32:85.

Cause: Broad-spectrum antibiotics, poor dental hygiene, smoking.
Pathophys: Elongation of filiform papillae.
Sx: Asx.
Si: Diffuse, fuzzy hairlike patch over anterior 1/2 or more; usually white, but often stained tan to black from food or smoking.

Crs: Persistent.

Rx: Re-evaluate need for antibiotics; improve dental hygiene; consider dental referral.

19.4.D. ORAL HAIRY LEUKOPLAKIA

Nejm 2000;343:481; J Am Acad Derm 1996;35:928. Ann IM 1996;125:485. Oral Surg Omop 1992;73:151.

Cause: Epstein-Barr virus.

Epidem: Immunosuppressed pts: most are HIV pos (occurs in 15% of HIV-pos pts) or had transplantation.

Sx: Asx or mild sx.

Si: Vertical, corrugated appearance w deep furrows and thickening; shaggy hair–like surface; mostly lateral surface of tongue but may be on other intraoral sites.

Crs: Persistent; pts have advanced immunosuppression.

Cmplc: May develop SCC; sign of progression to AIDS.

Lab: HIV serology.

Rx: Lesions may regress spontaneously or w antiretroviral rx; may respond to topical tretinoin, topical bleomycin (Cancer 1998;83:629), topical podophyllin (Arch Derm 1992;128:1659); consider referral to oral surgeon.

TONGUE, DEFORMED, CHRONIC

19.4.E. MEDIAN RHOMBOID GLOSSITIS

Summary: Rare; asx; raised mass; smooth; red, midline dorsum of tongue; *Candida* infection is probable cause (Br J Derm 1975;93:399); consider referral to oral surgeon to confirm dx and r/o cancer.

19.4.F. FISSURED TONGUE (SCROTAL TONGUE, GROOVED TONGUE)

Summary: Grooving or fissuring of surface of tongue; asx; persistent; 2% of normal, common in Down syndrome; r/o geographic tongue (see 19.4.g.); may occur in assoc w recurrent facial edema and facial paralysis (**Melkersson-Rosenthal syndrome**) (Derm Clin 1996;14:371); rx combination systemic CS and minocycline may be effective (J Am Acad Derm 1999;41:746) for acute attacks.

19.4.G. GEOGRAPHIC TONGUE (BENIGN MIGRATORY GLOSSITIS)

Summary: Irregularly shaped, red islands, pea to silver dollar sized; sharp, irregular edges; only occasional tenderness or pain; change in size and pattern wk to wk; episodic or persistent course; cause is unknown; r/o Reiter's syndrome, psoriasis, lichen planus; no rx.

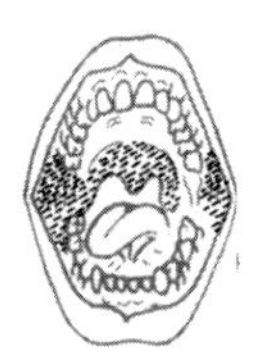

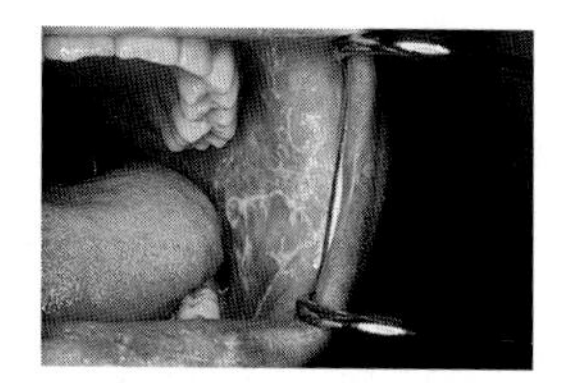

Lichen planus (see 19.1.i.)

CHEEKS OR SOFT PALATE, COLOR CHANGE—DARK

19.5.A. ADDISON'S DISEASE

Summary: Irregular bluish black or brownish spots or blotches on mucosal tissues, esp cheeks, gums, tongue, lips.

For additional details, see PIGMENT INCREASE, 22.5.a.

19.5.B. RACIAL PIGMENTATION

Summary: Tan to dark brown patches w/o other surface changes; persistent; common on mucosa, esp lips and gums, of blacks.

19.5.C. HEMANGIOMA OR HEMATOMA

Summary: Single; red to purple; congenital or may follow mouth trauma (see 19.2.b.).

19.5.D. NEVUS, MELANOCYTIC

Oral Surg Omop 1987;63:566, 676.

Summary: Round; tan to dark brown; flat to slightly raised; common but if recent onset, consider melanoma and refer to dermatologist or oral surgeon for dx or bx.

For additional details and rx, see GROWTHS, 11.1.a.

19.5.E. PIGMENTATION, METALS

Summary: Blue or black lines at gum line between gingiva and teeth; cause: deposition of heavy metals: silver, lead, mercury, bismuth; pica; occupational; distinguish from racial pigmentation; consider referral if assoc mood or sensory changes.

MOUTH

CHEEKS OR SOFT PALATE, COLOR CHANGE—LIGHT

19.5.F. FORDYCE SPOTS (OR GRANULES)

Summary: Multiple, sand grain sized, yellow or whitish, slightly elevated; mostly on buccal mucosa and lips; asx; lifelong; enlarged sebaceous glands; no rx except reassurance.

19.5.H. LINEA ALBA

Summary: Horizontal white line on buccal mucosa at bite line; asx; no rx.

19.5.J. WHITE SPONGE NEVUS (CANNON'S DISEASE)

Summary: White or gray, thickened or folded patch on buccal mucosa, palate, gums, floor of mouth; usually asx; resembles leukoplakia and *Candida* infection; persists but is benign; autosomal dominant; refer to confirm dx; no rx.

CHEEKS OR SOFT PALATE, PAINLESS GROWTH

19.5.K. EPULIS

Summary: Soft-tissue overgrowth from gingiva or hard palate inflammation; at borders of ill-fitting dentures; refer to dentist for confirmation and rx.

GINGIVA OR HARD PALATE, INFLAMMATION

19.6.A. ACUTE NECROTIZING ULCERATIVE GINGIVITIS (ANUG, TRENCH MOUTH, VINCENT'S GINGIVOSTOMATITIS)

Summary: Inflamed red gingiva, white pseudomembrane; tenderness in interdental space; pain, bad taste, fetid odor; multiple diet and bacterial causes; refer to dentist.

GINGIVA OR HARD PALATE, COLOR CHANGE

19.6.B. MISC

Summary: Racial pigmentation, melanocytic nevi, chemical pigmentation, amalgam tattoo, hemangioma.

- *KS*: most common oral neoplasia in HIV-pos pts; most common site is palate; usually not painful but superimposed infection, esp candidal, may cause pain; difficulty swallowing.

GINGIVA OR HARD PALATE, PAINLESS GROWTHS

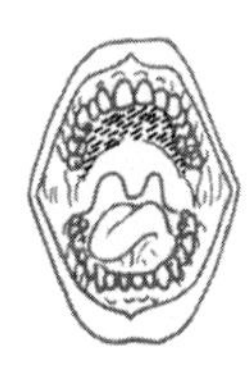

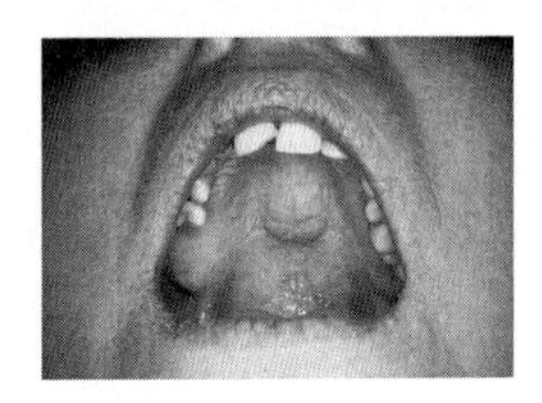

Torus palatinus

19.6.D. TORUS PALATINUS

Summary: Bony protuberance midline on hard palate, begins in early adulthood, asx; refer any pt w recent new growth to oral surgeon to r/o cancer.

19.6.E. PARULIS (GUM BOIL)

Summary: Mass of inflamed granulation tissue on gingiva; sinus tract from tooth or periodontal infection; may lead to cutaneous fistula; malodor and purulent drainage.

FLOOR OF MOUTH, PAINLESS GROWTHS

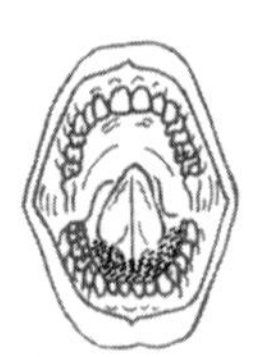

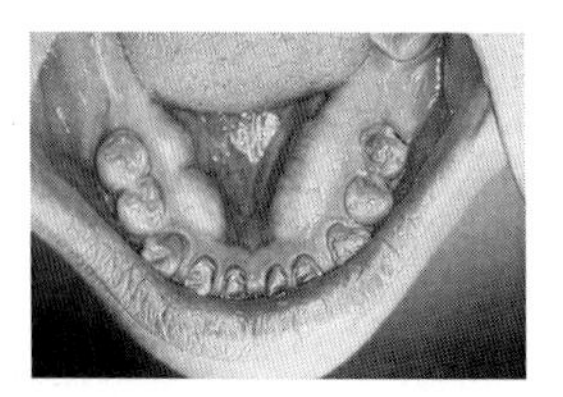

Torus mandibularis

19.7.A. TORUS MANDIBULARIS (RANULA)

Summary: If long-standing: **torus mandibularis**: bony protuberance below tongue and on hard palate; benign; asx; if recent **ranula**: bluish soft fluctuant swelling due to salivary gland cyst; benign; refer any pt w recent new growth to oral surgeon or ENT to r/o cancer.

LIPS, INFLAMMATION

19.8.A. HERPES SIMPLEX LABIALIS, RECURRENT

Oral Surg Omop 1989;68:701.

Summary: Groups of pinhead-sized blisters on lip, usually at vermilion border, w a hx of recurrence at same or nearly same site; rx: penciclovir cr (Denavir, 2 gm, Rx, $$) q 2 h while awake × 4 d.

For additional details and rx, see BLISTERS, 2.1.a.

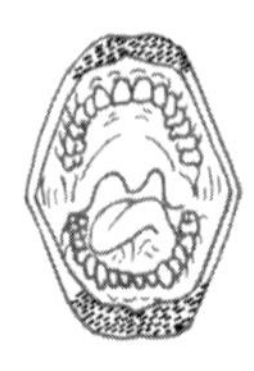

LIPS, BURNING AND/OR DRYNESS

19.8.E. ANGULAR CHEILITIS (PERLÈCHE, CHEILOSIS)

Cause: *C. albicans*, esp pts w removable or ill-fitting dentures w drooling or sagging cheeks; vitamin deficiency; allergic rxn to lipstick or toothpaste; HSV; syphilis (uncommon).

Si: Red, crusty, scaling, fissuring of commissures.

Rx: Nystatin cr or econazole cr hs covered w thick layer of ZnOx to protect lips from moisture; multivitamins may be indicated; consider lipstick or toothpaste elimination trials; refer to dentist for denture adjustment.

19.8.F. CHEILITIS

Summary: Dry, crusty, "chapped" lips may be persistent or intermittent:

- Persistent: consider **actinic cheilitis**: esp men, outdoor work, smoker; premalignant; white plaques of **leukoplakia** may need bx to r/o SCC; consider referral to ENT (see 19.2.e.).
- Intermittent: 1° irritation assoc w low humidity, wind, sun, lip licking; consider contact allergy to lipstick, mouthwash, toothpaste; refer to dermatology if not responding to simple lip balm.

LIPS, LIGHT SPOTS

19.8.G. FORDYCE SPOTS (OR GRANULES)

Summary: Multiple, sand grain sized, yellow or whitish, slightly elevated; mostly on buccal mucosa and lips; asx; lifelong; harmless normal but enlarged sebaceous glands; no rx except reassurance.

LIPS, PAINLESS GROWTH

19.8.I. MUCOCELE (MUCOUS RETENTION CYST)

Summary: Bluish soft, fluctuant, slightly elevated lump in lower lip, normal color if deep; persistent; size fluctuates, may ↑ at mealtime; salivary gland blockage; may need referral for excision.

19.8.J. VASCULAR LESIONS

Summary: Dark red or purple; may blanch w pressure; **congenital hemangioma** in child, typically involute; **traumatic hemangioma (venous lake)** in adult, persistent; **pyogenic granuloma** if new, elevated, red, bleeding growth, surgically excise or refer; small telangiectasias appear in **scleroderma** and **hereditary hemorrhagic telangiectasia**.

19.8.K. VERRUCA VULGARIS

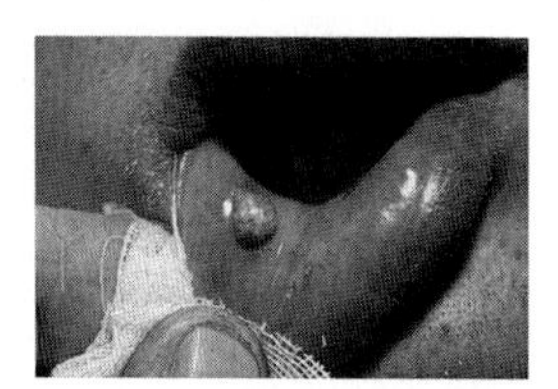

Verruca vulgaris

Summary: Raised; skin colored to white; single or multiple, often in cluster; lips or oral mucosa; asx or pain from irritation; caused by HPV 2, 4, or 40; autoinoculated from other areas, esp fingers; persists for yrs or removed by LN2; cautery; excision (Oral Surg Omop 1986;62:410).

For additional details and rx, see HANDS, 14.1.a.

20 Nails

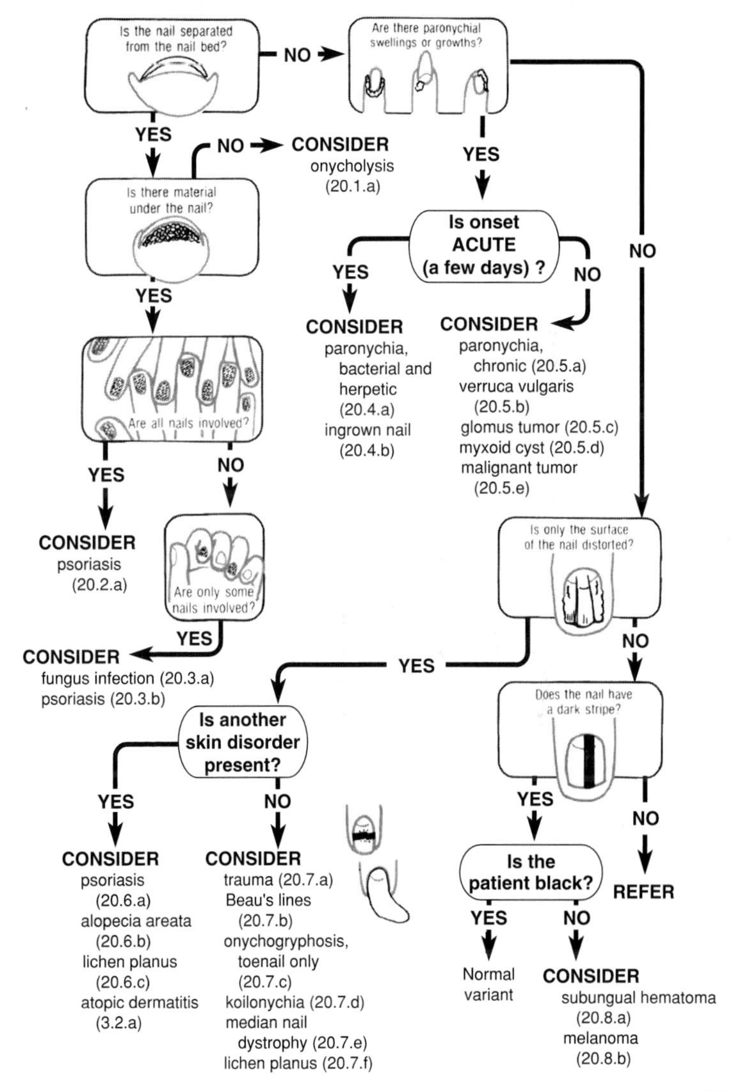

NAILS

SEPARATED FROM NAIL BED, NO DEBRIS UNDER NAIL

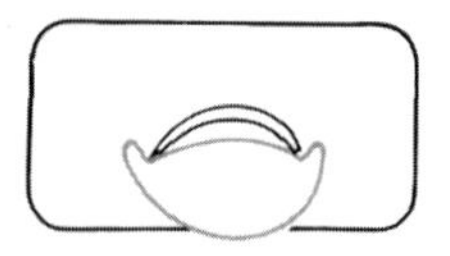

20.1.A. ONYCHOLYSIS

Peds 1998;102:979. Am J Contact Derm 1996;7:109.

Cause: Disruption of junction between nail and nail bed; most common cause: acrylic nail cement or polish; other: phototoxic or photosensitive drug rxn: esp cycline antibiotics, cancer-treating agents, sulfonamides, captopril, retinoids, thiazides, phenothiazines; rarely hyperthyroidism.

Epidem: Women >>> men; most have used professional manicurists.

Sx: Nail/nail bed may be tender and unsightly.

Si: Nail is separated and raised from nail bed; 1 to few nails involved; color: yellow to white; if green: infected w *Pseudomonas* species; if brown to black: infected w *Proteus* species.

Crs: New growth may attach to nail bed once cause is eliminated; no reattachment of existing separated nail and no reattachment if nail bed is scarred; as nails grow slowly, re-examine pts and measure new nail growth q 3 mo.

Lab: Culture not useful except to r/o tinea.

Rx: Advise clipping nail back to pink attached portion to ↓ trauma; toluene-free and formaldehyde-free nail polish may be less damaging: pt can buy and bring to manicurist; dc, if possible, photoactive drugs; try a combination of miconazole soln in AM and sulfacetamide sodium (Sulamyd 10%, Rx, $) hs under and around each affected nail to prevent infections while nail grows out; improvement will not be evident for mos.

SEPARATED FROM NAIL BED, DEBRIS UNDER NAILS, ALL NAILS

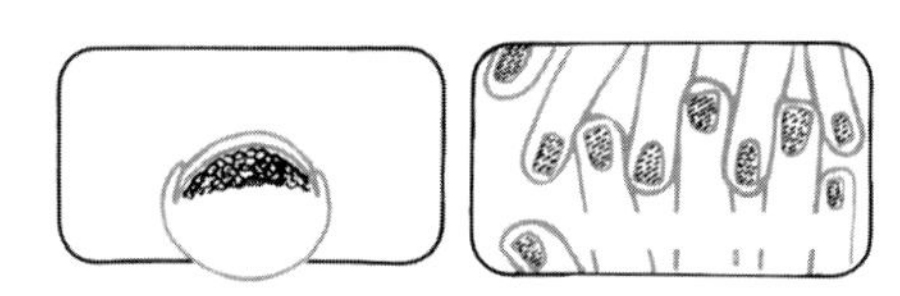

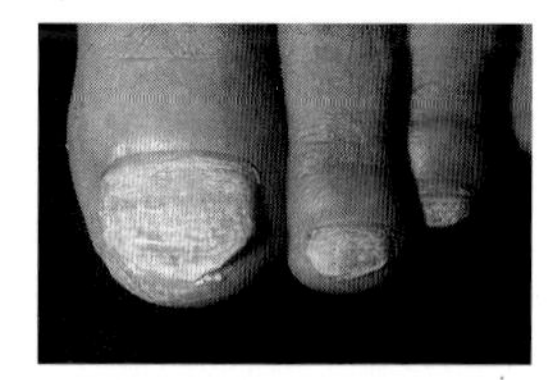

Psoriasis

20.2.A. PSORIASIS

Derm 1996;193:300.

Cause: Minute psoriatic lesions in nail matrix w focal damage to nail.

Epidem: About 1/2 of pts w moderate-severe psoriasis have nail dystrophy.

Si: Most common: sharply edged minute pits, resembling a pinprick; rippling; separation of nail from its bed w keratotic debris under nail; splinter hemorrhages from trauma to small capillaries in nail bed; look for si of psoriasis elsewhere.

Crs: Chronic and persistent.

Ddx: Commonly confused w fungus infection; usually involves all or most nails.

Rx: Poor; may respond to IL CS or PUVA.

For additional details and rx, see BODY, 3.1.d.

SEPARATED FROM NAIL BED, DEBRIS UNDER NAILS, SOME NAILS

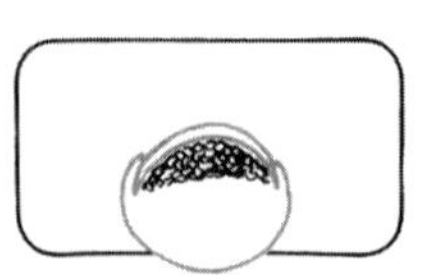
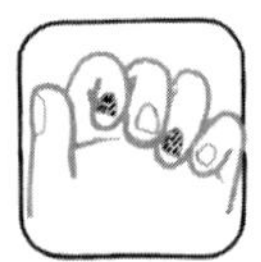
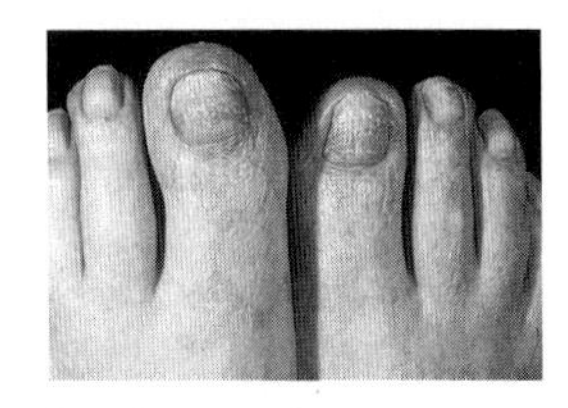

Onychomycosis

20.3.A. FUNGUS INFECTION (ONYCHOMYCOSIS)

Derm Clin 1997;15:121. J Am Acad Derm 1996;35:S2. J Am Acad Derm 1996;34:529.

Cause: *Toenails*: common due to moist, warm, dark condition in shoes; familial susceptibility; DM; *fingernails*: not common but manicurists blame fungus, rather than acrylics (see 20.1.a.); most common fungus in both: *Trichophyton rubrum*, but *Epidermophyton floccosum* and *T. mentagrophytes* also infect nails; incidence ↑ 3 × in HIV-pos pts (Arch Derm 1998;134:1216).

Sx: Painful if nail becomes distorted.

Si: Thickened and yellow nails w crumbly subungual debris; fingernail onychomycosis is nearly always assoc w toenail fungus infection; some nails or just 1 hand is involved.

Crs: Usually starts at lateral margin or tip and extends proximally over mos; may start proximal in immunosuppressed pts; some nails may clear spontaneously.

Lab: Confirm tinea w KOH exam or culture (see DX.3.) prior to starting systemic rx; tinea may be deep within debris and culture is often neg; obtain deep clippings or ask pt to gather subungual debris in a sterile tube for a wk or so and bring to office to be sent to a mycology lab.

Rx:

- Topical therapy of *onychomycosis*: ciclopirox (Penlac nail lacquer); first FDA-approved (late 1999) topical rx for nail fungal infections;

apply qd to affected nails and adjacent skin, recoat daily but file off and restart coats every wk, trim unattached nail wkly by pt and monthly by podiatrist as recommended by manufacturer; alternative: clearing w naftifine gel (Naftin gel) bid to nail has been reported (Cutis 1993;51:205).

Systemic antifungal agents give mycologic and clinical cure in about 70%, esp of fingernails (Jaad 2001;44:479), but recurrence is 30%–70% in 3 yr, meds are expensive; pts may have unrealistic expectations based on consumer advertising; pts > 65 yo usually do not respond as their nails grow too slowly to incorporate med, immunosuppressed pts usually do not respond; the FDA issued a **Public Health Advisory** in May, 2001 because of a rare risk of congestive heart failure and liver failure (see RX.11); to ↓ sx: pt may file nail plate parallel w its flat surface using a woodworker's file or rasp to thin nail and reduce pain from having an otherwise stiff nail press into soft corners of nail bed; if pts find nails difficult to trim, suggest podiatric referral; for details of systemic rx, see RX.11.

20.3.B. PSORIASIS

Summary: All nails tend to be involved in severe psoriasis, but only 1 or a few are dystrophic in mild cases (see 20.2.a. and BODY, 3.1.d.).

PARONYCHIAL SWELLINGS OR GROWTHS, ACUTE (FEW DAYS)

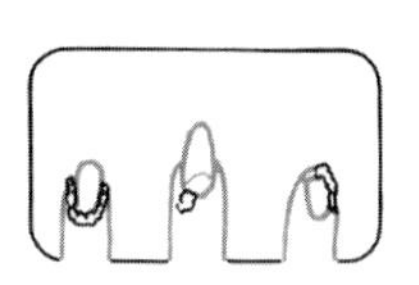

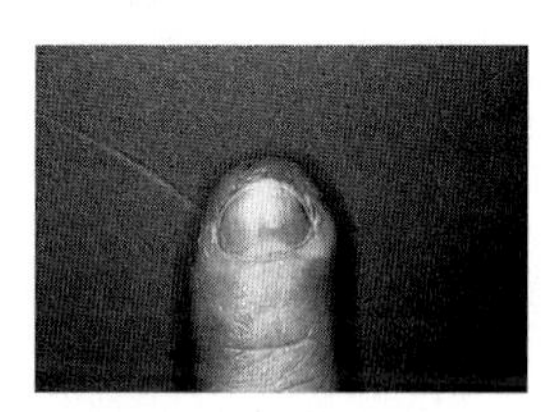

Paronychia—acute

NAILS

20.4.A.(1). PARONYCHIA, BACTERIAL

Cause: Usually *S. aureus*, but *Streptococcus* or a gram-neg organism sometimes is causal; may be initiated by injury or "hangnail," but usually pt does not recall trauma.

Epidem: Most common in housewives, beauticians, bartenders, and others w chronic exposure to hand irritants.

Sx: Acute pain from onset.

Si: Acute swelling w pain of a single fingertip; cuticle of affected nail usually is intact (see 20.5.a.); LN↑ may be present, but pts usually not febrile or toxic.

Crs: Starts acutely and develops rapidly.

Cmplc: Permanent damage to nerve endings and tendons of fingertip if severe and not promptly treated.

Lab: C + s of any drainage or material released by I&D.

Rx: Initiate rx before culture results; obtain early surgical consultation as antibiotics alone often are insufficient; start systemic antibiotic (dicloxacillin 125–250 mg qid).

20.4.A.(2). PARONYCHIA, HERPETIC

Cause: *Herpesvirus hominus*, either type 1 or 2.

Epidem: Susceptible persons, ie, nursing or dental students giving mouth care.

Sx: Painful.

Si: Similar to acute bacterial paronychia; multiple small vesicles; LN↑ may be severe; often febrile.

Crs: May be quite uncomfortable and disabled for 1–2 wk; recurrences seldom occur at same site.

Lab: Confirm w viral culture.

Rx: Reduce sx w analgesia, even opiates; I&D is not helpful; initiate antiviral rx as for 1° HSV (see BLISTERS, 2.1.a.); note that the infection is contagious to others.

20.4.B. INGROWN NAIL

Cause: Constricting shoes and clipping nails too short contribute; sharp corner of nail, esp hallux, pushes into fleshy fold lateral to nail.

Sx: Pain.

Si: Toenails >> fingernails; lateral nail fold is red, swollen, and tender; purulent material often expressed.

Crs: Discomfort develops over a few d; may become disabling; recurrences are common.

Lab: Culture not necessary.

Rx: Refer to podiatry or attempt to rx as follows: lift impinging edge of nail away from overlapping nail fold w a small hemostat; separate nail from wound by placing a small wad of cotton under nail; cut back protruding nail; local anesthesia may or may not be necessary; pt should compress the nail (see RX.2.) 20 min tid for a few d and leave cotton wad in place; for recurrences, refer to podiatrist who may permanently remove lateral portion of nail plate.

PARONYCHIAL SWELLINGS OR GROWTHS, CHRONIC (WEEKS OR MONTHS)

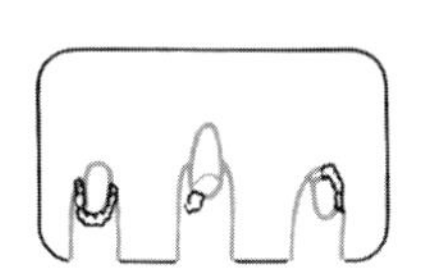

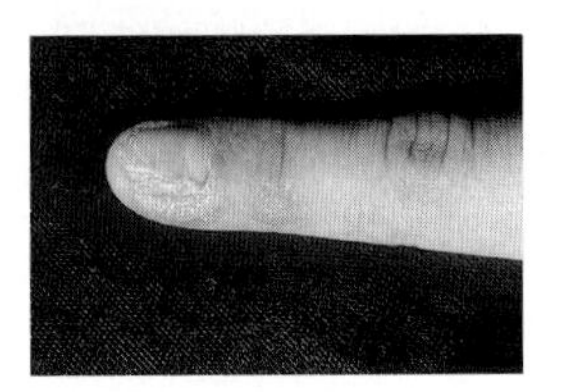

Verruca—periungual

20.5.A. PARONYCHIA, CHRONIC

Cutis 1996;58:397.

Cause: Usually *C. albicans*; typical pt has damaged cuticles allowing moisture and colonization by microorganism of space between distal nail fold and nail plate; common causes: manicuring w pushing back cuticle or maceration from wet work, ie, nurses, bartenders, new mothers; if blue-green under nail: *Pseudomonas* species, may be confirmed by culture or bluish-green fluorescence under Wood's light.

Sx: Painful but not acute as w bacterial or viral paronychial infection (see above).

Si: Boggy, red, crusty; around 1 or several fingernails; women >> men; present for many wk to mos; nail plate is distorted and ridged; purulent material sometimes can be expressed.

Crs: Persistent unless inducing conditions are controlled; time that infection started can be estimated from length of dystrophic nail (4–6 mo for damage to push out to tip).

Lab: Examine expressed material w KOH for hyphae (see DX.3.) or send swab to mycology lab; note on request form that *Candida* species is suspected; otherwise lab may use culture media that suppresses yeast "contamination."

Rx: Maintain dry conditions w protective gloves; fluconazole (Diflucan, 100 mg, Rx, $$$) 3–5 d qd or itraconazole (Sporanox, 100 mg, Rx, $$$) 1–2 wk bid reduces infection and pain quickly; application of 4% thymol in alcohol to nail fold after each water exposure reduces moisture under fold; topical anticandidal medication, ie, nystatin cr or suspension, or a broad-spectrum topical antifungal (see RX.10.) bid may speed resolution and reduce recurrence.

20.5.B. VERRUCA VULGARIS (COMMON WARTS)

Summary: Single to multiple; surface is raised, rough, cauliflower like; pinhead to dime sized; most are on hands, feet, face; usually painless unless periungual or fingertip; nails may be distorted by growing wart or by disturbance of nail matrix; periungual warts tend to become worse in habitual nail biters and tend to be persistent.

For additional details and rx, see HANDS, 14.1.a.

20.5.C. GLOMUS TUMOR

Summary: Solitary tumors; usual location is periungual skin, fingertip fat pad, nail bed; pinhead to a BB in size; blue to pink if visible; typically radiating pain triggered by pressure, heat, or spontaneous.

For additional details and rx, see HANDS, 14.4.d.

20.5.D. MYXOID CYST (MUCOID CYST)

Summary: Pea-sized swelling; skin colored to glistening in color; usually on dorsum of finger near tip or about nail; painless; if cyst impinges on nail plate, a depression or crease in nail may develop.

For additional details and rx, see HANDS, 14.4.c.

20.5.E. MALIGNANT TUMORS

Summary: Rare on finger or toe, but if enlarging single tumor mass develops that is not a wart, consider a malignant or metastatic tumor; pigment streak in nail may be an early si of melanoma (Clin Exp Derm 1996;21:377) (see GROWTHS, 11.4.b.).

SURFACE IS DISTORTED, OTHER SKIN DISORDER PRESENT

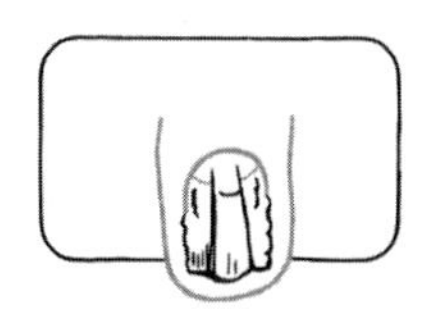

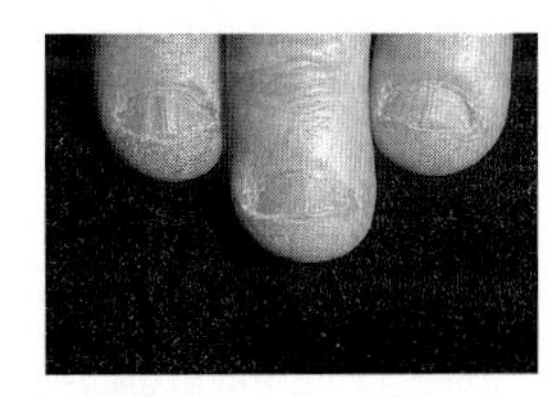

Lichen planus

NAILS

20.6.A. PSORIASIS

Summary: Nail pits, distal onycholysis, splinter hemorrhages, subungual debris are frequent clinical si of psoriasis and help confirm dx in presence of a skin eruption (see 20.2.a. and BODY, 3.1.d.).

20.6.B. ALOPECIA AREATA

Summary: Some or all finger and toe nails; pits or longitudinal and transverse striations; surface may appear roughened, as if deeply scratched; nails are not shed; no debris under nail; no inflammation; course follows hair loss of alopecia areata (see HAIR DECREASE, 12.3.a.).

20.6.C. LICHEN PLANUS

Summary: Several or all nails; surface of nails is rippled and pitted; nail does not separate from bed; no debris under nail; no inflammation; pterygium may cover nail bed if scarring develops; course is chronic, often w scarring; look for lichen planus elsewhere (see BODY, 3.3.n.); bx may confirm dx; generally refer pts to dermatologist or podiatrist to confirm dx; rx not effective (J Am Acad Derm 1995;33:903).

For additional details and rx, see BODY, 3.3.n.

SURFACE IS DISTORTED, OTHER SKIN DISORDER ABSENT

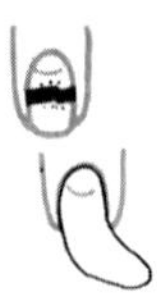

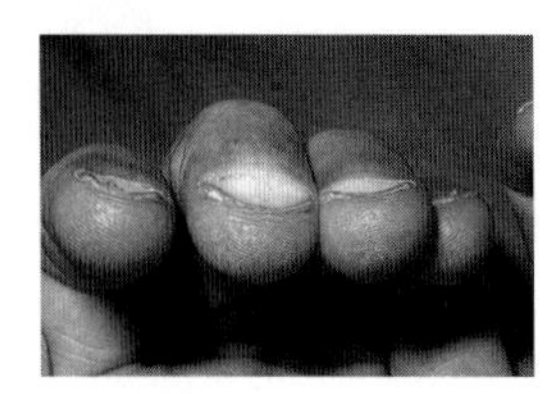

Koilonychia

20.7.A. TRAUMA

Summary: Most common on thumb; also called **median nail dystrophy** and **habit tic**; ridging from repeated rubbing or grinding of nails against other nails or objects; harmless tic; rx not effective if habit continues (see 20.7.e.).

20.7.B. BEAU'S LINES

Summary: Transverse grooves in 1 or more nails; appear as nail grows out; induced by trauma, ie, serious systemic illness, high fever, traumatic accident; date event measuring distance from growing matrix to ridge (fingernails grow about 3 mm/mo) (Int J Derm 1994;33:545).

20.7.C. ONYCHOGRYPHOSIS

Summary: Long, curved toe nails; older persons unable to care for their feet; interfere w footwear and walking; refer to podiatrist for trimming if pt unable to cut them.

20.7.D. KOILONYCHIA (SPOON NAILS)

Summary: Nails thinned and curved like a spoon; mostly cosmetic; rare assoc w iron deficiency anemia and esophageal webs (**Plummer-Vinson syndrome**); consider tests of iron levels and iron-binding capacity.

20.7.E. MEDIAN NAIL DYSTROPHY

Summary: Usually thumb nail, 1 or both; partial or complete split or firlike appearance; runs from free edge as far as cuticle; may persist for yr or may resolve and recur; considered 2° to chronic trauma, esp habit tic; if trauma is to cuticle, may lead to washboard appearance of nail; no rx (Int J Derm 1995;34:799).

20.7.F. LICHEN PLANUS

Summary: Several or all nails; surface of nails is rippled and pitted; nail does not separate from bed; no debris under nail; no inflammation; pterygium may cover nail bed if scarring develops; course is chronic, often w scarring; look for lichen planus elsewhere (see BODY, 3.3.n.); bx may confirm dx; generally refer pts to dermatologist or podiatrist to confirm dx; rx not effective; for details, see 20.6.c. and BODY, 3.3.n.

DARK STRIPE

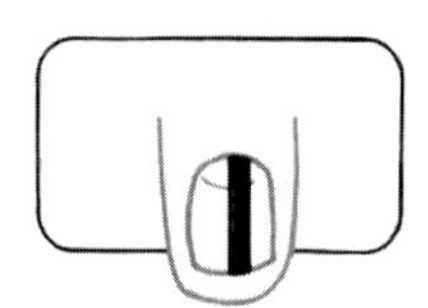

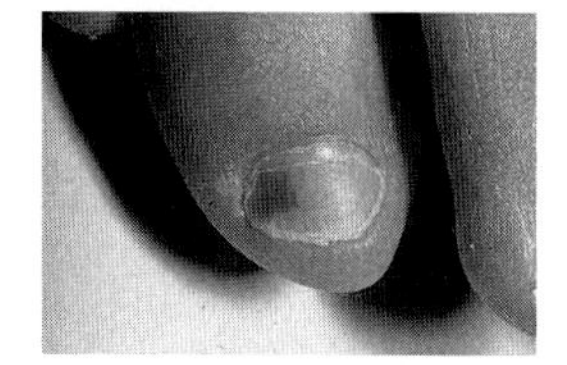

Nail pigment

20.8.A. SUBUNGUAL HEMATOMA

Summary: Sudden onset; may be painful; most common on hallux; dark purple to black patch or line; common running injury in tennis players and joggers; if acute and painful, relieve pressure w heated end of an opened paper clip pushed slowly through nail plate.

20.8.B. MELANOMA

Summary: If develops in nail matrix, presents as dark stripe running from base to tip as pigment deposits into nail; no cases of melanoma reported in pts <16 yo (J Am Acad Derm 1999;41:17); blacks: finger nail stripes are common and melanomas are rare; **zidovudine (AZT) nail**: azure blue lunulae; longitudinal and transverse dark bands; thumbs most common; blacks >> whites; refer pt w *new* black-brown stripe in nail, not on AZT, to dermatologist or surgeon for possible bx.

For additional details and rx, see GROWTHS, 11.4.b.

NAILS

21 Pigment Decrease

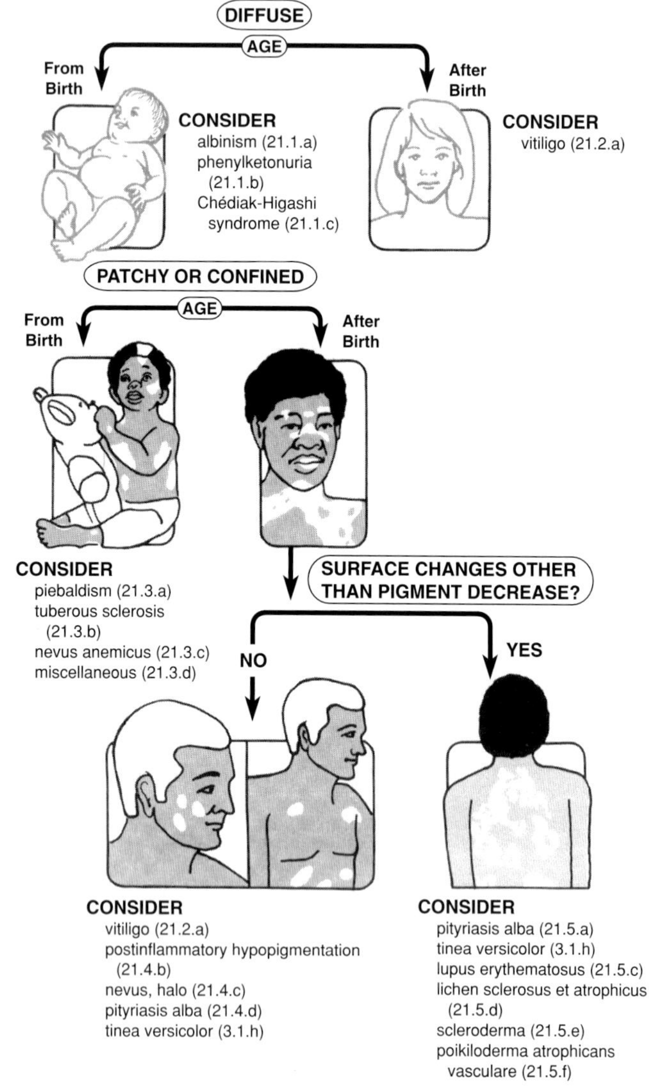

DIFFUSE DECREASE, PRESENT AT BIRTH

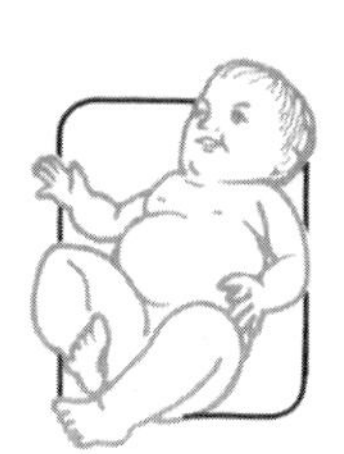

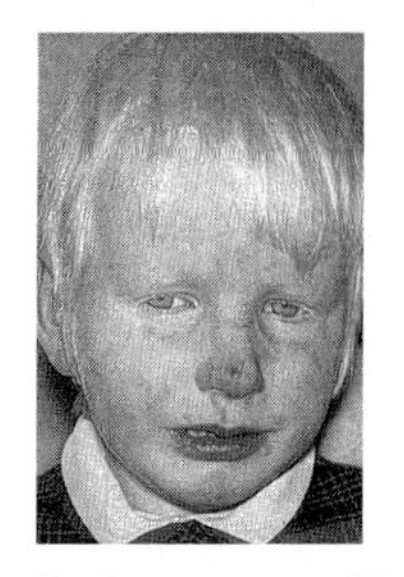

Oculocutaneous albinism

21.1.A. ALBINISM

Cutis 1996;57:397. Semin Derm 1995;14:27.

Cause: *Oculocutaneous*: autosomal recessive; subtypes: severe type: melanocytes lack tyrosinase; mild type: tyrosinase is present; number of melanocytes is normal in both types; *ocular*: rarer; sex-linked recessive

Epidem: Equal in all races.

Sx: Photosensitivity.

Si: *Severe type* (tyrosinase neg): near total depigmentation w golden white hair and light blue irises; nystagmus; a few pigmented nevi; *mild type* (tyrosinase pos or *P* gene mutation): some pigmentation develops w age; less eye damage; a few nevi; *ocular type*: eye changes only.

Crs: Lack of pigment is evident at birth and persists through life; nystagmus develops because of sunlight damage to unpigmented retina.

Cmplc: ↓ vision is the most devastating cmplc; skin develops chronic sun damage, actinic keratoses, skin cancers.

Ddx: Generalized vitiligo, phenylketonuria, homocystinuria.

Lab: Skin bx: absence of melanin confirms dx; tyrosinase staining is available.

Rx: None known; pts need regular eye exams and skin exams; stress UV protection measures (see RX.16.); provide genetic counseling.

21.1.B. PHENYLKETONURIA

BMJ 1993;306:115.

Summary: Moderate and diffuse hypopigmentation w light hair and blue eyes; other si: "mousy" odor, photosensitivity, eczema, mental retardation, seizures; autosomal recessive; ↓ conversion of phenylalanine to tyrosine, which is a precursor of melanin; early dx usually is made by routine newborn urine testing.

21.1.C. CHÉDIAK-HIGASHI SYNDROME

Derm Clin 1995;13:65.

Summary: Partial oculocutaneous albinism; rare; autosomal recessive; lethal; ↑ susceptibility to infection; hematologic and neurologic abnormalities; melanocytes contain large melanosomes.

DIFFUSE DECREASE, NOT PRESENT AT BIRTH

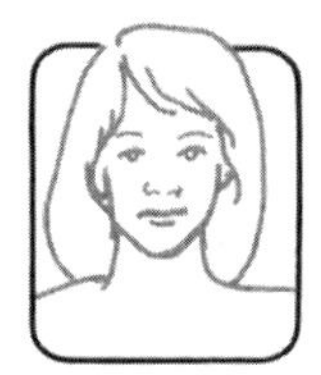

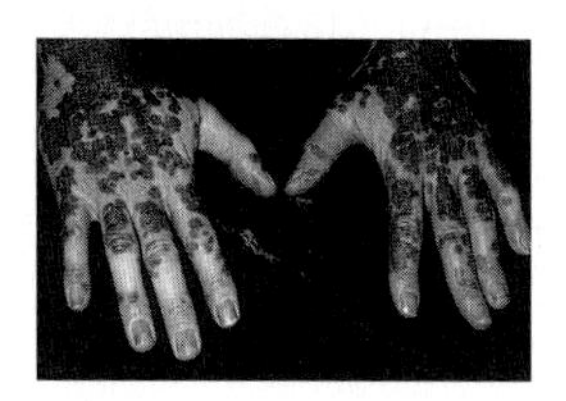

Vitiligo

21.2.A. VITILIGO

J Am Acad Derm 1998;38:647. Ped Clin N Am 1991;38:991. J Am Acad Derm 1987;16:948.

Cause: Unknown but probably immunologic; 1/4 have relative w vitiligo.

Epidem: ↑ frequency of vitiligo in pts w thyroid disease, Addison's disease, pernicious anemia, alopecia areata; although most noticeable in darker races, frequency is equal in all races; about 1–2 million are affected in U.S.

Pathophys: Inflammation about melanocytes, ↓ melanin synthesis, disappearance of melanocytes.

Sx: Psychologic effects; ↑ sun sensitivity.

Si: Nearly chalk-white patches w sharp edges devoid of scale or texture changes; most often over joints and about orifices: mouth, eyes, nose.

Crs: Onset usually early adulthood; variable and unpredictable; vitiligo may stop w a few patches, become generalized, or clear spontaneously.

Ddx: If limited to hands, consider occupational exposure to phenolic cleaning compounds.

Lab: Bx unnecessary; thyroid antibodies frequent but rx of thyroid does not improve vitiligo.

Rx: None alters course; *small areas*: high-potency (class I) TCS for a few wks to mos, watching for atrophy and ↓ pigmentation of surrounding normal skin, then taper to class IV–V (Derm Clin 1993;11:325); consider covering cosmetics or stains, esp in women; *cosmetics*: Covermark (Lydia O'Leary 800.524.1120); Dermablend (800.345.1515); *stains*: Chromelin (Summers 800.533.7546); Dy-O-Derm (Galderma 817.263.2600); Vitadye (ICN 800.556.1937); also try self-tanning creams available at cosmetic counters; use broad-spectrum sunblock w high SPF (see RX.16.) to ↓ sun burning of involved patches and to ↓ darkening of adjacent normal areas that would only further ↑ color contrast; *large areas*: repigmentation w PUVA (see RX.15.) sometimes works, but process is slow and costly; skin grafts w melanin-producing skin are feasible for small areas; sometimes used: permanent bleaching of residual normally pigmented skin w monobenzyl ether of hydroquinone (Derm Clin 1993;11:27).

Contact National Vitiligo Foundation (611 South Fleishel, Tyler, TX 75701; 903.531.0074; www.nvfi.org or www.vitiligofoundation.org) for pt support information.

PATCHY DECREASE, PRESENT AT OR NEAR BIRTH

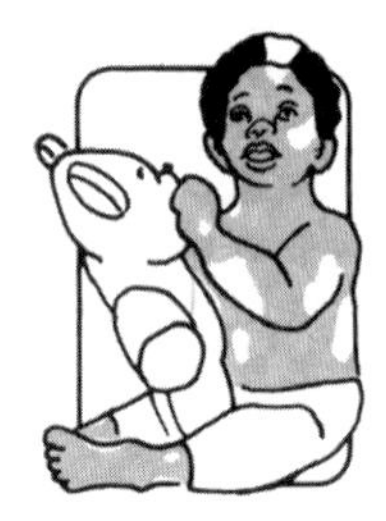

Tuberous sclerosis

21.3.A. PIEBALDISM

Summary: White forelock, forehead, and sometimes elsewhere; autosomal dominant; affected persons otherwise normal; consider **Waardenburg's syndrome**: piebaldism w eye, ear, and systemic abn.

21.3.B. TUBEROUS SCLEROSIS (EPILOIA)

Arch Dis Child 1995;72:471. Arch Derm 1994;130:348. Ped Clin N Am 1991;38:991.

Cause: Autosomal dominant; 1/2 cases are new mutations (Science 1997;277:805).

Epidem: Males = females.

Si: *Ash-leaf macules*: light-colored, oval, ash leaf–shaped patches (Arch Derm 1968;98:1); lesions of *adenoma sebaceum*: resembles acne vulgaris but not painful or pustular; 1–4-mm growths; firm; flesh colored to red; mid part of face; *shagreen patch*: rough thickened pigskin-like patch on back; also: epidermal nevi, periungual fibromas or angiomas.

Crs: Ash-leaf macules are only cutaneous si present at birth: other skin si develop later and ↑ at puberty; most die <50 yo from neurologic complications.

Cmplc: Numerous, esp benign tumors of viscera; 60% of children <18 yo have cardiac rhabdomyomas by echocardiography; seizures; mental retardation appears and worsens during early childhood, although some persons affected have normal intelligence (Mayo Clin Proc 1991;66:792).

Rx: Multidisciplinary: genetic counseling; control of seizures; surgical removal of visceral tumors if they interfere w function; perhaps cosmetic surgery to reduce facial papules and periungual fibromas.

Contact National Tuberous Sclerosis Foundation (8181 Professional Place/#110, Landover, MD 20785; 800.225.6872 or 301.459.9888; www.ntsa.org) for pt support information.

21.3.C. NEVUS ANEMICUS

Summary: Rare; congenital; irregularly shaped patch of lightened skin; persists; disorder of blood vessels; no rx available.

21.3.D. MISCELLANEOUS

Numerous other rare disorders of hypopigmentation exist; some are congenital, ie, incontinentia pigmenti; some are infectious, ie, pinta; some are acquired, ie, Vogt-Koyanagi-Harada syndrome.

PATCHY DECREASE, NOT PRESENT AT BIRTH, NO OTHER SURFACE CHANGE

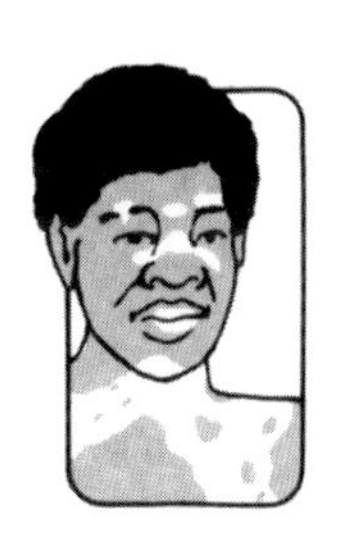

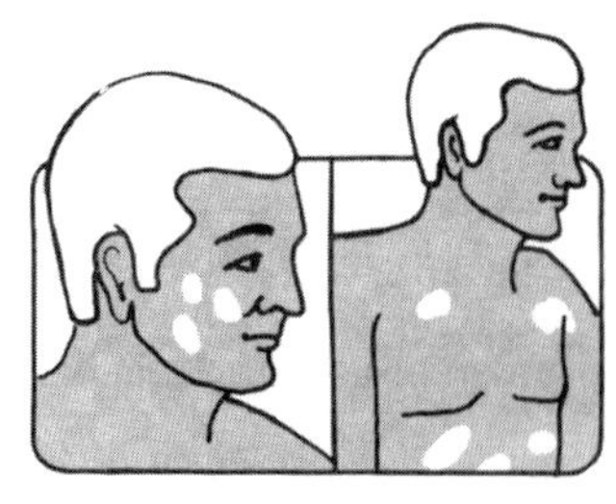

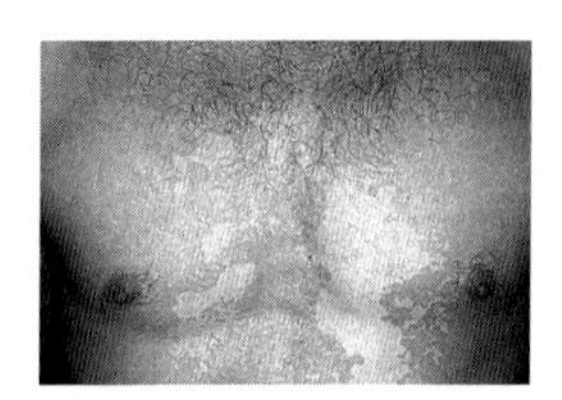

Tinea versicolor

21.4.B. POSTINFLAMMATORY HYPOPIGMENTATION

Summary: Pigmentation may ↑ or ↓ following almost any inflammatory dermatosis; if ↓ pigment: light but not ivory-white color of vitiligo; pigment returns after many wks to mos; sun exposure may speed up pigmentation.

21.4.C. NEVUS, HALO

Summary: Depigmentation around a pigmented melanocytic nevus produces a halo; most are in children and young adults; rarely halos develop around melanomas; halo nevi do not require excision unless central nevus is suspicious for melanoma.

21.4.D. PITYRIASIS ALBA

Arch Derm 1963;88:88.

Cause: Unknown; may be a manifestation of atopic dermatitis, esp if pt has "dry" patches elsewhere (Ped Derm 1996;13:10).

Epidem: Blacks = whites; boys = girls; mostly children and teens (Semin Derm 1995;14:15; Arch Derm 1960;82:183).

Sx: None.

Si: Slightly scaly or powdery; light colored but not white; few in number; 1–6 cm; mostly face, upper arms, neck, shoulders.

Crs: Persists for many mo; resolves by puberty.

Ddx: Tinea versicolor sometimes appears on face, esp in blacks, but is uncommon before puberty; consider atopic dermatitis.

Rx: Moisturizers; 1%–2.5% HC cr; reassure parents that condition is harmless, will eventually clear, will not scar.

PATCHY DECREASE, NOT PRESENT AT BIRTH, OTHER SURFACE CHANGES PRESENT

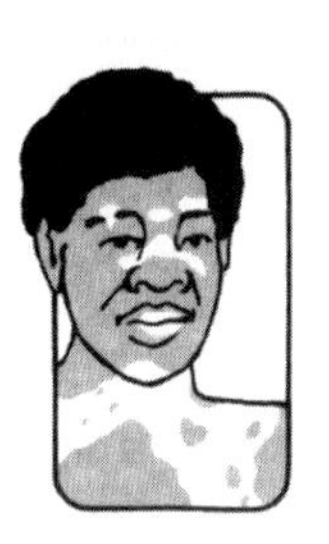

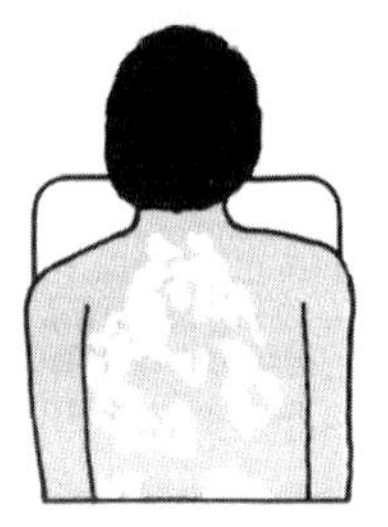

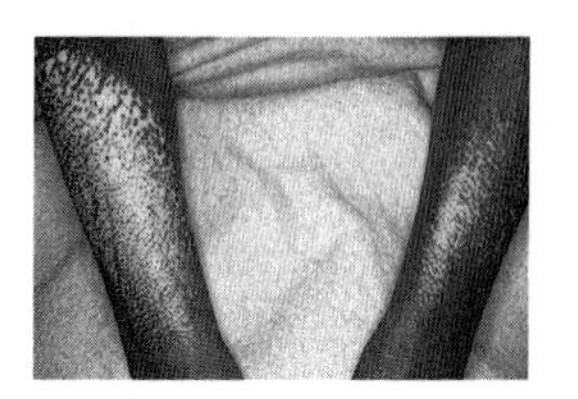

Scleroderma

21.5.A. PITYRIASIS ALBA

Summary: Light-colored patches are slightly scaly or powdery and are asx; usually restricted to face and upper part of torso in children (see 21.4.d.).

21.5.C. LUPUS ERYTHEMATOSUS (LE)

Summary: Sharply demarcated, pink to red, slightly scaly, coin-shaped plaques; develop areas of atrophy w shiny, depressed, depigmented, hairless skin.

For additional details and rx, see FACE, 6.2.c.

21.5.D. LICHEN SCLEROSUS ET ATROPHICUS

Summary: Initial: pink, inflamed, occas blisters; late: atrophic w light color, shiny surface, lack hair follicles; in groin or perianal: painful atrophy may develop.

For additional details, see GENITAL, 9.4.c.

21.5.E. SCLERODERMA (MORPHEA)

Summary: Light-colored patches; atrophic, depressed, hairless; not assoc w systemic sclerosis; dx confirmed by bx; refer to dermatology for confirmation.

For additional details, see FEVER, 8.3.c.

21.5.F. POIKILODERMA ATROPHICANS VASCULARE

Summary: Uncommon; light-colored patches speckled w pigment and fine telangiectasias; resembles radiation dermatitis; may be assoc w lymphoma, including Hodgkin's disease and mycosis fungoides; refer suspected cases to a dermatologist for confirmation.

22 Pigment Increase

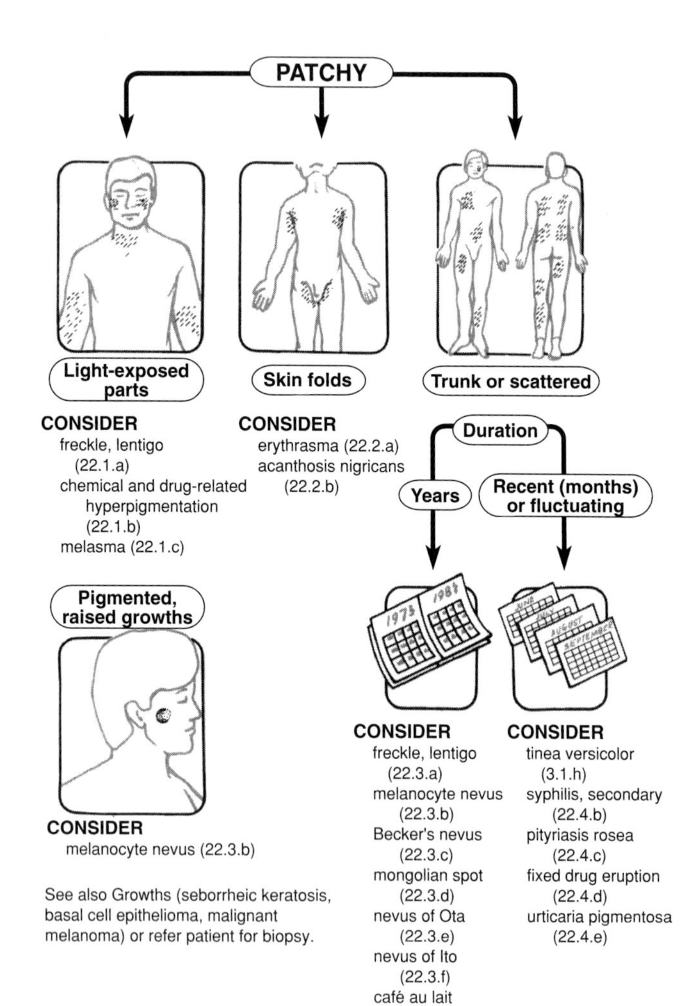

DIFFUSE

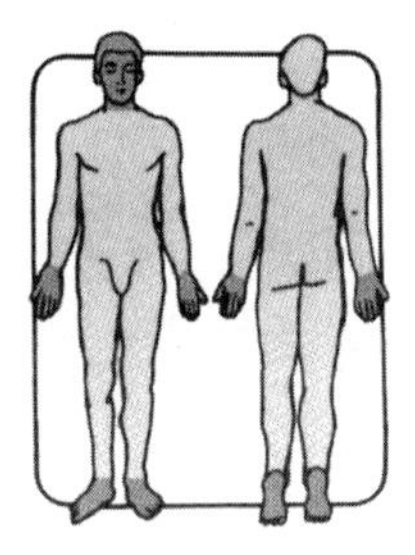

May be darker on light-exposed parts

CONSIDER

miscellaneous uncommon disorders (22.5)
Addison's disease (22.5.a)
hemochromatosis (22.5.b)
tumors (22.5.c)

Also see Cushing's syndrome, porphyria cutanea tarda, scleroderma, drug-induced reaction, biliary cirrhosis, melanoma and melanomatosis, vitamin B deficiency, and Wilson's disease in the appropriate sections.

PATCHY, LIGHT-EXPOSED PARTS ONLY

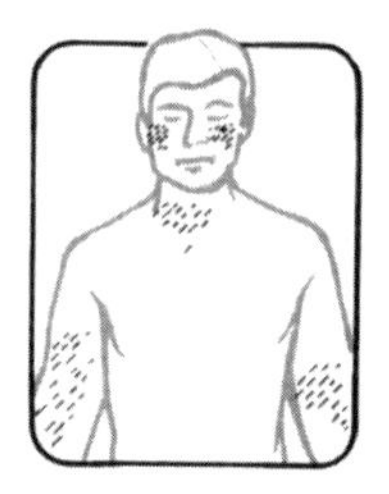

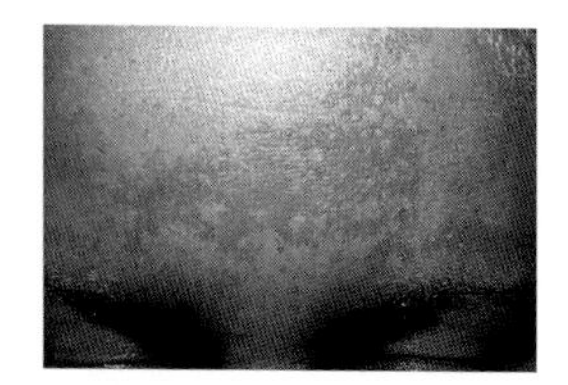

Melasma

22.1.A. FRECKLE/LENTIGO

Summary: *Freckle*: common; 1–3 mm; multiple; brown; flat; genetically determined on face; presence on trunk and arms indicates past intense sun exposure; not premalignant; rx not necessary or practical; *lentigo*: smaller and darker than freckle; fewer in number; not confined to sun-exposed areas; bx occasionally warranted to r/o melanoma.

For additional details and rx, see GROWTHS, 11.7.a.

22.1.B. CHEMICAL- AND DRUG-RELATED HYPERPIGMENTATION

Summary:

- Pigmentation limited to light-exposed areas; most common are photosensitizing drugs: imipramine and desipramine, phenothiazines, barbiturates, antimalarials, hydantoin, some cytotoxic agents: bleomycin, busulfan, cyclophosphamide, doxorubicin, 5-FU, hydroxyurea, mithramycin; others: amiodarone, tetracycline and similar antibiotics, sulfonamides, zidovudine (AZT), nicotinic acid, bcp's.
- Deposits of drug or metabolite directly in skin; pigmentation is generalized but often worse in light-exposed areas; heavy metals: silver, gold, bismuth, mercury, arsenic.

For additional details and rx, see LIGHT REACTIONS, 18.1.b.

22.1.C. MELASMA (CHLOASMA)

Med Clin N Am 1998;82:1185. Arch Derm 1995;131:1453.

Cause: Photosensitivity w hormonal changes usually assoc w pregnancy or bcp's; r/o photosensitizing drugs (see LIGHT REACTIONS, 18.1.b.).

Epidem: Women only.

Si: Brown; symmetric; patchy; mostly sun-exposed areas: forehead, cheeks, temples, upper lip.

Crs: Slowly fades many mo after delivery or after bcp's are dc'd; may persist indefinitely; worsens each summer w UV exposure.

Rx: Minimize UV exposure (see RX.16.); hydroquinone (Eldoquin, Melanex, Solaquin, Lustra, Rx, $$) hs, sometimes w topical tretinoin, may be tried, although hydroquinone is potentially sensitizing and may induce uneven lightening; consider referral to dermatology.

PATCHY, SKINFOLDS ONLY

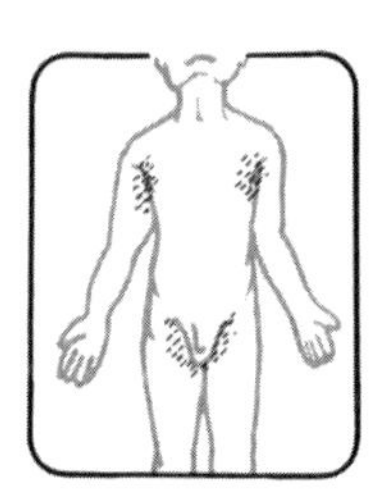

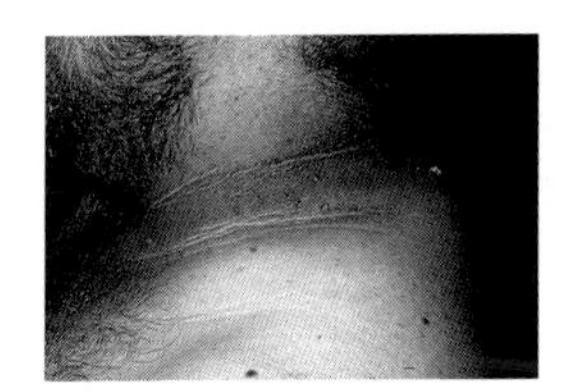

Acanthosis nigricans

22.2.A. ERYTHRASMA

Summary: Brown scaly rash; asx; pt often obese; look for similar eruption in toe webs, groin, perianal regions; bacterial infection; confirm by coral-red fluorescence w Wood's light if available (DX.4); does not respond to antifungal meds.

For additional details and rx, see GROIN RASH, 10.3.a.

22.2.B. ACANTHOSIS NIGRICANS

J Am Acad Derm 1994;31:1. Arch Derm 1992;128:941.

Cause: *Benign form*: most pts are obese; may have endocrinopathy, ie, DM, esp insulin resistant (Nejm 1976;294:739), pituitary or adrenal adenoma, Stein-Leventhal syndrome, chronic hepatitis, Cushing's syndrome, stilbestrol, or nicotinic acid (J Am Acad Derm 1994;31:1); *malignant form*: pt is thin; >40 yo; recent origin; most common assoc w abdominal adenocarcinoma, esp stomach (Am J Med 1995;99:662).

Epidem: Blacks >> whites (Am J Med 1989;87:269).

Sx: Asx.

Si: Brown to black; velvety texture; pedunculated FEPs often are present; most common sites are axillae, neck, groin; symmetric.

Crs: Most pts are young and obese and have had pigmentation for mos to yrs; eruption may clear w weight loss or correction of underlying endocrine or malignant disorder.

Lab: Consider pituitary, adrenal, or gonadotrophic cause in obese pt, esp if present for yrs; w/u for underlying malignancy of older thin pt, esp if recent onset.

Rx: Local rx not effective.

PATCHY, TRUNK OR SCATTERED, CHRONIC (YEARS)

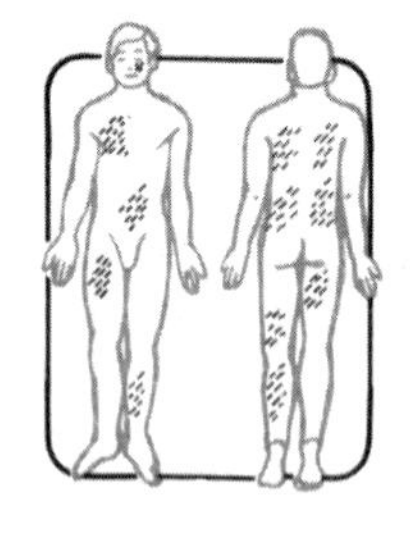

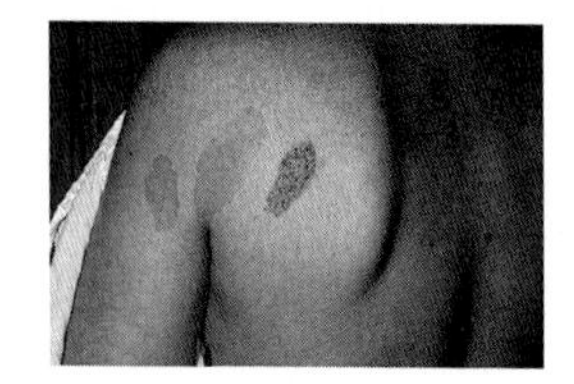

Café au lait spots

22.3.A. FRECKLE/LENTIGO

Summary: *Freckle*: common; 1–3 mm; multiple; brown; flat; genetically determined on face; presence on trunk and arms indicates past intense sun exposure; not premalignant; rx not necessary or practical; *lentigo*: smaller and darker than freckle; fewer in number; not confined to sun-exposed areas; bx occasionally warranted to r/o melanoma.

For additional details and rx, see GROWTHS, 11.7.a.

22.3.B. NEVUS, MELANOCYTIC (MOLE—JUNCTIONAL, COMPOUND, AND INTRADERMAL)

Summary: Round; tan to dark brown; sharply outlined, present since young adulthood; average white adult has 20; prophylactic removal of all nevi is neither possible nor necessary; excise or bx a nevus that has changed, bled, or is irregular or black.

For additional details and rx, see GROWTHS, 11.1.a.

22.3.C. BECKER'S NEVUS

Arch Derm 1965;92:249.

Summary: Localized; persistent; hairy patch; usually upper part of trunk; normal skin colored or light brown; most in adult men; no malignant potential; no rx needed.

22.3.D. MONGOLIAN SPOT

Summary: Common at birth or during first few wk; blue-black; flat; single or multiple; lumbosacral region, buttocks, or back; never malignant; usually disappear by 5 yo; no rx needed.

22.3.E. NEVUS OF OTA

Summary: Congenital but onset may be delayed until puberty; flat patch; dark brown to black; limited to 1st and 2nd branches of trigeminal nerve: unilateral (bilateral in 5%) over forehead, upper cheek, eye, often including sclera; most are female and Asian or black; never disappears; ↑risk of choroidal melanoma; no rx available.

22.3.F. NEVUS OF ITO

Summary: Congenital but onset may be delayed until puberty; unilateral; blue-black; limited to supraclavicular and brachial cutaneous nerves: neck and shoulder; no rx available.

PATCHY, TRUNK OR SCATTERED, RECENT (MONTHS) OR FLUCTUATING

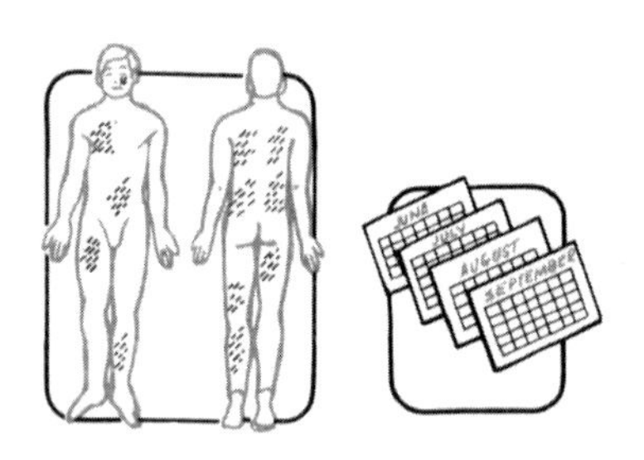

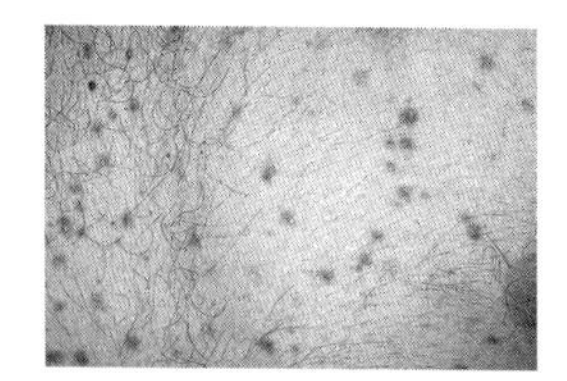

Urticaria pigmentosa

22.4.B. SYPHILIS, SECONDARY

Summary: Many patterns; most common: widespread, slightly scaly, tan, copper-colored, nonitchy patches, lesions on palms and/or soles; recent or healing genital ulcer; moist, wartlike genital growths (condylomata lata); painless oral erosions and mucous patches; "moth-eaten" scalp hair loss; mild or absent constitutional si and sx; LN↑, esp epitrochlear nodes; no blisters except in newborn; 2° lesions appear few wk after 1° rash disappears.

For additional details, see BODY, 3.1.f.

22.4.C. PITYRIASIS ROSEA

Summary: Pink to tan; round to oval; scaly patches; often distributed in a fernlike pattern; often starts w single larger patch (herald patch); asx or itchy; spreads from trunk to extremities, then recedes over 4–8 wk; r/o secondary syphilis w RPR.

For additional details and rx, see BODY, 3.1.c.

22.4.D. FIXED DRUG ERUPTION

Arch Derm 1984;120:520.

See color plate section.

Cause: Drug-induced local rxn; most common: bcp's, barbiturates, aspirin, NSAIDs, allopurinol, antibiotics, laxatives, or wines containing phenolphthalein.

Sx: Itchy and painful w exacerbations.

Si: One to few; patches are red and thickened w flare and deeply pigmented between flares; color darkens w each flare.

Crs: Recurs within 1 d after re-exposure.

Lab: Consider re-exposure to prove association; no danger of anaphylaxis.

Rx: Stop offending agent; TCS (class II–III); pigmentation may not subside for many mo.

22.4.E. URTICARIA PIGMENTOSA

Summary: About pencil eraser in size; tan; flat to slightly raised; often numerous; lesions become raised, reddened, and itchy, like a small hive, after rubbing or a hot shower (*Darier's sign*); systemic: flushing, palpitations, headache, tachycardia, syncope, hypotension, GI.

For additional details, see ITCH, 16.5.c.

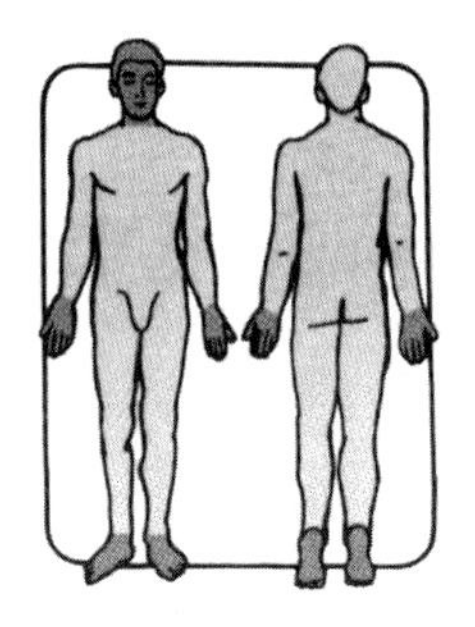

22.5. MISCELLANEOUS UNCOMMON DISORDERS

Summary: A variety of systemic disorders and systemic meds may induce diffuse hyperpigmentation but such cases encountered in clinical practice are few: Addison's disease (see 22.5.a.), biliary cirrhosis, Cushing's syndrome (see HAIR INCREASE, 13.2.), hemochromatosis (see 22.5.b.), malignancy (see 22.5.c.), melanoma (see GROWTHS, 11.4.b.), PCT (see LIGHT REACTIONS, 18.1.c.), scleroderma (see FEVER, 8.3.c.(1).), vitamin deficiency (see LIGHT REACTIONS, 18.3.d.), Wilson's disease.

22.5.A. ADDISON'S DISEASE

Am J Surg 1997;174:280. Endo Metab Clin N Am 1993;22:303.

Summary: Diffuse hyperpigmentation; darkest on sun-exposed parts, body folds, palmar creases, elbows, knees, oral mucosa, recent scars; hair thinning is common; pts often are thin and gaunt; up to 15% have vitiligo; course may be rapidly progressive and even fatal; deficiency of adrenocortical hormones from 1° adrenal insufficiency or 2° to pituitary insufficiency; only Addison's from adrenal failure leads to pigmentation; screen suspected pts w serum cortisol in early AM and 4 PM to detect either low baseline or absence of normal diurnal change (Review: Arch Dis Child 1999;80:330); consider referring suspected cases to endocrinology; pts may require cortisone and mineralocorticoid to prevent sudden circulatory collapse while evaluation is in progress.

22.5.B. HEMOCHROMATOSIS

BMJ 1998;316:125. Gastroenterol 1996;110:1107.

Cause: Genetic (Jama 1998;280:172): autosomal recessive w 1 in 10 persons a heterozygous carrier; iron overload, eg, thalassemia major; or dietary overload; ↑ dietary iron is rarely a factor in the U.S. but has been assoc w iron overload in the Bantu; most of skin darkening results from melanin, apparently induced by iron deposited in tissues.

Epidem: Women << men because of blood loss w menstruation.

Sx: Weakness, fatigue, abdominal pain, arthralgia.

Si: Diffuse darkening; deeper in sun-exposed regions; metallic gray to golden bronze hue; look for si of chronic liver disease: ↑ liver size, palmar erythema, spider angiomas.

Crs: Depends on underlying cause, which can be hereditary, hematologic, or hepatic; all cmplc worsen w age so younger pt may appear normal.

Cmplc: Diabetes (*bronze diabetic*); liver disease; heart disease, arthritis, hypogonadism; early rx prevents.

Lab: Screen: serum ferritin and iron-binding capacity are ↑; liver enzymes are usually abn; serum glucose is usually ↑ (Nejm 1993;328:1616).

Rx: Phlebotomy is 1° rx; obtain suitable consultations.

22.5.C. TUMORS

Rarely, pigmentation is associated w internal malignancy: esp carcinoma of lung due to production of pigment-stimulating hormones; metastatic melanoma due to uncontrolled melanin production.

23 Pregnancy Rashes

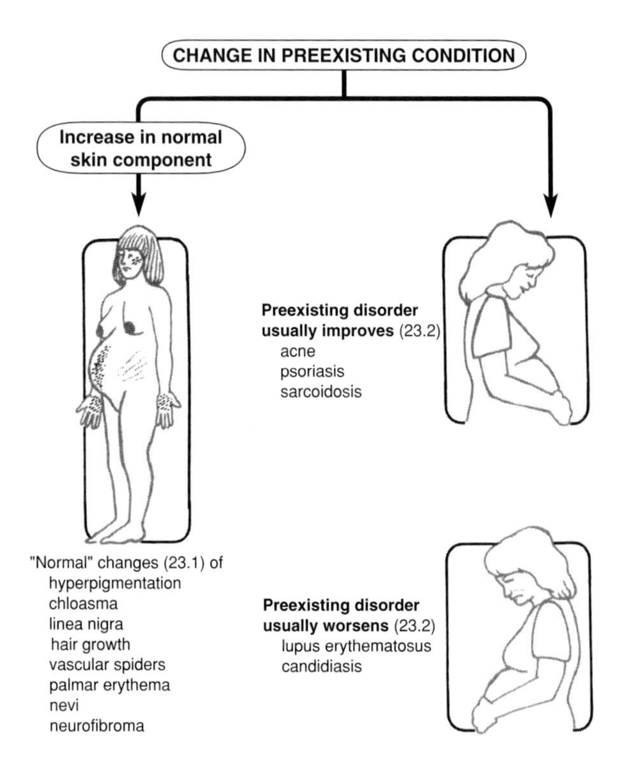

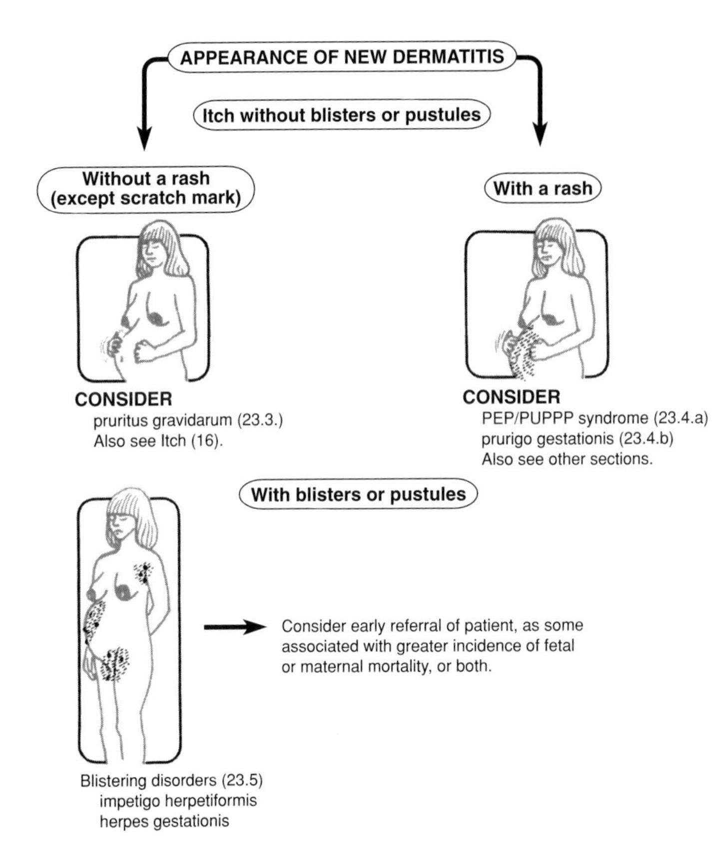

Also see Blisters (varicella, zoster, impetigo).

J Am Acad Derm 1999;40:233. J Am Acad Derm 1989;20:1. J Am Acad Derm 1983;8:405.

CHANGE IN THE APPEARANCE OF A PREEXISTING CONDITION

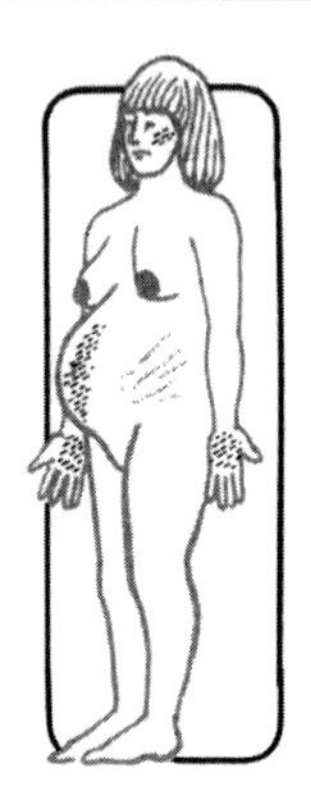

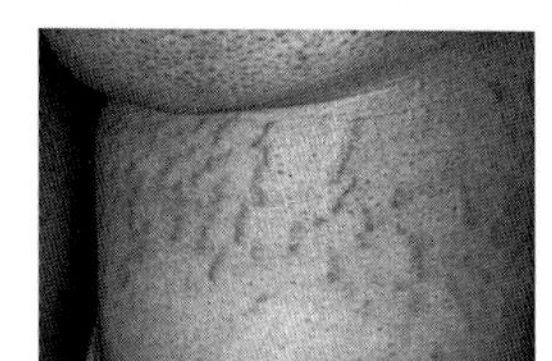

Striae

23.1. "NORMAL" PHYSIOLOGIC CHANGES OF PREGNANCY

Cause: Hormonal stimuli induce numerous physiologic changes during pregnancy.

Si:

- Hyperpigmentation: common (90%); usually 1st trimester: *linea alba* becomes *linea nigra*; freckles and nevi appear or darken; masklike facial pigment (70%), *chloasma*, worsens after UV exposure.
- Hair: temporarily ↑; moderate hair thinning often occurs about 3 mo after delivery (see HAIR DECREASE, 12.1.a.).
- Other: new atrophic *striae* on abdomen and breasts (90%); *vascular spiders* on face and upper trunk; *palmar erythema*; oily skin; *seborrhea*, common in late pregnancy; previously present growths, ie, *nevi*, *skin tags*, and *neurofibromas* are stimulated to grow; new nevi and skin tags appear.

Crs: May persist after delivery: chloasma, vascular spiders, striae, growths.
Rx: Generally avoid rx during pregnancy or while nursing.

23.2. CHANGE IN PREEXISTING SKIN DISORDER

Epidem/compl:

- Worsen: SLE; neurofibromas grow; some chronic infections flare, inc warts and candidal infection.
- Improve: acne, psoriasis, sarcoid.
- No change or no consistent effect: atopic dermatitis, scleroderma, or dermatomyositis (J Am Acad Derm 1998;20:100).

APPEARANCE OF A NEW SKIN CONDITION, ITCH WITHOUT A RASH (EXCEPT SCRATCH MARKS)

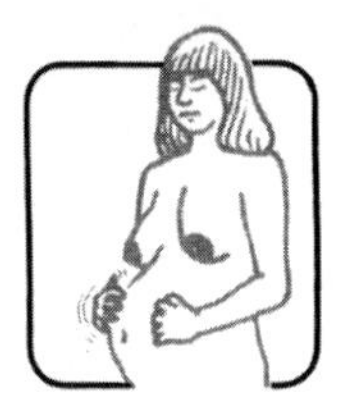

23.3. CHOLESTASIS OF PREGNANCY (PRURITUS GRAVIDARUM)

J Am Acad Derm 1998;20:100. BMJ 1994;309:1243.

Cause: Unknown; pos fhx in 50%.
Epidem: If appears in pregnancy, may develop later if taking bcp's.
Pathophys: Sx related to intrahepatic cholestasis and accumulation of bile salts (J Am Acad Derm 1998;20:100).
Sx: Intensely itchy; may be generalized but often worse on trunk.

Si: No skin lesions, except scratch marks.
Crs: Itching develops in 3rd trimester and tends to recur earlier in each subsequent pregnancy; usually clears shortly after delivery.
Cmplc: May have ↑ fetal distress.

- R/o other causes of liver insufficiency, eg, biliary stone or hepatitis; liver bx occasionally is necessary; for further evaluation of itching w/o skin rash in nonpregnant pts (see ITCH, 16.).

Lab: Although alkaline phosphatase is ↑ 2–4 × during pregnancy, it may be ↑ 7–10 × in this disorder.
Rx: Cholestyramine (Questran, 9 gm bid–qid) may relieve itching; probably safe during pregnancy because it is not absorbed, but no studies have been performed to prove safety; drug interferes w absorption of fat-soluble vitamins so give supplementation (J Am Acad Derm 1998;20:100); UVB helpful.

APPEARANCE OF A NEW SKIN CONDITION, ITCH WITH A RASH

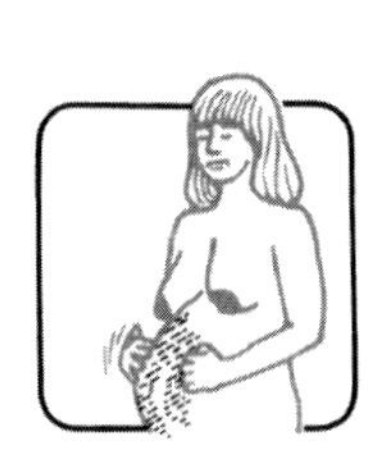

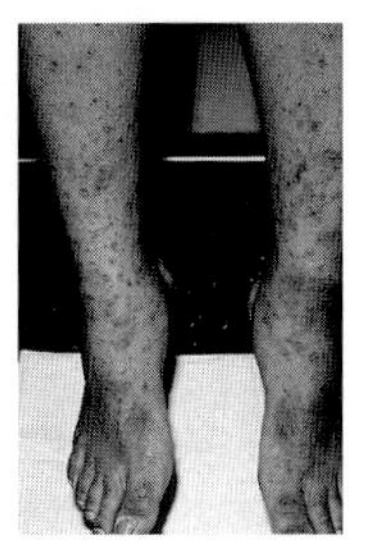

Prurigo gestationis

23.4.A. POLYMORPHIC ERUPTION OF PREGNANCY (PEP) OR PRURITIC URTICARIAL PAPULES AND PLAQUES OF PREGNANCY (PUPPP)

J Am Acad Derm 1998;39:933. J Am Acad Derm 1998;20:100. J Am Acad Derm 1984;10:473.

Cause: Unknown.
Sx: Pruritus.
Si: Discrete, itchy bumps and hivelike patches that suddenly appear over abdomen, esp in abdominal striae; later spread to thighs; spares umbilicus; no blisters.
Crs: Common; starts in primigravidae in late 3rd trimester; clears slowly in days to wks following delivery; seldom recurs in subsequent pregnancies; ↑ if carrying twins or more.
Cmplc: No ↑ fetal or maternal mortality (Jama 1979;241:1696).
Lab: No specific lab or bx changes.
Rx:

- Topical antipruritic, ie, calamine lotion, is safest rx and is partially effective.
- If additional relief is needed, add 2.5% HC oint.
- More potent TCS, ie, triamcinolone oint 0.1%, may be necessary.
- Discomfort occas necessitates use of systemic CSs in dose of 20–40 mg qd tapered over 2 wk.

PREGNANCY RASHES

23.4.B. PRURIGO GESTATIONIS

Cause: Unknown.
Epidem: Common; latter half of pregnancy (J Am Acad Derm 1998;20:100); often assoc w atopy.
Sx: Pruritus.
Si: Small, scratched papules, intermingled w scratch marks; generally confined to extensor surfaces of arms, legs, abdomen; if severe, also may involve trunk.
Crs: Both itch and rash clear shortly after delivery; may persist for mos; recurs w subsequent pregnancies.
Cmplc: No ↑ fetal or maternal cmplc; r/o: insect bites, drug eruptions, dermatitis herpetiformis, and other dermatoses of pregnancy.

Lab: No abn.

Rx:

- Topical antipruritics, ie, calamine lotion w 0.025% menthol, are safe and partially effective.

APPEARANCE OF A NEW SKIN CONDITION, BLISTERS OR PUSTULES

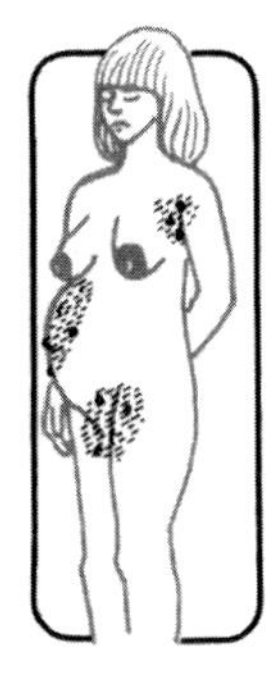

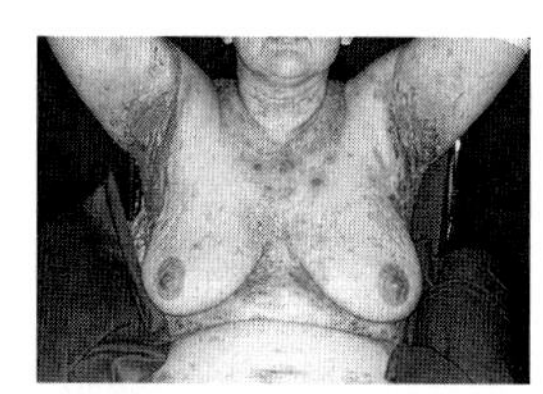

Impetigo herpetiformis

23.5. BLISTERING DISORDERS

Cause: Blisters or pustules are serious si; all disorders w blisters need prompt dx and rx (J Am Acad Derm 1998;20:100).

Cmplc: R/o:

- Infection, ie, bacterial impetigo, HSV, HZ.
- Blistering disorder not assoc w pregnancy (see BLISTERS, 2.).
- Rare condition assoc w pregnancy:

Impetigo herpetiformis: resembles pustular psoriasis; assoc w hypocalcemia; severe systemic sx and si; ↓ fetal survival; recurs w subsequent pregnancies (Arch Derm 1982;118:103).

Pemphigoid ("herpes") gestationis: starts as pruritus; later urticarial plaques w tense small and large blisters; 2nd–3rd trimesters; recurs w subsequent pregnancies and w periods, bcp's; may flare at delivery; dx confirmed w bx; some infants borne to mothers w condition have temporary blistering (Derm 1994;189(S1):50; Am J Ob Gynec 2000;183:483).

Rx: Consultation is almost always necessary; distinguishing between disorders may be difficult; some have potentially serious consequences, inc ↑ fetal and/or maternal mortality; get early dermatology consultation.

24 Scalp

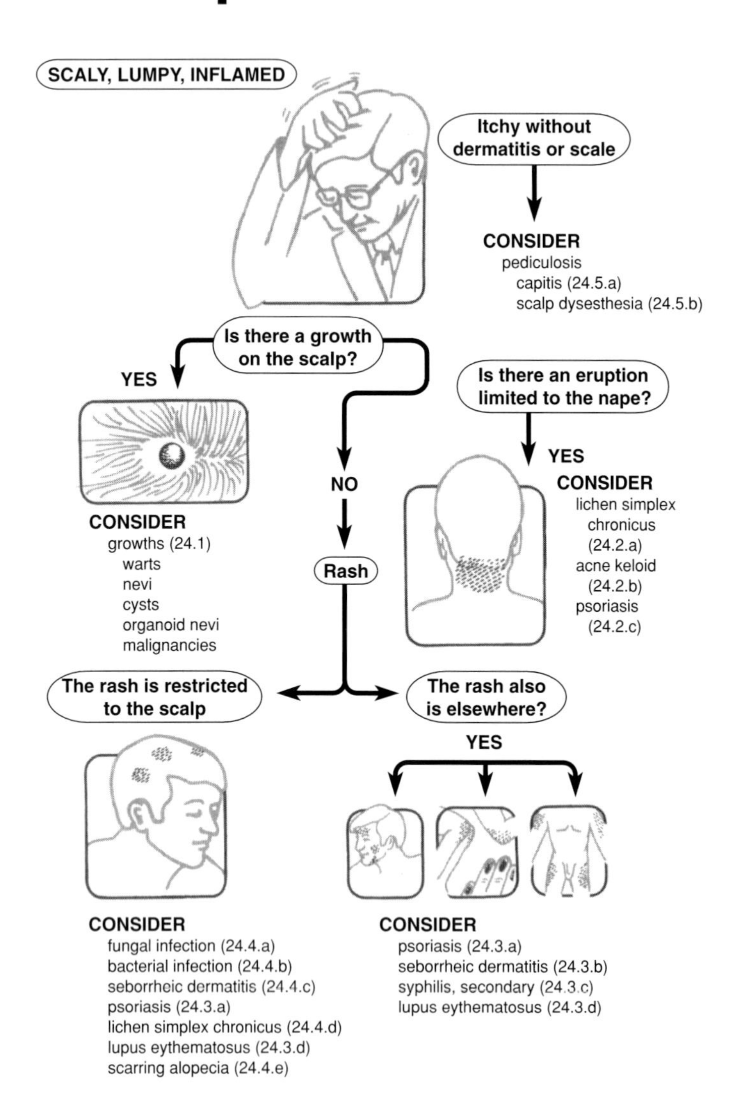

CONSIDER

fungal infection (24.4.a)
bacterial infection (24.4.b)
seborrheic dermatitis (24.4.c)
psoriasis (24.3.a)
lichen simplex chronicus (24.4.d)
lupus eythematosus (24.3.d)
scarring alopecia (24.4.e)

CONSIDER

psoriasis (24.3.a)
seborrheic dermatitis (24.3.b)
syphilis, secondary (24.3.c)
lupus eythematosus (24.3.d)

GROWTH

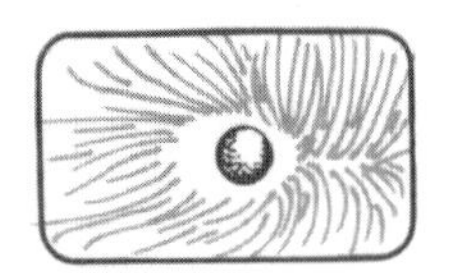

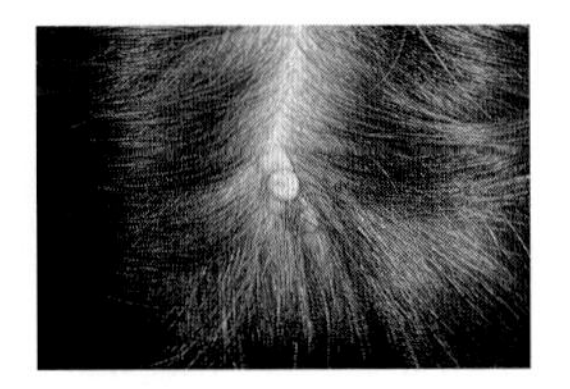

Organoid nevus

24.1. GROWTHS

Cause: Most common are *benign*: **warts** (see HAND, 14.1.a.), **nevi** (see GROWTHS, 11.1.a.), and **cysts** (see GROWTHS, 11.3.a.); *premalignant*: **organoid nevus** (nevus sebaceus); *malignant*: uncommon because of relative protection from UV light damage given by hair; *metastatic*: frequent site due to profuse blood supply, esp from breast, lung, renal.

Sx: None unless large or irritated.

Si: Large tumors, benign or malignant, may lead to localized hair loss, either by replacing hair-bearing skin or by damaging hair follicle from underlying pressure; organoid nevus: congenital; plaque; scalp or forehead; pebbly, hairless, yellow-orange-brown plaque; about 15% evolve into BCE during adulthood.

Lab: Bx occasionally needed to establish dx (see DX.7.).

Rx: Wart: LN2 (see RX.18.) or D&C (see RX.17.); rx of other scalp lesions depends on dx: see appropriate section after dx is established or refer pt to a dermatologist for confirmation and rx.

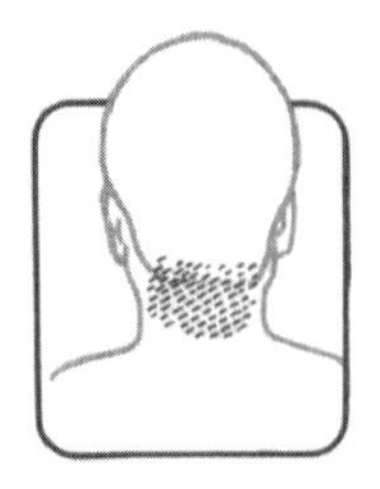

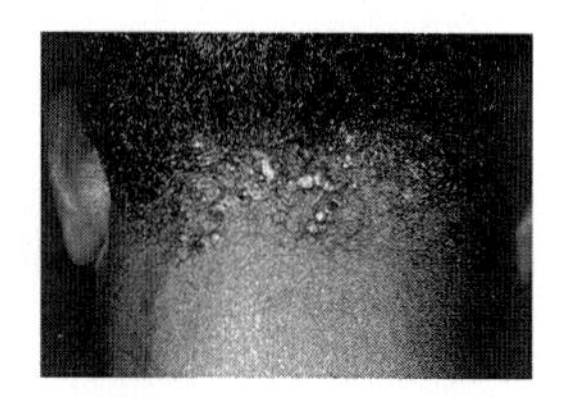

Acne keloid

24.2.A. LICHEN SIMPLEX CHRONICUS (LOCALIZED NEURODERMATITIS)

Summary: **Executive scalp syndrome**; single or a few; excoriated papules that heal and recur; may be a quite itchy, persistent patch; itches more during unoccupied evening hrs and at times of emotional stress; pts tend to be "high strung" and intense; appears anywhere on scalp but often at nape; chronic but waxes and wanes; resembles psoriasis.

For additional details and rx, see LEG RASH, 17.1.a.

24.2.B. ACNE KELOID

Cause: Hair appears to push into or re-enter scalp, inciting an inflammatory foreign body rxn, similar to that of pseudofolliculitis barbae (see FACE, 6.3.a.); close shaving of nape w a razor may trigger the condition.

Epidem: Nearly restricted to persons and races w tight curly hair.

Sx: Asx, itchy, or painful.

Si: Pustules and abscesses scattered among firm papules at back of the head or nape; fibrous keloidal plaques and scarring alopecia may develop eventually.

Crs: Chronic; responds poorly to rx.

Rx: Results are disappointing; may benefit from long-term systemic antibiotic, ie, erythromycin (500 mg qd–bid, $) or cephalexin

(500 mg qd–bid, $$); TCS (class I) gel or soln ($$$) (see RX.5.); IL CS (triamcinolone acetonide, 10 mg/mL repeated each mo × 3) (see RX.7.); topical retinoic acid (Retin-A cr 0.5% bid, $$) sometimes helps; severe: laser removal, surgical resection, or temporary epilation w x-ray has been used w variable success; refer extensive or resistant cases to a dermatologist.

24.2.C. PSORIASIS

Summary: A single patch of psoriasis may be restricted to nape but usually appears on other parts as well; examine other areas of scalp and elbows, knees, fingernails, umbilicus, and gluteal cleft to confirm dx.

For additional details and rx, see 24.3.a. and BODY, 3.1.d.

SCALY, LUMPY, OR INFLAMED, RASH ELSEWHERE AS WELL

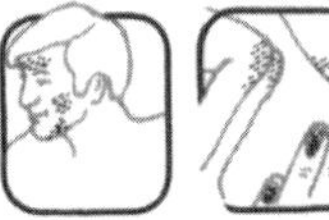

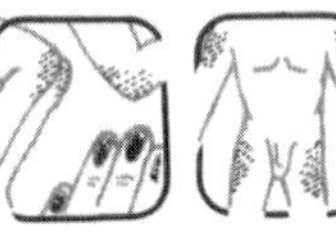

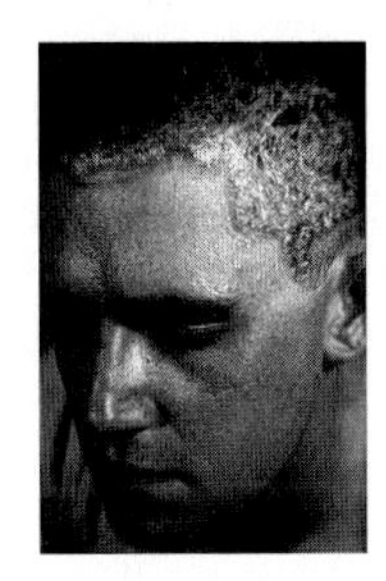

Psoriasis

SCALP

24.3.A. PSORIASIS

Summary: Scalp scaling may be patchy or may cover entire scalp; margins of plaques typically extend up to hairline, like a helmet; does not cause permanent balding, but scratching and resultant hair shaft breakage may lead to temporary thinning; look for other si of psoriasis, ie, round, reddened patches w dense, silvery, nongreasy scale on elbows, knees, coccyx, umbilicus, shins; also shallow pinpoint nail pits and separation of tip of nail from nail bed.

Rx: Psoriasis of scalp does not respond well to topical rx; may precede appearance of psoriasis elsewhere for yrs and persist long after psoriasis elsewhere has improved; try TCS (class II–III) lotions or soln bid (see RX.5.); if resistant, add topical calcipotriene (Dovonex soln, Rx, $$$) hs and continue TCS in AM; refer widespread or resistant cases to a dermatologist.

For additional details and rx, see BODY, 3.1.d.

24.3.B. SEBORRHEIC DERMATITIS

Cause: Probably *Pityrosporum ovale* infection or sensitivity.

Epidem: Common; often worse w stress and changes of season.

Sx: Itchy.

Si: Usually diffuse on scalp but may be patchy; mild erythema; scale is yellowish, greasy; **dandruff**, common term for scale w/o redness, is present; look for similar greasy scale and erythema at ear canals, behind ears, eyebrows, nasolabial folds; does not cause permanent balding, but scratching and resultant hair shaft breakage may lead to temporary thinning.

Crs: Chronic but fluctuating; most pts have mos of relative clearing and mos of relative worsening; often appears during infancy, clears in childhood, reappears in puberty, and may persist into old age.

Lab: None, although if extensive and recent onset, consider HIV infection (see HIV, 16.).

Rx:

- Mild or dandruff only: regular shampooing often provides sufficient control and reduces visible scale; daily shampooing is not harmful; if OTC "dandruff" shampoos containing zinc pyrithione are not

sufficient, try 1% OTC or 2% Rx ketoconazole shampoo (Nizoral shampoo, $$) twice wkly, or fluocinolone shampoo (Capex shampoo, $$) daily.
- Severe or does not respond to shampooing: continue ketoconazole shampoo and add TCS (class IV–V) lotion or soln to scalp after shampooing or bid, while scalp is still slightly damp (see RX.5.); consider psoriasis (see 24.3.a.) if condition continues to prove resistant to rx and consider dermatology referral.

For details and rx of seborrheic dermatitis of face, see FACE, 6.2.a.

24.3.C. SYPHILIS, SECONDARY

Summary: Scalp is not obviously inflamed, but patchy "moth-eaten" alopecia may be present.

For further details, see HAIR DECREASE, 12.3.b., BODY, 3.1.f., and GENITAL, 9.2.a.

24.3.D. LUPUS ERYTHEMATOSUS (LE)

Summary: Scalp may be only site; look for lesions on face, other light-exposed areas, in ear canals; DLE: patchy hair loss; SLE: patchy or diffuse loss.

For additional details and rx, see FACE, 6.2.c., and FEVER, 8.3.a.

SCALP

SCALY, LUMPY, OR INFLAMED, RESTRICTED TO THE SCALP

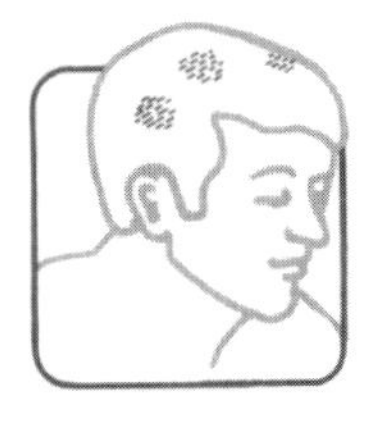

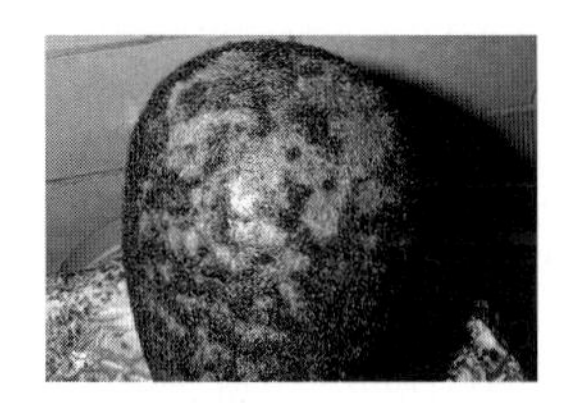

Tinea capitis

24.4.A. FUNGUS INFECTION (RINGWORM, TINEA CAPITIS)

Jaad 2000;42:1; J Am Acad Derm 1996;34:290. Derm Clin 1996;14:23.

Cause: Most common is *Trichophyton* species, esp *T. tonsurans*; *Microsporum* species had been common in past.

Epidem: Most occur in prepubertal children, often in minor epidemics.

Sx: Itchy; may be painful if *kerion*, a boggy, purulent inflammatory rxn, develops.

Si: Patches of thinned and broken scalp hairs, sometimes leaving only stubble of black dots; scalp is variably inflamed and may be scaly, resembling seborrheic dermatitis, or may be crusted or pustular; kerion may lead to permanent hair loss; cervical LN↑, esp w kerion.

Crs: Persistent and spreading, but inflammatory lesions eventually heal or "burn out."

Lab: Submit scaly debris and several plucked hairs for mycology culture; if a Wood's light is available (see DX.4), look for greenish yellow hairs indicating *Microsporum* infection, but this fungus has become uncommon; interpretation of a KOH exam of hair is difficult (see DX.3); inflammatory fungal infections may mimic bacterial folliculitis or cellulitis, but bacterial culture may be misleading.

Rx: Systemic griseofulvin in adequate doses (microsized, 20 mg/kg/d in children and 0.5–1.0 gm/d in adults, $$) in 2 or 3 divided doses after meals × 8 wk (see RX.11.); alternatives: terbinafine (250 mg, Lamasil, $$) 1/4 tab if < 20 kg, 1/2 tab if 20–40 kg, 1 tab if > 40 kg, all pc × 2 wk (*T. tonsurans* only) (J Am Acad Derm 1999;41:60), itraconazole (5 mg/kg/d × 1 mo, Sporanox, $$) (J Am Acad Derm 1998;39:216); fluconazole (1/2 tsp/20 kg/d × 3 wk, Diflucan, $$) (Ped Derm 1998;15:229); ketoconazole or selenium sulfide shampoo helps reduce numbers of infective spores; topical antifungal rx alone is inadequate.

24.4.B.(1). BACTERIAL INFECTION

Summary: Crusty and oozy yellow patches scattered about and on scalp w an unpleasant odor and cervical LN↑; suspect an underlying cause: pediculosis capitis (see 24.5.a.) or a fungus infection (see 24.4.a.); chronic scalp pyoderma may be assoc w hidradenitis suppurativa of axilla and groin (see AXILLA, 1.3.b.); consider dissecting perifolliculitis (see 24.4.b.(2).), esp in black male; refer pts w chronic scalp infection to dermatologist.

24.4.B.(2). DISSECTING PERIFOLLICULITIS OF THE SCALP (PERIFOLLICULITIS ABSCEDENS ET SUFFODIENS)

Cause: Unknown; mixed bacteria flora can be cultured from lesions, but condition is not primarily a bacterial infection.

Epidem: Generally restricted to black males.

Sx: Pain and pressure localized to lesions.

Si: Chronic, painful nodules, cysts, sinus tracts of scalp in a black male; assoc w scarring alopecia in patches at sites of lesions; often assoc w cystic acne or chronic hidradenitis suppurativa (see AXILLA, 1.3.b.).

Crs: Chronic and recalcitrant.

Lab: Not helpful; bacterial c + s sensitivities may be obtained prior to a course of antibiotics.

Rx: Unsatisfactory; some lesions may be relieved w IL triamcinolone acetonide (Kenalog, 10 mg/mL) (see RX.7.) or LN2 cryotherapy (see RX.18.); some extensive and resistant cases respond to temporary x-ray epilation; refer pts to dermatology to confirm dx and attempt control.

24.4.C. SEBORRHEIC DERMATITIS

Summary: Usually diffuse but may be patchy; yellowish greasy scale; mild redness and itching; similar scale and itching often present in ear canals, retroauricular areas, eyebrows, nasolabial folds.

For additional details and rx, see 24.3.b. and FACE, 6.2.a.

24.4.D. LICHEN SIMPLEX CHRONICUS

Summary: **Executive scalp syndrome**; single or a few excoriated papules that heal and recur; may be a quite itchy, persistent patch; itches more during unoccupied evening hrs and at times of emotional stress; pts tend to be "high strung" and intense; appears anywhere on scalp but usually at nape; chronic but waxes and wanes; resembles psoriasis.

For additional details and rx, see LEG RASH, 17.1.a.; also see SCALP DYSESTHESIA, 24.5.b.

24.4.E. SCARRING ALOPECIA

Summary: Acute phase: inflammation; later phase: shiny, atrophic, devoid of hair follicle openings; causes: DLE, lichen planus, sarcoid, pseudopelade, scleroderma, neoplasms; refer pt w scarring alopecia promptly to a dermatologist for dx and rx.

ITCHY, NO DERMATITIS OR SCALE

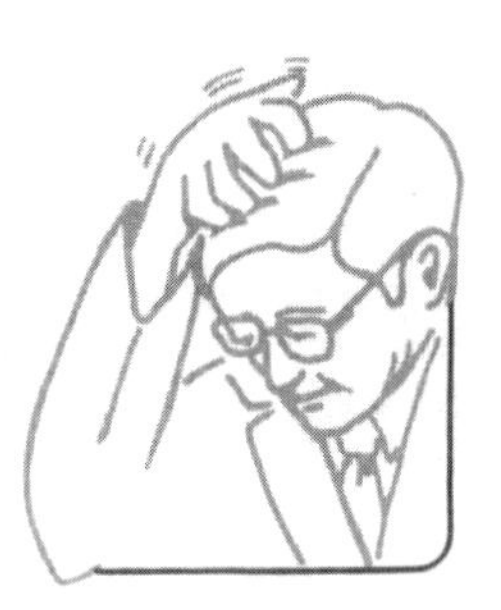

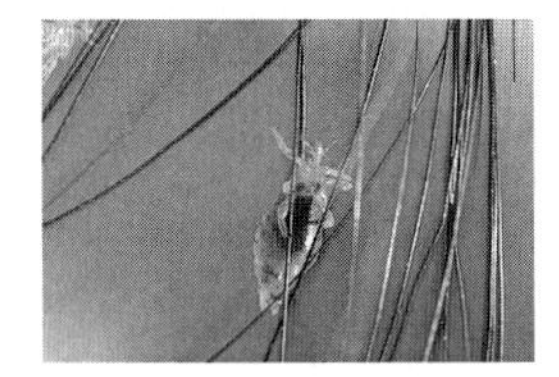

Louse on hair

24.5.A. PEDICULOSIS CAPITIS (HEAD LICE)

J Am Acad Derm 1998;38:979. Arch Dis Child 1996;75:471.

Cause: *Pediculus humanus capitis.*

Epidem: Spread by sharing clothing or combs; casual contact is not enough; involves all socioeconomic groups.

Sx: Persistent itching.

Si: Constant scratching w crusting and oozing; worse at nape; 2° bacterial infection common; lice resemble grains of wild rice, ie, brown and longer than wide; attached to scalp or loosely adherent to hair; prolonged infestation: *nits*, or egg cases, appear along hair shaft as adherent white granules, smaller than a pinhead; frequent cervical LN↑.

Crs: As nits are deposited at scalp level, estimate duration of infestation by measuring distance of nits above scalp w each cm representing about 1 mo of hair growth.

Cmplc: Persistent scratching may lead to emotional irritability, impetigo, furuncles.

Rx: Inform camp, school, or daycare center of infestation; permethrin (Nix cream rinse, OTC, $; Elimite or Acticin, Rx, $$) is preferred over lindane, which is neurotoxic: directions for use of permethrin: shampoo 1st w regular shampoo; rinse and towel dry; shake lotion; wet hair, scalp, behind ears, nape w lotion and leave on 10 min; rinse thoroughly and dry w clean towel; may use fine-toothed comb to remove dead lice and eggs; wash hairbrushes, combs, toys in very hot soapy water and do not share; vacuum furniture, floors, rugs; machine wash all clothing and bedding in very hot water and dry on hot cycle for 20 min; if not washable (hats, stuffed toys), dry-clean or seal in airtight plastic bag for 2 wk; pyrethrin w piperonyl butoxide (RID, A-200, OTC, $) is safe alternative but is not ovicidal and requires re-rx 1 wk later; malathion lotion (Ovide, 60 mL, Rx): kills lice and ova; safe for children and adults but not approved for neonates or infants; use for head lice that recur or resist other rx (Arch Derm 2001;137:287).

24.5.B. SCALP DYSESTHESIA

Summary: Itchy; burning; stinging; often "pins-and-needles"; "band" around head; most cases are in women; many also have anxiety, somatization; does not wake pt from sleep; may show mild hair thinning from chronic trauma; most respond to doxepin or amitriptyline (Arch Derm 1998;134:327); also see 24.4.d., Executive scalp syndrome.

25 Ulcer—Leg

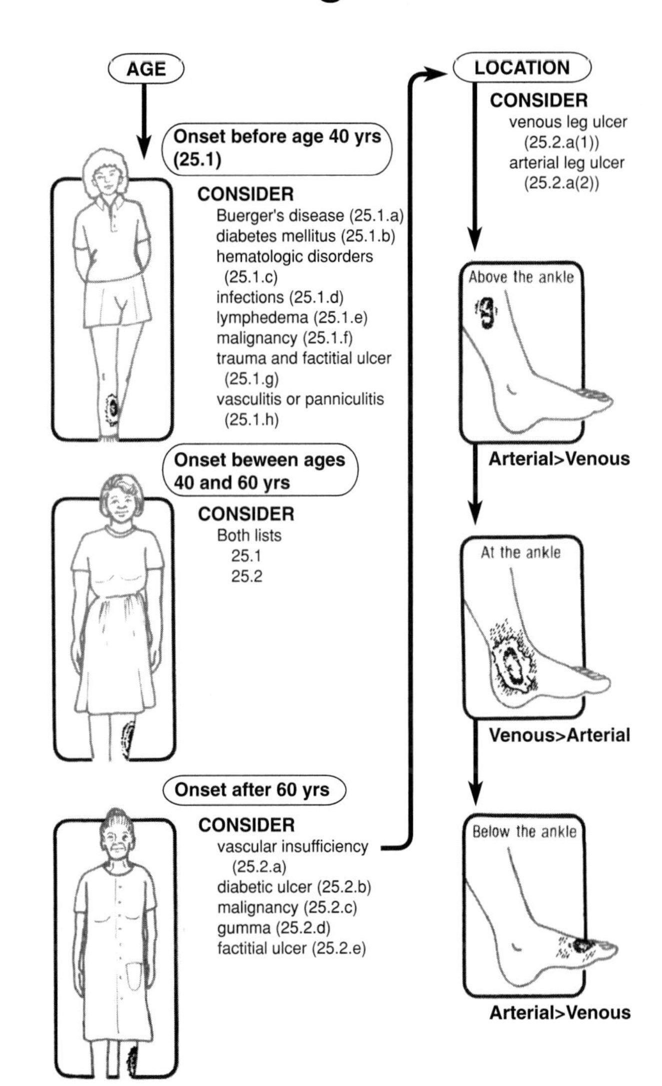

AGE
Onset before age 40 yrs (25.1)
CONSIDER
Buerger's disease (25.1.a)
diabetes mellitus (25.1.b)
hematologic disorders (25.1.c)
infections (25.1.d)
lymphedema (25.1.e)
malignancy (25.1.f)
trauma and factitial ulcer (25.1.g)
vasculitis or panniculitis (25.1.h)
Onset beween ages 40 and 60 yrs
CONSIDER
Both lists
25.1
25.2
Onset after 60 yrs
CONSIDER
vascular insufficiency (25.2.a)
diabetic ulcer (25.2.b)
malignancy (25.2.c)
gumma (25.2.d)
factitial ulcer (25.2.e)
LOCATION
CONSIDER
venous leg ulcer (25.2.a(1))
arterial leg ulcer (25.2.a(2))
Above the ankle
Arterial>Venous
At the ankle
Venous>Arterial
Below the ankle
Arterial>Venous

AGE <40 YEARS OLD

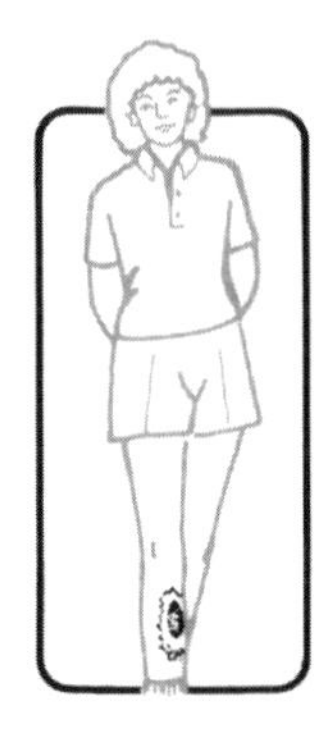

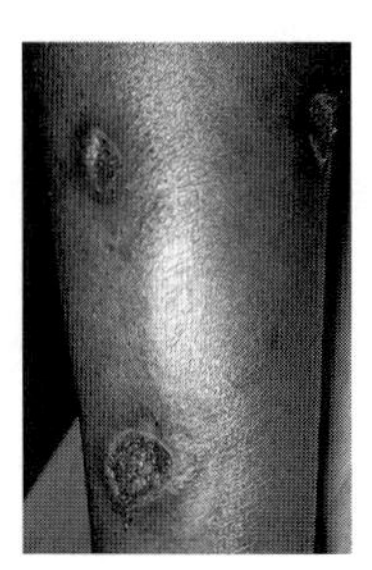

Vasculitis

25.1.A. THROMBOANGIITIS OBLITERANS (BUERGER'S DISEASE)

Cause: Usually addictive smoking; ↑ incidence of HLA-B5 and -A9 antigens.

Epidem: Men >>> women; 20–40 yo; heavy smokers; more common in Asians and persons of eastern European descent (Circ 1990;82:IV-3).

Pathophys: Occlusive vascular disorder of small and medium-sized arteries and veins, esp distal parts of legs and arms, but all vessels may be involved.

Sx: Claudication is early sx, 1st of foot, then calf.

Si: Raynaud's phenomenon; migratory superficial vein thrombophlebitis; ulceration develops w advanced disease; ↓ posterior tibial and dorsalis pedis pulses; hair loss on dorsa of feet; ulcers on fingers; skin atrophy; dependent rubor.

Crs: Progressive, esp if smoking is continued.

Ddx: Buerger's disease more likely than arteriosclerosis if serum lipids WNL, no DM, upper extremities involved, pt <40 yo.

Lab: Arteriography shows occluded small arteries w smooth-walled larger vessels w/o irregular plaques in large arteries assoc w arteriosclerosis; bx of vessel confirms dx.

Rx: No specific rx except dc tobacco products; obtain consultation w vascular surgeon (Nejm 2000;343:864).

25.1.B. DIABETES MELLITUS

Summary: Often deep; punched out; toes, plantar surface or over malleoli; painful unless neuropathy is severe; results directly from occlusion of small arterioles or indirectly following loss of local sensation from occlusion of vessels supplying nerve fibers; pedal pulses often remain normal; rx is difficult; rx as arterial ulcers (see 25.2.a.(2).); consider ulcerated necrobiosis lipoidica (see LEG RASH, 17.6.e.); seek early surgical consultation.

25.1.C. HEMATOLOGIC DISORDERS

Summary: Tend to be deep; punched out; persistent; result from sludging of blood and small-vessel occlusion; disorders: sickle cell disease, hemoglobin SC disease, thalassemia minor, hereditary spherocytosis, polycythemia vera, macroglobulinemia, cryoproteinemia, cold hemagglutinins α1-antitrypsin deficiency.

25.1.D. INFECTIONS

Summary: Tend to have heaped-up margins that spread outward, leaving a purulent and necrotic center; chronic infections, ie, tbc, gumma, may have areas of scarring from partial healing; **septic emboli** appear similar to **cholesterol emboli**: emboli released from ulcerated atherogenic plaque or from fragmenting atrial myxoma; diseases or organisms leading to leg ulcers include:

animal bites (*Pasteurella*)
anthrax
blastomycosis
clostridial abscess
diphtheria
fungi, deep

glanders (equine source)
mycobacteria and tbc
Pseudomonas infection, inc meliodosis
rat-bite fever (*Streptobacillus*)
schistosomiasis
staphylococcal infections
streptococcal infections
syphilis, tertiary
tularemia (*Francisella tularensis*)
Attempt dx by culture and bacterial and fungal staining of skin bx from edge of ulcer.

25.1.E. LYMPHEDEMA

Summary: *Congenital*: may be present at or near birth (**Milroy's disease**) or develop during early adulthood (**lymphedema praecox**); affects 1 or both legs; soft, pitting, painless, progressive; *acquired*: follows blocking of lymphatics by recurrent painful bouts of bacterial cellulitis or lymphangitis leading to further swelling, firm nonpitting edema, and dusky, pebbly surface; consider pelvic malignancy.

25.1.F. MALIGNANCY

Summary: Less likely cause of leg ulcer if pt <40 yo (see 25.2.c.).

25.1.G. TRAUMATIC AND FACTITIAL ULCER

Summary: Dx difficult: ulcer may have bizarre outline; may remain unchanged after extensive efforts at rx; may be in region of old scars; *physical factors*: previous x-ray rx, old thermal burns, cold injury, chrome toxicity, factitial or neurotic scratching; look for continuing source of injury, either self-induced for emotional or physical gain or from inadvertent irritating methods of care, ie, heating pad; r/o underlying vascular disease.

25.1.H. VASCULITIS OR PANNICULITIS

Cause: Ulcers may be deep, indolent; assoc w SLE, scleroderma, dermatomyositis; **pyoderma gangrenosum**: starts as pustule or red-blue nodule that ulcerates and forms a rolled, undermined violaceous border that expands, sometimes to many cm; assoc w inflammatory bowel disease in 1/2; others may have RA, paraproteinemia, malignancy, esp leukemia or lymphoma (J Am Acad Derm 1996;34:1047).

Si: Skin lesions usually are palpable and purpuric; usually multiple; if systemic: may have arthralgias, fatigue, GI and/or renal sx.

Lab: May include bx of ulcer edge for histology stains and culture, hgb electrophoresis, serum protein electrophoresis, cryoprotein levels, serum amylase, urine and stool specimens for blood; obtain dermatology and vascular consultation.

Rx: Treat specific cause when identified; cleanse w compressing and control bacterial contamination (see 25.2.a.(1).); rx of pyoderma gangrenosum may include systemic CS, immunosuppressants (J Am Acad Derm 1996;34:1047), cyclosporine, thalidomide (J Am Acad Derm 1998;38:490); consider referral of unresponsive leg ulcers to dermatology or wound center.

For additional details, see FEVER, 8.1.n.

AGE >60 YEARS OLD

25.2.A. VASCULAR INSUFFICIENCY (VENOUS, ARTERIAL, BOTH)

Cause of >90% of leg ulcers; most due to incompetent veins w chronic venous hypertension, rather than occluded arteries; persons w leg ulcers >60 yo have both venous and arterial insufficiency, but often 1 component predominates and affects rx and outcome.

25.2.A.(1). VENOUS LEG ULCER (VENOUS INSUFFICIENCY, VARICOSE ULCER, STASIS ULCER)

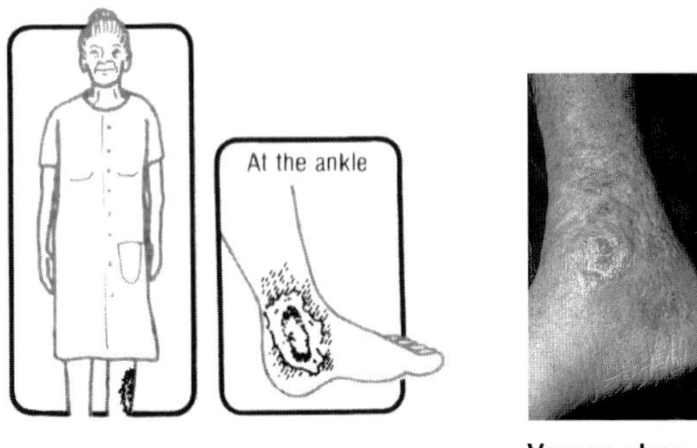

Venous ulcer

Cause: Veins widen w age as surrounding supportive tissue weakens; then valves become incompetent and blood pools, further dilating veins, leading to episodes of phlebitis, which further damage valves, leading to leakage of serum and rbc's through dilated and damaged vessel walls, leading to edema, hemosiderin deposits, which lead to inflammatory rxn and then pigmentation and fibrosis.

Sx: Painful but not so severe as to interfere w sleep; pain of arterial insufficiency is worsened by elevation; that from venous insufficiency is worsened by dependency.

Si: Leg edema; brown, speckled pigmentation from hemosiderin; dry scaling and itching precede ulcer; *ulcer*: usually single; located on medial side of ankle or lower third of shin; tends to be wide rather than deep; usually irregular undulating edge and clean base; ulcers >3 cm usually venous rather than arterial; leg or foot is warm; palpable pedal pulses suggest venous rather than arterial cause; varicosities nearly always present.

Crs: Preceding circulatory stasis; healing is slow; recurrences are common; eventually, skin becomes fibrotic and indurated.

Lab: Specialty evaluation usually not needed unless correctable arterial disease is suspected; special assessment may be noninvasive:

venous plethysmography and venous Doppler studies; or more definitive, but invasive, phlebography.

Rx: (Review: Jaad 2001;44:401).

- Control factors that interfere w healing, esp leg edema, anemia, poor nutrition, infection, DM, irritating topical meds.
- Maintain a clean ulcer base w saline or aluminum acetate compresses (see RX.2.) 20 min qid; if ulcer has a greenish purulent exudate and a foul, mousy odor: consider *Pseudomonas* species and compress w 2% acetic acid, made by adding 5 tsp household white vinegar to 2 cups lukewarm tap water; whirlpool, available in physical therapy units at most hospitals, also speeds up debridement.
- Cover ulcer after cleansing w thick coat of silver sulfadiazine cream (Silvadene, $) or mafenide acetate cream (Sulfamylon, $$); finally, pt covers ulcer w dry, sterile gauze; dressings that assist in cleansing and re-epithelialization: Bioclusive, DuoDerm, Op-Site, Tegaderm, Vigilon left in place for several d; these dressings accumulate drainage material and are difficult for pts to use themselves.
- Obtain c + s if ulcer not healing or purulent.
- If ulcer is clean and dry, consider an *Unna boot*: zinc oxide/gelatin dressing (Dome Paste) for protection and support; follow package instructions to apply; leave in place for a wk unless there is excessive drainage.
- Support stockings provide compression of superficial veins, as well as protection from minor injury; *defer their use until ulcer has fully healed*; the best are labeled as supplying 20–40 mm of pressure but are expensive ($70, not covered by most insurers) and difficult to put on, but an acceptable alternative can be purchased in local pharmacies for about $20 (Jobst, Medi USA, and Sigvaris).

25.2.A.(2). ARTERIAL LEG ULCER (HYPERTENSIVE ISCHEMIC, ARTERIOSCLEROTIC ULCER)

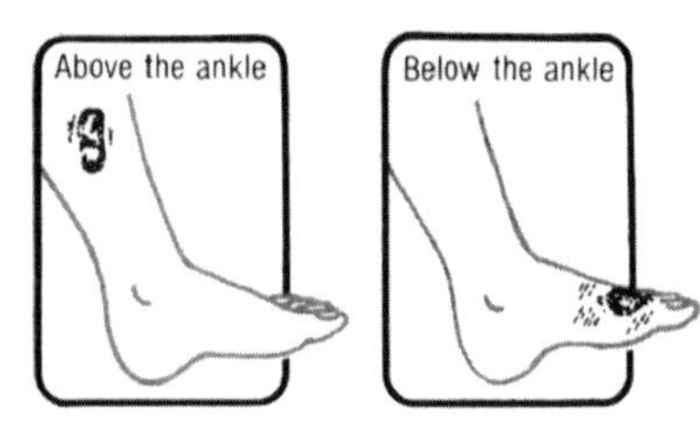

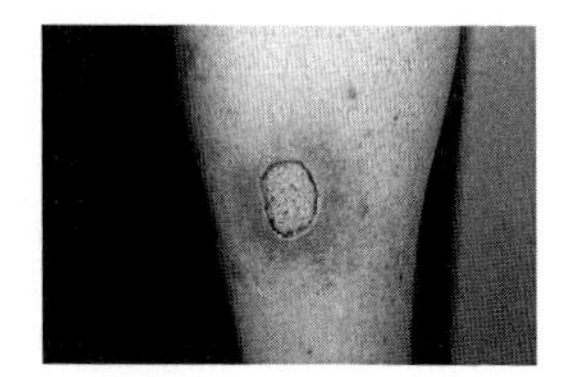

Arterial ulcer

Cause: Arterial obstruction in major or both large and small arteries: atherosclerosis; small arteries: esp w DM or in heavy smokers (Review: Jaad 2000;43:1001).

Sx: Often excruciatingly painful, even at rest; more likely to interfere w sleep than venous ulcers; pain of arterial insufficiency is worsened by elevation; that from venous insufficiency is worsened by dependency.

Si: Usually lateral side of ankle or calf or over heel; if severe may cause ulcers or gangrene of distal part of foot or toes; mottled brown pigmentation of venous stasis dermatitis is not present; leg edema is minimal or absent; hair on dorsum of foot is absent; not as large as venous ulcers but are deeper w a more sharply "punched-out" edge and a more necrotic base; pulses often are absent and foot is cold in pts w large-artery occlusion, but these si are unreliable indicators of small-artery occlusion, esp in pts w DM.

Crs: Ulcers heal slowly or not at all; may precede other si of major arterial insufficiency, inc gangrene of toes.

Lab: Doppler flow studies are justified in pt w absent or diminished pulses, esp if in groin or popliteal space, as a surgically correctable large-artery occlusion may be present.

Rx:

- Because of diminished blood supply, ulcers 2° to arterial insufficiency do not heal well, only about 1/3 respond to conservative rx (Acta Derm Venereol 1995;75:133); emphasize need to quit smoking; vasodilator drugs are of little value.
- Leg elevation is harmful, as this diminishes tissue perfusion; pt may benefit from moderate exercise, ie, dangling legs over the bed and successively flexing the foot in dorsal and plantar direction, starting w 5 min tid; seek surgical or vascular evaluation early if suspect arterial insufficiency.

25.2.B. DIABETIC ULCERS

Summary: Often deep; punched out; toes, plantar surface, or over malleoli; painful unless neuropathy is severe; result directly from occlusion of small arterioles or indirectly following loss of local sensation from occlusion of vessels supplying nerve fibers; pedal pulses often remain normal; rx is difficult; rx as arterial ulcers (see 25.2.a.(2).).

25.2.C. MALIGNANCY

Summary: Most are from *local skin tumors*: BCE, SCC, melanoma, KS; *systemic tumors*: ulcers less common than phlebitis; phlebitis tends to be migratory, may appear anywhere, not just legs; most assoc w carcinoma of pancreas; obtain skin bx (see DX.7.) of edge.

For additional details, see LEG RASH, 17.

25.2.D. SYPHILIS, TERTIARY (GUMMA)

Summary: Chronic "punched-out" ulcer; border may be bizarre w some regions showing scarring while others are spreading into circles or arcs; feels deeply infiltrating; resembles malignancy; usually single; all occur in older persons; underlying bone may show destructive changes; skin and bone most common, but any organ may be involved; *T. pallidum* may be recovered in lesion; STS often neg but FTA is pos; late syphilis is now rare; responds to penicillin; for other infections, see 25.1.d.

25.2.E. FACTITIAL

Summary: Consider possibility of factitial injury in any pt w chronic leg ulcers that do not respond to rx.

26 DX—Diagnostic Procedures

DX.1. BACTERIAL SMEARS AND CULTURES

Purpose: To identify and classify bacterial infections into gram-pos and gram-neg bacilli or cocci; to visualize some yeasts; Gram's stain: easy, assists selection of initial rx, is more quantitative than routine cultures in which minor organisms may overgrow the dominant one.

Sampling: Obtain specimen from unopened pustule or abscess, where possible.

Method: CLIA rules now make it difficult to perform Gram's stain in practitioner's offices; therefore, details of the method are not included; submit material for Gram's stain to a commercial laboratory.

Pitfalls: Culture of open, scaly, or eczematous skin or culture of tissue or blood through such areas may reveal irrelevant and contaminating bacteria, not the true pathogen.

DX.2. CYTOLOGIC (TZANCK) SMEAR

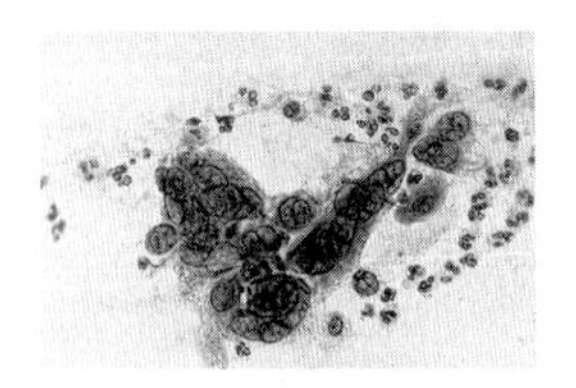

Multinucleated giant cells

Purpose: To rapidly identify some herpesvirus infections and to distinguish pemphigus vulgaris from other bullous disorders.

Sampling: Ideal source of cells: base of intact blister, but multinucleated cells of a herpesvirus infection sometimes may be identified from a herpetic erosion or crust; unroof blister w scissors or No. 10 or 15 scalpel blade; gently scrape base of blister w edge of blade and roll debris gently onto microscope slide; spray w PAP fix, if available; submit for Tzanck smear, usually performed w Giemsa stain.

Method: CLIA rules now make it difficult to perform Tzanck stain in practitioner's offices; therefore, details of the method are not included; submit material for Tzanck or Giemsa stain to a commercial laboratory to be read by a pathologist or dermatopathologist.

Pitfalls: Late or crusty lesions usually yield neg smears.

DX.3. POTASSIUM HYDROXIDE (KOH) EXAMINATION

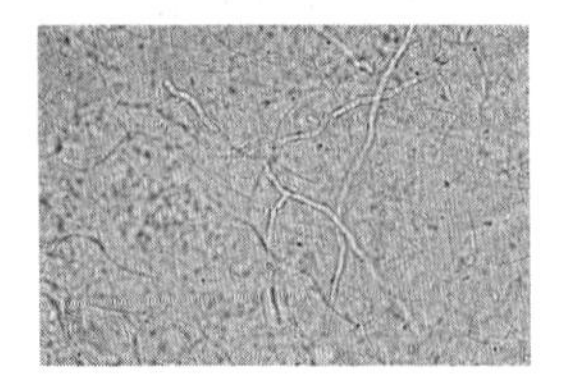

Hyphae of dermatophyte

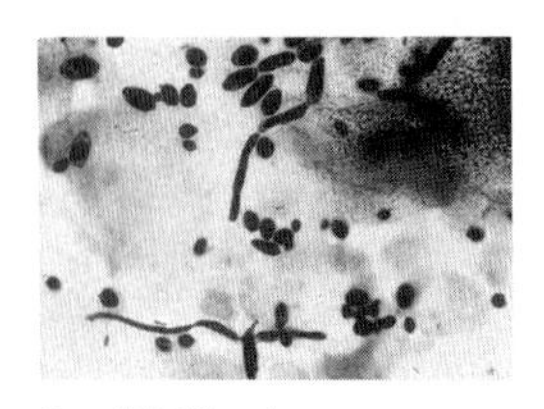

Candidal hyphae

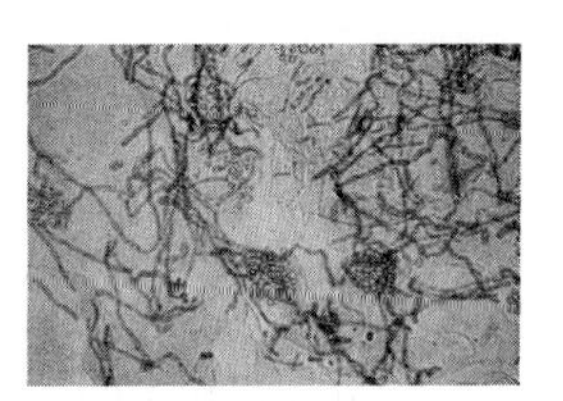

Tinea versicolor hyphae

DX

Purpose: To identify fungal and yeast organisms; KOH dissolves epidermal cells but not fungal elements, allowing hyphae to be visualized more easily among cell walls.

Sampling: *Scaly rash*: cleanse skin w an alcohol swab to remove surface lipids and hold scale together; scrape lesion w edge of No. 10 or 15 blade, catching scale directly onto microscope slide; *blister*: unroof w scalpel blade; put blister roof, blister side up, on slide; *hair*: infected hair tends to break off at scalp level so pluck short hairs, which may appear as black "dots" in thinned areas of scalp, w forceps.

Method: CLIA rules now make it difficult to perform KOH exams in practitioner's offices; therefore, although details of the method are provided here, generally the PCP must submit material in a sterile dry tube to a commercial laboratory for a KOH exam or refer pt to a dermatologist, most of whom are CLIA certified for the exam.

- Put 1–3 drops 10% KOH solution on specimen and cover w a coverslip; gently warm slide over a low flame for 5–10 sec to speed dissolving of epidermal cells; locate suggestive hyphae w low-power objective and confirm w high-dry; refractile differences between hyphae and epidermal cells ↑ if light intensity is ↓ and microscope condenser is racked to its lowest position; clean microscope objective and stage to avoid etching instrument with KOH.

Interpretation: Hyphae of *dermatophyte* infections are thin, long, and branched, extending over many epidermal cell diameters; *candidal* hyphae are easily broken and often shorter, typically w clusters of spores; hyphae of *tinea versicolor* are short, only as long as a few cell diameters, stubby, curved, usually numerous and are accompanied by small spores, giving an appearance of spaghetti and meatballs.

Pitfalls: Fibers and threads resemble hyphae but are thicker and more irregular; epidermal cell walls may line up to resemble hyphae: sufficient warming and time will cause these walls to disappear; scraping may not have been deep enough: scrape deeply enough to *almost* draw blood; ask pt about antifungal agents, as even use for a few d often precludes a pos result on KOH exam.

DX.4. WOOD'S LIGHT EXAMINATION

Purpose: To identify *erythrasma*, an infection of *Corynebacterium minutissimum*; *tinea capitis* caused by *Microsporum* species; *Pseudomonas* infection; hypopigmented lesions of *tinea versicolor*; *vitiligo*; ash-leaf spots of *tuberous sclerosis;* fluorescence of urine from pts w PCT.

Materials: A Wood's light w an output in the 360-nm range can be purchased from a medical, laboratory, or hobby supply shop as a "black light" for $50–$75.

Method: Output of a Wood's light is low; perform exam in a completely darkened room, bringing light within 1–2 inches (2.5–5 cm) of area being examined.

Interpretation: *Erythrasma*: bright coral-red color in deeper skin folds; *tinea capitis*: blue-green fluorescence if caused by *Microsporum* species but is nonfluorescent in more common inflammatory form caused by *Trichophyton* species; *Pseudomonas aeruginosa* infections: yellow-green: *tinea versicolor*, *vitiligo*, and *tuberous sclerosis*: do not fluoresce, but Wood's light causes them to appear lighter or distinct from background skin color; *PCT*: may have sufficiently high urinary levels of porphyrins to show a coral-red fluorescence.

Pitfalls: False neg if room is too light or if lamp is not placed close enough to lesion; most cases of tinea capitis do not show fluorescence; a more sensitive screening procedure must be used if porphyria is suspected and Wood's light exam is neg; cosmetics and topical meds often are fluorescent.

DX.5. HAIR TESTS

HAIR PULL

Purpose: To determine if hair loss is actively occurring.
Method: Grasp a hank of 20 or so hairs between thumb and forefinger, gently squeeze and pull away from scalp.
Interpretation: *Normal*: 1 or 2 hairs come away from scalp; *active hair loss*: 5 or more hairs come out, most often occurs w telogen effluvium and at edge of a patch of still-expanding alopecia areata.

HAIR COLLECTION

Purpose: To determine if abn numbers of hairs are being shed.
Method: Pt collects scalp hair each d for 7 consecutive d, including hairs collected from comb, brush, sink and tub, pillows; counts them and places them in separate *clear* plastic sandwich bags labeled w number of hairs and whether hair was shampooed that d.
Interpretation: Normal hair loss is 50–100/d; this may be several hundred/d w active telogen effluvium.

HAIR SHAFT EXAM

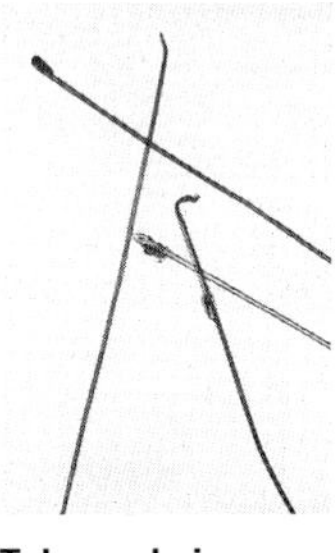

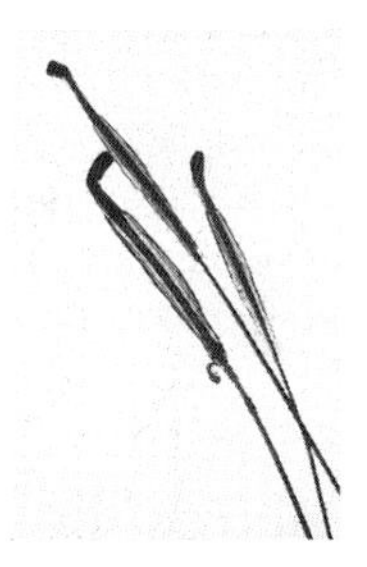

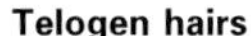

Telogen hairs **Anagen hairs**

Purpose: To determine if shed hairs are normal or abn.
Method: Exam proximal ends, distal ends, and shaft of a representative number of hairs; this is done conveniently by examining hairs while still in their clear plastic bags as brought in by pt as described above; use low-power microscope objective or an inverted eyepiece.

Interpretation:

- **Proximal ends**: *telogen* hairs are bulbous "clubs"; *anagen* hairs have a long sheath along proximal end and should be infrequent; *broken ends*: suggestive of hair shaft abn often due to excessive perms or straighteners.
- **Distal ends**: most hairs will be neatly squared off from hair cutting; distal ends that are frayed or look like broom straws result from recent exogenous trauma, esp hair care, or an endogenous hair shaft abn, generally present for yrs.
- **Hair shaft**: partially broken hairs, frayed segments indicate the same damage as w frayed distal ends; a mixture of numerous hairs of narrow diameter and normal-sized hairs may indicate androgenic alopecia (pattern balding).

DX.6. PATCH TESTING

Purpose: To identify substances to which pt has developed an allergy.

Materials: A kit of 24 test items set in 2 easily placed multiwell test strips for office patch testing (T.R.U.E. Test Allergen Patch Test, Glaxo Wellcome; 800.878.3837); $250/5 test kits; individual antigens, ie, components of latex gloves, cosmetics, industrial chemicals, household cleaners, and hobby materials, in a form or concentration suitable for patch testing, are no longer easily obtained due to recent stringent FDA requirements on purity of components; testing generally requires referral to a dermatologist who specializes in contact allergy or to specialized occupational medicine or contact allergy clinics in teaching centers.

Method: As allergy patch testing is generally impractical for the PCP and even most dermatologists and allergists, and since most pts w significant problems that require patch testing will be referred to specialty centers, no details on methods or interpretation are provided here; however, method for use of T.R.U.E. test may be obtained from Glaxo Wellcome (800.334.0089).

- *USE TEST*: often an inciting antigen can be identified by a simple elimination protocol that can be done in the office (see BODY, 3.1.a.).

Pitfalls: Discovery of 1 allergy-inducing product does not eliminate all others, as multiple products may contain the same antigenic agent; a false-pos result may result from nonspecific erythema induced by occlusion and pressure of the patch test; pos patch rxns may be delayed for 1–2 d; people are exposed to thousands of chemical products every yr and only a handful are available for testing, so if rxn is neg, the right chemical or concentration may not have been tested; high doses of systemic CS may depress patch test results.

DX.7. SKIN BIOPSY

Purpose: To obtain a small amount of tissue for histologic examination; 3 methods of skin bx are commonly used: punch, TSR, incision (excision); methods for punch and shave bx are outlined here; the purpose of incisional or excisional bx is to remove a larger area or to remove the entire lesion for dx and is a larger surgical procedure not covered in this text; "what" to bx is more important than "how to" bx and the physician who performs bx must be able to interpret histopathologic findings (Ann IM 1999;130:617).

PUNCH BIOPSY

Purpose: Punch bx is simple and quick and can yield a plug of skin that extends into sc fat.

Materials: Sterile disposable circular skin punches in diameters of 1–8 mm (generally, use 2 mm on face and 4 mm elsewhere); available from Acuderm, Inc., Ft. Lauderdale, FL 33309 (954.733.6935) or Fray, Miltex, Sklar, or others through distributor, at a cost of about $1.50 each.

Method: Cleanse skin w an antiseptic; inject sufficient volume of local anesthetic; twirl punch in a circular motion deep enough to reach sc layer; either pluck loose plug out w a forceps or lift it and snip it off at base of bx specimen; drop into fixative; close wound w suture, a small piece of Gelfoam, or just apply pressure and cover w tape.

TANGENTIAL SHAVE REMOVAL (TSR)

Purpose: TSR removes only epidermis and upper part of dermis but is sufficient if pathology is superficial.

Materials: Double-edged razor blade broken in half and sterilized.

Method: Hold razor blade between thumb and forefinger; bend it into a slight curve; slice off a layer of skin extending down into dermis; stop any bleeding w light pressure, electrodesiccation, or application of Monsel's solution or aluminum chloride (Drysol) on a cotton-tip applicator; although anticoagulants or salicylates cause ↑ bleeding, a skin bx may still be performed on pts taking either med.

Pitfalls of skin bx:

- Bx newly appearing or infiltrated lesions rather than scratched or infected sites.
- Bx edge of large lesions rather than a central scarred or necrotic area.
- Obtain 2 or 3 specimens if lesions are in varying stages.
- Bx blisters by incision or excision w scalpel, rather than punch, as twisting of punch usually disrupts blister roof.
- Do not include normal skin in specimen; the technician may have oriented specimen so that only normal area is sectioned; furthermore, the pathologist knows what normal skin looks like.

27 RX—Therapy

RX.1. MOISTURIZERS

Purpose: Use moisturizers to relieve itch and discomfort of chronic, scaly, noninflamed skin conditions; avoid them or use them only as an adjunct in acute or subacute conditions presenting w oozing, crusting, or pain.

Mechanism: Moisturizers slow evaporation of water, thus hydrating skin, making it more supple; use moisturizers in conjunction w ↓ use of soap and overlong or overfrequent bathing or hand washing, which leaches skin lipids and prevents retention of moisture (see Bathing Instructions for Dry Skin).

Preparations: Moisturizers are of 2 general types: white cr, ie, cold cr, and clear oints, ie, petrolatum; crs are more easily removed w water and feel less thick and sticky than oints; medicinals in oints are better absorbed than those in crs; in general, use oints for maximal moisturizing and hs; use crs for daytime use; numerous moisturizers are available, but plain petrolatum remains most effective; others are listed in Bathing Instructions for Dry Skin (feel free to photocopy, enlarge, and distribute to pts).

RX.2. COMPRESSES (WET DRESSINGS)

Purpose: Use compresses—repeated applications of moist dressings—for either acute or chronic skin conditions that are crusty, oozy, or swollen; compresses are cooling, suppress inflammation, and provide gentle debridement.

Mechanism: Compresses differ from soaks, or immersion, of the affected part; soaks are not effective for skin conditions as they produce maceration of crusts, rather than debridement; use *cool compresses* for acute inflammation w crusting, swelling, and itch, ie, acute poison ivy dermatitis; use *warm compresses* for chronic conditions, ie, dirty or crusty leg ulcers.

Preparations: Salt water: least expensive and most convenient; prepare by dissolving a tsp of table salt in 2 cups of tap water; ulcers contaminated w gram-neg organisms, ie, *Pseudomonas* species, can be cleansed w 2% acetic acid made by adding 5 tsp of household white vinegar to 2 cups of warm tap water; follow directions in pt handout, Wet Compresses (feel free to photocopy, enlarge, and distribute to pts):

- Note: if pt cannot manage compressing alone and if nursing assistance is limited, the affected area can be wrapped w moist dressings, covered w dry dressings, left undisturbed for an h or 2, and repeat the process; debridement is less complete w these “wet-to-dry” dressings than w true compresses.

BATHING INSTRUCTIONS FOR DRY SKIN

Dry and itchy skin develops when the air is dry, particularly during the winter in heated homes, but also in the summer in air-conditioning. Dryness is worsened with excessive bathing, which removes natural oil the skin needs to retain moisture, particularly as people grow older and their skin makes less oil. The instructions here will help you bathe without depriving yourself of the protective oil you need. In addition, you will benefit during the winter from using a humidifier installed on the furnace (about $200) or a smaller room unit for your bedroom (about $35).

Follow this 2-STEP procedure, keeping the 2 steps separate because soap reduces the effectiveness of bath oil.

STEP 1: Soap Cleansing: Use soap *only* on the armpits, groin, buttocks, and feet, and shampoo your hair, if desired. Any soap brand is fine as long as you confine its use to these areas. If you have a ***shower/tub*** combination, use the shower for this soap step. If you have a ***tub*** only, let the soapy water run out, then refill the tub for the next step.

STEP 2: Oil Cleansing and Moisturizing: This step uses bath oils, which contain emulsifiers that clean but do not extract natural oils.

If using a ***shower***, sprinkle a capful of any nonperfumed bath oil (such as RoBathol Alpha-Keri, Lubath, Domol, or pharmacy generic) or a shower gel (such as Rainbath by Neutrogena) over your shoulders and use the oily water to rinse the rest of your body. **Note:** Mineral oil or baby oil will not mix with water and will not work.

If using a ***tub*** (often best for *severe* dryness), fill the tub with a few inches of comfortably warm, not hot, water. Add 1/2 ounce (usually about 2 capfuls) of any bath oil listed above. Use this oily water to sponge bathe.

Be careful when stepping out of the slippery tub or shower.

Pat your skin dry. Do not rub.

While your skin is still damp, apply a lubricating cream to trap moisture in the skin. Popular moisturizers include (alphabetically): Alpha Keri, Aquaphor, Complex-15, Curel, Eucerin, Lubriderm, Moisturel, Ultra Sensitive Skin Cream (J&J), Vanicream, or any other fragrance-free product.

We suggest that older persons troubled by dry skin bathe only *two* times a week with only touch-up washing on the other days.

Please come to see us again if these steps do not relieve your itching and dryness.

WET COMPRESSES

What is compressing?

"Compressing" is the application of a moist cloth to the skin, not the immersion of the skin in the container of solution. The purposes of using compresses are to cool and cleanse the skin and to reduce oozing and inflammation.

Method:

1. Find any soft, clean, lightweight cloth, such as thin kitchen towels, cotton handkerchiefs, washcloths, or torn pieces of cotton sheeting.
2. Mix fresh solution each time. Use 1 tsp of table salt *per pint* of cool or lukewarm tap water.
3. Moisten dressings in the solution and then wring them out so they are wet, but not dripping.
4. Apply by laying on or wrapping the inflamed area loosely with 2 or 3 layers of the moist dressings.
5. Leave the dressings in place for 2 to 3 minutes, then remove and rinse them in the soaking solution, squeeze out as before, and reapply. As the debris softens, gently wipe it away.

Do this for 20 minutes every _____ hours or _____ times a day.

After compressing: apply ________________________

At bedtime: apply ________________________

Compressing eventually leads to drying, which may be excessive if continued too long. When the skin is no longer inflamed or oozy, which usually takes 2 to 4 days, stop compressing, but continue to apply the medication as prescribed.

After compressing: pt may apply an antimicrobial preparation, ie, a topical antibiotic (see RX.9.), topical silver preparation (see ULCER —LEG, 25.2.a.(1).), or plain petrolatum; cover area w clean gauze pad or cotton sheet; if ulcer is oozing apply thick layer of ZnOx paste (see RX.4.), which absorbs oozing and makes next compressing easier.

RX.3. SHAKE LOTIONS

Purpose: So named because they must be shaken before use; cooling; soothing; use for acute itching conditions, ie, poison ivy dermatitis, sunburn, acute drug eruptions, viral exanthems, urticaria.

Preparations: Most common: calamine lotion (OTC), a suspension of 8% ZnOx and iron oxide (for color) w glycerin and calcium hydroxide in water; 0.5% menthol improves antipruritic properties; avoid using calamine lotion w diphenhydramine, ie, Caladryl, or topical anesthetics, as both are sensitizing.

Directions: As often as desired.

RX.4. PASTES

Purpose: Acute and subacute oozing dermatitis, ie, diaper dermatitis, intertrigo, pruritus ani, acute dyshidrotic eczema.

Mechanism: Pastes provide protection, absorb serous drainage, are somewhat occlusive.

Preparations: ZnOx, either paste or oint, Lassar's paste, is readily available OTC, generally 1 oz and 1 lb.

Directions: Apply paste thickly, like icing cake, w a butter knife or tongue blade; bid or reapplied if wiped off, as in the perianal area; residual paste can be removed easily w cotton balls or tissues moistened w mineral oil.

RX.5. CORTICOSTEROIDS, TOPICAL

Purpose: For inflammatory subacute or chronic skin disorders; low potency formulations of 0.5% and 1% HC are available OTC.

Mechanism: Anti-inflammatory.

Preparations: Numerous TCSs; most available in cr, oint, lotion, soln forms in several strengths; all are expensive ($5–$30/oz); triamcinolone (15–240 gm, Rx): the least expensive generic TCS of medium potency, is the TCS most often recommended in this book; on occasion, a TCS from a higher-potency group appears to work where a weaker one did not, but the most common reason that a TCS proves ineffective is that it is given for the wrong dx or in too small an amount.

Classes **of TCSs arranged by potency** (modified from Onion D, The little black book of primary care, 3rd ed, Blackwell Science, Malden, MA, 1999:125–127). Classes II and III, IV and V, and VI and VII have been combined to simplify the tables as potency differences within each of the combined classes are not clinically important.

Class		Generic
I	**ULTRA HIGH POTENCY**	
	Cormax cr/lotion/oint	Clobetasol propionate*
	Diprolene oint/AF cr/gel/lotion	Betamethasone diproprionate*
	Emboline	Clobetasol propionate*
	Psorcon oint	Diflorasone diacetate*
	Temovate cr/oint/scalp/E/gel	Clobetasol propionate*
	Ultravate cr/oint/soln	Halobetasol propionate
II–III	**HIGH POTENCY**	
	Aristocort oint 0.5%	Triamcinolone acetonide*
	Cyclocort cr/lotion/oint	Amcinonide
	Diprosone cr/oint	Betamethasone dipropionate*
	Elocon oint	Mometasone furoate
	Florone cr/oint	Diflorasone diacetate*
	Halog cr/oint/soln	Halcinonide
	Lidex cr/gel/oint/soln	Fluocinonide*
	Maxiflor cr/oint	Diflorasone diacetate*
	Maxivate cr/lotion/oint	Betamethasone dipropionate*
	Topicort cr/gel/oint	Desoximetasone*
	Valisone oint	Betamethasone valerate*
IV–V	**MEDIUM POTENCY**	
	Aristocort cr/oint 0.1%	Triamcinolone acetonide*
	Cordran cr/oint 0.05%	Flurandrenolide*

Class		Generic
	Cutivate cr/oint	Fluticasone propionate
	Diprosone lotion	Betamethasone dipropionate*
	Elocon cr/lotion	Mometasone furoate
	Kenalog cr/lotion/oint 0.1%	Triamcinolone acetonide*
	Locoid cr/oint	Hydrocortisone butyrate
	Pandel cr	Hydrocortisone buteprate
	Synalar cr/oint 0.025%	Fluocinolone acetonide*
	Topicort LP cr 0.05%	Desoximetasone
	Tridesilon oint 0.05%	Desonide*
	Valisone cr/lotion	Betamethasone valerate*
	Westcort cr/oint	Hydrocortisone valerate*
VI–VII	**LOW POTENCY**	
	Aclovate cr/oint	Alclometasone dipropionate
	Aristocort cr/oint 0.025%	Triamcinolone acetonide*
	DesOwen cr/lotion/oint	Desonide*
	Hytone cr/lotion/oint 1.0%–2.5%	Hydrocortisone*
	Kenalog cr/lotion 0.025%	Triamcinolone acetonide*
	Locoid soln	Hydrocortisone butyrate
	Locortan cr	Flumethasone pivalate
	Pramosone cr/lotion/oint 1.0%–2.5%	Hydrocortisone/Pramoxine
	Synalar cr 0.01%/soln	Fluocinolone acetonide*
	Tridesilon cr	Desonide*
	others containing dexamethasone, flumethasone, prednisolone, or methylprednisolone	

** Indicates available size of 120 gm or more, usually 225 and 450 gm; all TCSs are available in at least 2 or 3 of the following sizes: 15, 30, 45, 60 gm. Do not try to remember the size of the tube, just order an amount that seems appropriate and let the pharmacist dispense an amount closest to the size you ordered.*

% of active steroid is given only if the product comes in >1 strength.

Choice of Vehicle:

- *Cream*: acute and subacute dermatitis w redness or oozing.
- *Ointment*: chronic dermatitis w scale and itching; absorption of TCS from oint > cr; spreads further than cr but feels greasy.
- *Solution, lotion, gel*: best in hairy skin, intertriginous regions, ear canals.

Directions: Do not underestimate amount required; 1 oz is needed to cover the entire body surface once; eg: to estimate amount needed to rx both thighs and legs (about 1/3 total skin surface) tid for 3 wk = 30 gm × 0.33 × 3×/d × 21 d = 630 gm (1.5 lb), an amount far more than most practitioners dispense; volume of TCS may be ↓ if applied when skin is slightly damp, which allows thinner spreading, and by restricting its use to inflamed parts only; use a moisturizer (see RX.1.) elsewhere, since pts often use TCS for lubrication unless instructed otherwise; consider using TCS w plastic wrap occlusion at bedtime (see RX.6.).

Warnings: Potent TCSs may mask si of underlying skin infections, contact allergies, and even cutaneous lymphoma; local complications following long use of high- or intermediate-potency TCSs include persistent erythema and telangiectasias, acneiform eruptions, interference w healing, induction of atrophic striae, and easy bruising; glaucoma and cataracts have developed from use of TCS about the eyes; absorption of TCS occurs, but systemic effects are difficult to demonstrate in adults unless steroids are occluded w plastic film applied over 1/2 the body; systemic effects from absorbed TCS include ↑ BP, ↑ glucose intolerance in DM, glaucoma, salt retention, and ↓ pituitary-adrenal responsiveness; growth retardation and hypertension have been reported in small children after use of potent TCS, even w/o occlusion.

RX.6. TOPICAL CORTICOSTEROIDS (TCSs) WITH OCCLUSION

Purpose: Use TCSs w occlusion for chronic, nonoozy dermatitis confined to small areas, ie, plaques of psoriasis on elbows and knees, lichen simplex chronicus on ankle or nape, or chronic hand dermatitis; overnight occlusion often is more effective and certainly is less expensive than several applications of CSs w/o occlusion during the d.

Mechanism: Effectiveness of TCS is ↑ when covered w occlusive plastic film or tape; med is held in place better; hydration of horny layer improves absorption.

Preparations: Use cr > oint as cr is less likely to induce miliaria and folliculitis; an occlusive tape w TCS incorporated in a waterproof, transparent adhesive (Cordran tape, 60/200 cm, Rx, $$) is convenient for use in small areas.

Directions: Vary form and type of plastic occlusion according to site: thin plastic paint gloves or small kitchen food storage bags for hands; kitchen plastic wrap for larger areas, ie, trunk or legs; keep plastic film in place w elastic or gauze bandages or clothing, ie, underwear, cotton gloves, or cutdown panty hose, rather than tape, which may induce skin irritation.

Warnings: See RX.5.

RX.7. INTRALESIONAL CORTICOSTEROIDS

Purpose: Shrink inflamed acne cysts; reduce hypertrophic scars and keloids; other disorders sometimes treated w injections: lichen simplex chronicus, alopecia areata, granuloma annulare, psoriasis, DLE.

Mechanism: Anti-inflammatory; ↓ fibroblast proliferation.

Preparations: Triamcinolone acetonide (Kenalog, 10 mg/mL) is most widely used; material is crystalline, dissolves slowly, and benefits accrue over wks; 10 mg/mL can induce atrophy (see Warnings).

Directions: Use IL CS at full-strength (10 mg/mL) only for scar reduction; for all other applications: dilute steroid to about 2.5–3.5 mg/mL to lessen skin atrophy: 1 mL of 10 mg/mL triamcinolone given less frequently than q 3 wk does not induce adrenal suppression; inject material within lesion or just below it, rather than into sc tissue to prevent wide dispersal of med; a hand-operated air injection gun is available (Dermojet, Medijet), causes less pain, disperses CS more widely than syringe and needle.

Warnings: Local: atrophy or dimpling; ↓ pigment; rarely skin necrosis; dimpling usually resolves in 6–12 mo.

RX.8. SYSTEMIC CORTICOSTEROIDS

Purpose: *Short term*: acute poison ivy dermatitis, postscabies rx, acute atopic dermatitis, acute dyshidrotic eczema; avoid if cause of rash is unclear or as a means to suppress drug rxn w/o dc of med; *long term*: SLE, pemphigus generally require specialty consultation.

PREDNISONE SCHEDULE

Directions:

☐ Take the tablets divided into 2 or 3 doses at meal times OR
☐ Take the tablets all at one time in the early morning with breakfast.

Take _____ each day for _____days
Then _____ each day for _____days
Then _____ each day for _____days
Then _____ each day for _____days
Then _____ each day for _____days

Sun	Mon	Tue	Wed	Thu	Fri	Sat

Preparations: Most widely used: prednisone: inexpensive, absorbed quickly and completely, 2-h half-life.

Directions: Depends on purpose; *acute, self-limited* eruption in adult, ie, poison ivy dermatitis: 40 mg/d prednisone; maintain dose until eruption is noticeably improved (few d); taper by about a tab q few d, depending on response; *chronic* disorder, ie, pemphigus, sarcoid, SLE: may be controlled by a single early AM dose given on alternate d; long-term complications (see Warnings) are reduced.

Warnings: Complications of long-term systemic CSs are numerous and potentially serious: salt retention w edema, high BP, glucose intolerance, osteoporosis, pituitary-adrenal suppression, cataract formation, ↑ susceptibility to infection; alternative-d rx mitigates all except cataract formation; obtain a PPD before starting long-term rx; consider alendronate sodium (Fosamax 5 mg qd or 35 mg q week) (Nejm 1998;339:292) to prevent osteoporosis.

RX

RX.9. ANTIBIOTICS, TOPICAL

Purpose: Overused; efficacy not well documented; superficial bacterial infections usually respond as well to simple cleansing w soap/water; deep infections do not respond to topical antibiotics; use for limited impetigo, intranasal suppression of carrier state, occas superficial bacterial infections, occas chronic leg ulcers; widely used to rx acne vulgaris (see FACE, 6.1.a.).

Preparations: Numerous OTC preparations contain bacitracin, polymyxin, neomycin, or combinations; mupirocin (Bactroban, $$) used for staphylococcal and streptococcal impetigo (see FACE, 6.6.a.) and nasal carrier state (see FACE, 6.6.a.); numerous topical *acne* preparations (see FACE, 6.1.a.); *burns*: silver sulfadiazine cr (Silvadene) or mafenide acetate cr (Sulfamylon); *rosacea*: topical metronidazole (see FACE, 6.1.c.); when used: apply 3–6 ×/d.

Warnings: Resistance develops quickly; potential to sensitize, esp neomycin; inflammation around chronic leg ulcer that is being treated w topical antibiotics may be contact dermatitis, not infection; rare cases of bone marrow suppression w topical chloramphenicol.

RX.10. ANTIFUNGAL AGENTS, TOPICAL

Purpose: Topical rx of common superficial fungal infections: *dermatophytes*: *Trichophyton* species, *Microsporum* species, *Epidermophyton* species; or *yeast*: mostly *Candida albicans*; most involve warm moist areas, ie, feet, groin; for details, see Index for area of body involved; topical agents are not sufficient for deep-seated or widespread superficial fungal infections, tinea capitis, fungal infections in immunosuppressed hosts, nail fungal infections.

Mechanism: Most inhibit synthesis of ergosterol, essential fungal cell wall component; fungistatic.

Preparations:

- Topical *broad-spectrum* antifungal preparations, effective against *both dermatophytes and yeast*, include, alphabetically: butenafine (Mentax, Rx), ciclopirox (Loprox, Rx), clotrimazole (Lotrimin, Mycelex, OTC), econazole (Spectazole, Rx), miconazole (Monistat-Derm, Rx; Micatin, OTC), naftifine (Naftin, Rx), oxiconazole (Oxistat, Rx) (Derm Clin 1992;10:799).
- Topical agents effective for *dermatophytes, but not Candida*, include terbinafine (Lamasil, OTC), tolnaftate (Tinactin, OTC).
- Topical agents effective for *Candida, but not dermatophytes*, include nystatin (rx), amphotericin B (Fungizone, rx); amphotericin B and, to a lesser extent, nystatin, have been supplanted by the *broad-spectrum* antifungal agents listed above.

Directions: Apply sparingly bid; yeast infections in diaper area: re-rx w each diaper change; add measures to ↓ moisture, ie, cotton underclothing and socks, open shoes, liberal use of talcum powder, and, if moist, ZnOx paste.

Warning:

- Clearing of fungal infections is slow; tell pts to expect to use topical rx for 1 wk before responding fully.
- Avoid combinations w TCS (ie, Lotrisone), which may hide an underlying allergic or irritant dermatitis and allow fungus infection to worsen while suppressing assoc inflammation; if fungal infection is suspected, consider a trial w broad-spectrum antifungal agent above.

RX.11. ANTIFUNGAL AGENTS, SYSTEMIC

Purpose: Systemic rx of some superficial fungal infections: tinea capitis, onychomycosis, tinea corporis too extensive for topical rx, some candidal infections, any resistant superficial fungal infection in immunocompromised pts; rx of systemic fungal infections is not discussed.

Preparations:

- *Griseofulvin*: Microsized; 250–500-mg tab/cap (Fulvicin-U/F, Grifulvin-V, Grisactin, Rx, $$); pediatric suspension (125 mg/tsp, Rx, $$).
- *Ketoconazole* (Nizoral, Rx, $$): 200-mg tab.
- *Itraconazole* (Sporanox, Rx, $$$): 100-mg cap; Sporanox oral soln: 10 mg/mL (150 mL).
- *Terbinafine* (Lamasil, Rx, $$$): 250-mg tab.
- *Fluconazole* (Diflucan, Rx, $$$$): 50-, 100-, 150-, 200-mg tab; 150-mg tab for vaginal *Candida*; oral suspension: 10 and 40 mg/mL (35 mL).

Indications:

- *Griseofulvin*: some superficial dermatophytes; *not* tinea versicolor, onychomycosis, candidal infection; mainly now used for tinea capitis in children.
- *Ketoconazole*: not recommended for onychomycosis as safer drugs are available; shampoo usually sufficient for tinea versicolor but systemic use may be considered (see BODY, 3.1.h.); mucocutaneous candidal infection; *Pityrosporum* folliculitis (see BODY, 3.1.g.); FDA approved for use in candidal infection, certain systemic fungal infections, and severe cutaneous dermatophyte infections not responsive to topical rx or griseofulvin.
- *Itraconazole*: onychomycosis, extensive tinea corporis, tinea capitis, *Pityrosporum* folliculitis, tinea versicolor; oral soln for oral and/or esophageal candidiasis; FDA approved for use in blastomycosis, histoplasmosis, aspergillosis, onychomycosis.
- *Terbinafine*: onychomycosis not candidal infection; extensive tinea corporis; tinea capitis.
- *Fluconazole*: mucocutaneous candidal infection, candidal onychomycosis.

Directions:

- *Griseofulvin*: dose: children w tinea capitis: 15–20 mg/kg/d × 2 mo; most failures to respond are due to too low a dose;

RX

this dose is > dose used in past because of ↑ drug resistance; absorption ↑ w fatty meal or milk.

- *Ketoconazole*: 1–2 tab qd, depending on condition, ie, 1–2 wk for candidal infection; absorption ↑ w acidic carbonated beverage.
- *Itraconazole*: *onychomycosis*: pulse-dose w 2 cap bid for 1 wk, then do not rx for 3 wk; repeat for another pulse for fingernail involvement (total of 2 pulses); pulse rx not FDA approved for toenails; use 2 cap qd × 12 wks for toenail involvement; absorption ↑ if taken w full meal; *oral and/or esophageal candidiasis*: oral soln: 10 mL bid, vigorously swished in mouth for several sec and then swallowed.
- *Terbinafine*: fingernail onychomycosis: 1 tab qd × 6 wk; toenail onychomycosis: 1 tab qd × 12 wk; drug may be taken w or w/o food.
- *Fluconazole*: 2 × 100-mg tab on 1st d, then qd until resolution (few d to 2 wk, depending on situation); onychomycosis: nonstandard usage of 100-mg tab/wk for 9–12 mo; may be taken w or w/o food but avoid antacids.

Warnings:

- *Griseofulvin*: metabolized by liver; *side effects*: GI upset, headaches; *do not use:* during pregnancy, men advised to wait 6 mo before fathering a child, liver failure, porphyria; *interactions*: warfarin (Coumadin); barbiturates; ROH; possibly ↓ bcp effectiveness; *lab*: abn are rare; obtain CBC if high dose for long time as ↓ wbc has been reported.
- *Ketoconazole*: metabolized by liver, cytochrome P450; *side effects*: 2%–5% get ↑ liver enzymes; rare serious hepatotoxicity but some fatal; *do not use in* pregnancy, breast-feeding, pts w known liver disease; *interactions*: antacid ↓ absorption, AZT, calcium-channel blockers, cholesterol-lowering agents, cimetidine ↓ absorption, cisapride, coumarin, cyclosporine, digoxin, DM oral agents, digoxin, isoniazid, midazolam (triazolam, diazepam), phenytoin, ROH (disulfiram-like rxn), quinidine, rifampin; *lab*: follow LFTs, esp if pt taking long term; transient minor ↑ is common.
- *Itraconazole*: metabolized by liver; *side effects*: reversible abn liver enzymes; *do not use in*: pregnancy, breast-feeding, pts w known liver disease; *interactions*: benzodiazepines (midazolam, triazolam, diazepam), buspirone, busulfan, calcium-channel blockers,

cholesterol-lowering agents, cimetidine ↓ absorption, cisapride, coumarin, cyclosporine, digoxin, DM oral agents, digoxin, HIV protease inhibitors, isoniazid, phenytoin, quinidine, rifampin (J Am Acad Derm 1999;41:237; J Am Acad Derm 1997;37:765.); *lab*: follow LFTs, esp if pt taking long term; transient minor ↑ is common; *FDA Public Health Advisory*, May, 2001: rare risk of congestive heart failure (58 cases) and death (13 cases) and rare risk of liver failure (24 cases) and death (11 cases).

- *Terbinafine*: metabolized by liver; *side effects*: rare ↑ liver enzymes; ↓ wbc; *do not use in*: pregnancy, breast-feeding; *interactions*: terbinafine < ketoconazole or itraconazole; caffeine; cimetidine; cyclosporine; rifampin; theophylline (J Am Acad Derm 1999;41:237); *lab*: none required in absence of known liver disease but up to 4% abn LFTs have been reported (Br J Derm 1992;126:36) as has liver failure (Nejm 1999;340:1293); *FDA Public Health Advisory*, May, 2001: rare risk of liver failure (16 cases) and death (11 cases).
- *Fluconazole*: cleared unchanged by kidneys; *side effects*: rare ↑ liver enzymes, ↓ wbc; *do not use in*: pregnancy, breast-feeding; *interactions*: tricyclic antidepressants, AZT, benzodiazepines (midazolam, triazolam, diazepam), cimetidine, cisapride, coumarin, cyclosporine, DM oral agents, phenytoin, rifampin, theophylline, thiazides (J Am Acad Derm 1999;41:237); *lab*: none required in absence of known liver or kidney disease.

RX.12. ANTIHISTAMINES, SYSTEMIC

Purpose: Control of allergic disorders mediated by histamine, esp urticaria, angioedema, allergic rhinitis; suppress non-histamine-induced itching because of sedating side effects (J Am Acad Derm 1991;25:176).

Mechanism: Antihistamines occupy histamine receptor sites on cell membranes of mast cells, basophils, platelets, and some gastric and nerve endings, competing and interfering w actions of histamine; 2 classes: classic H1 blockers and H2 blockers, which also decrease gastric acid secretion; 1st-generation H1 blockers: onset of action within 30 min, peak action is 2 h, metabolism mainly by liver; 2nd-generation, low-sedating H1 blockers: onset of action within 2 h, effects last up to 1 d, metabolism variable (see below).

Preparations: 1st-generation H1 antihistamines comprise 6 chemical classes; some pts respond better to 1 class than another, but if antihistamines from 2 classes used at adequate dosage are ineffective, changing to another usually is futile; within each class some are more sedating than others.

1ST-GENERATION H1 BLOCKERS (SOME EXAMPLES)

1. Alkylamine class	1. Chlorpheniramine maleate (Chlor-Trimeton, 4/8/12 mg, OTC); brompheniramine (Dimetane, 4/8/12 mg, OTC)
2. Aminoalkyl ether class	2. Diphenhydramine (generic or Benadryl, 25 mg, OTC; 50 mg, rx), clemastine (Tavist, 1.3/2.7 mg, OTC)
3. Ethylenediamine class	3. Tripelennamine (PBZ, 25/50/100 mg, rx)
4. Phenothiazine class	4. Promethazine (generic or Phenergan, 12.5/25/50 mg, rx); trimeprazine tartrate (Temaril, 2.5 mg, rx)
5. Piperidine class	5. Cyproheptadine (Periactin tabs, 4 mg, or syrup, 2 mg/5 mL, rx)
6. Piperazine class	6. Hydroxyzine (generic, Atarax or Vistaril, 10/25/50/100 mg or syrup, 10/25 mg/mL, rx)

2ND-GENERATION H1 BLOCKERS

Low sedating and less anticholinergic side effects; cetirizine (Zyrtec, 5/10 mg, rx), fexofenadine (Allegra, rx), loratadine (Claritin, rx) (Derm Clin 1993;11:87).

Directions: Start antihistamines at low or moderate dosage; ↑ dose until sufficient improvement occurs or troublesome side effects develop; duration of action is 3–6 h, except for newer long-acting forms; w 1st-generation H1 blockers: start w tid or qid; if pruritus is predominantly in evening or if pt works or drives during d, prescribe for use at dinner or hs.

Warnings: Sedation, the most common side effect, usually lessens within few d of use; avoid antihistamines in pregnancy and breast-feeding; older persons: watch for CNS side effects: confusion, dizziness, syncope; watch for anticholinergic effects: urinary retention, dry mouth, blurred vision; do not use 1st-generation antihistamines if pts work around machinery or drive; warn about additive depressive effects of ROH and barbiturates; antihistamines may induce hyperactivity paradoxically in children; w the exception of topical doxepin (Zonalon, 30/45 gm, Rx), which can ↓ itch in atopic dermatitis (J Am Acad Derm 1994;31:613); topical antihistamines are only minimally effective; *2nd-generation antihistamines*: cetirizine may be used w liver and renal disease; fexofenadine may be used w liver but not renal disease; loratadine may be used w renal disease but not liver disease.

H2 BLOCKERS

Cimetidine, ranitidine, famotidine, nizatidine; sometimes used in combination w H1 blockers for urticaria and angioedema but not effective when used alone.

Warnings: Although generally considered safe, H2 blockers may cause mental confusion, esp in elderly; headache; dizziness; drowsiness; GI complaints; rare, even fatal, ↓ wbc.

RX.13. ANTIPARASITE MEDICATIONS

Purpose: Eradicate pediculosis capitis (scalp), pediculosis cruris (groin), pediculosis corporis (body), scabies.

Preparations: Permethrin 5% dermal cream (Elimite, or Acticin, Rx): safe and effective; may be used in children and pregnancy; for pediculosis and scabies; permethrin cr rinse (Nix, OTC): pediculosis capitis and cruris but not scabies as concentration is too low; γ-benzene hexachloride lotion or shampoo (lindane, Kwell, Rx): not for use in children or pregnant/nursing women because of potential neurotoxicity (Arch Derm 1996:132:901); effective for pediculosis and scabies; ivermectin (Stromectol, 3 and 6 mg, Merck, Rx, $$): po, 200 μg/kg (Nejm 1995;333:26; Arch Derm 1999;135:651); ivermectin appears to be safe, even in elderly pts (Arch Derm 1999;135:352; Lancet 1997;350:215).

Directions: For details of rx for pediculosis pubis, see GROIN RASH, 10.5.a.; for pediculosis capitis, see SCALP, 24.5.a.; and for scabies, see BODY, 3.1.e.; fomites (clothing, bed linen, furniture) may be contaminated; esp w scabies and pediculosis corporis; fomites must be disinfected by washing and dried on hot cycle; or put in clothes dryer for 20 min on hot cycle; or hot iron, esp over clothing seams; or dry-cleaning.

RX.14. TAR

Purpose: Dermatologists sometimes still use tar preparations for resistant chronic, itchy, and scaly disorders, ie, chronic eczematous dermatitis, seborrheic dermatitis, psoriasis; usually used after failure of TCSs or as an adjuvant; as it is unlikely that the PCP will utilize tar preparations when very little is used even by dermatologists, no further discussion on preparations or specific directions will be provided except in certain special cases in the text.

RX.15. ULTRAVIOLET (UV) LIGHT

Purpose: Most uses: rx of psoriasis; vitiligo; CTCL; some pts w atopic dermatitis; lichen planus; granuloma annulare; urticaria; no longer used for acne because it is potentially carcinogenic and is only minimally and temporarily effective.

Equipment: UV light units are available in at least 2 wavelength ranges:

- UVB: short wave; UV lights sold in drug and department stores as sun lamps emit mostly UVB; UVB causes sunburning and most of the long-term solar damage, esp fine wrinkling, freckling, most skin cancers; UVB has been effective to rx pruritus of renal and liver failure and HIV pruritus (see ITCH, 16.1.a.–16.2.e.).
- UVA: long wave; emitted by special medical units; also the predominant UV spectrum in commercial suntan centers; tanning >> burning.
- PUVA: UVA plus topical or oral psoralen, a drug that binds to DNA and sensitizes it to UVA; PUVA penetrates more deeply than UVB and has major medical uses; rx is provided in specialized centers and in some dermatologists' offices.

Warnings: *Skin cancers*: ↑ risk of SCC (Arch Derm 1999;134:1582), esp scrotal skin cancer (Nejm 1990;322:1093); 4 fold ↑ risk of melanoma in pts beginning 15 yr after first exposure to PUVA and who have had >200 treatments (Jaad 2001;44:755); ↑ benign keratoses; ↑ skin aging; *eye damage*: follow stringent guidelines to protect eyes, esp w protective eye shields and regular eye exams but no case of cataracts and retinal damage has been proven to be due to PUVA.

RX.16. SUNSCREEN AGENTS, TOPICAL

Purpose: Protection from acute and chronic damaging effects of UV radiation; *acute effects*: caused by burning short wavelengths, UVB (290–320 nm); *chronic effects*: caused by chronic exposure to UVB and, to a lesser extent, longer-wavelength UVA tanning rays (320–400 nm); leads to fine wrinkling, degenerative elastosis, actinic keratoses, skin cancers; *UVA effects*: most light-induced drug rxns, solar urticaria, porphyria rxns, polymorphic light eruptions; tolerance to UV light depends on amount of melanin present: light-complexioned, redheaded, blue-eyed Celtic people burn, rather than tan, and develop acute and chronic rxns, while darker-complexioned or black people tan, rarely develop skin cancers, and develop less sun-induced wrinkling (J Am Acad Derm 1990;22:1).

Preparations: Most important elements of sun protection: 1st: protective clothing, ie, hat, shirt, and 2nd: avoidance of sun between 10 AM and 3 PM; the 3rd element: apply sunscreen; clouds and beach umbrella reduce radiation by only about half and do not prevent severe sunburns; sun protective factor (SPF): the multiple by which the product extends period of exposure to reach rxn that would have taken place w/o sunscreen; eg, if sunburn would have developed from a 30-min exposure, a sunscreen w SPF of 15 extends that time to 7.5 h (30 m × 15); an SPF of 15 is adequate and anything > 30 is probably marketing hype; most sunscreens, esp those containing only PABA, are less effective in blocking UVA than UVB, but newer "broad-spectrum" sunscreens, containing avobenzone (Parsol 1789), benzophenone, or padimate-O have partial UVA-blocking properties; for more complete protection, use sunscreens that also contain opaque blockers, ie, titanium dioxide or ZnOx (Clinique Continuous Coverage, RVPaque) (Jaad 2001;44:505).

Directions: Apply sunscreens 1–2 h before exposure to allow time for absorption into horny layer; all sunscreens are soluble and are washed away by sweating or swimming, although some products are more resistant than others; advise pts to follow package label directions for reapplications; some stain white fabrics; may cause allergic contact dermatitis.

RX.17. DESICCATION AND CURETTAGE (D&C)

Purpose: Alternative to surgical excision for destruction of benign or superficial malignant lesions; *most suitable*: verrucae, seborrheic keratoses, molluscum contagiosum, actinic keratosis, BCE; *not suitable*: SCC, melanoma, any nodule of uncertain pathology w/o prior bx.

Equipment:

- Curette: loop-shaped cutting edge placed at tip of a handle; size varies, but 4-mm diameter is most useful; available in stainless steel or disposable (Acuderm, Ft. Lauderdale, FL; 954.733.6935).
- *Electrosurgical unit*: delivers high-frequency alternating current that generates heat as current passes through electrically resistant skin; the electrode does not itself become hot; numerous manufacturers ($1000–$2000).

Method: *Cleanse* area w nonalcoholic antiseptic, ie, chlorhexidine (Hibiclens) or iodophor (Betadine or povidone); avoid ROH, which may be ignited by the electrosurgical unit; *inject* local anesthetic (J Am Acad Derm 1988;19:599); *bx* by TSR or punch (see DX.7.) prior to D&C provides a better specimen for pathologic exam than shredded curettements; *curettage* should be vigorous so that it extends down to resistant and gritty-feeling normal tissue; if lesion is thought to be benign and superficial, ie, actinic keratosis or seborrheic keratosis (J Am Acad Derm 1986;15:697): lightly *desiccate* the base so as not to deeply scar; for BCEs: desiccate extensively until wound retracts slightly; repeat D&C once or twice for suspected malignant lesions; leave the final desiccated wound open; advise saline *compresses* for 20 min tid–qid for 1st few d until oozing stops and a dry crust forms; petroleum jelly may be used until scab comes off; final result after 2–4 mo: usually is a slightly depressed, light-colored, cosmetically acceptable scar; cure rate in experienced hands for superficial skin cancers is similar to that of surgical excision (about 95%); *f/u* at intervals for 2 yr.

Warnings: Electrosurgery is hazardous in pts w pacemakers; infection after D&C is uncommon.

RX.18. CRYOSURGERY

Purpose: To destroy benign growths, ie, warts, seborrheic keratoses; superficial premalignant or malignant growths, ie, actinic keratoses, Bowen's disease, superficial BCEs; damage is restricted to superficial levels of skin because rich blood supply of dermis reduces penetration of freezing (J Am Acad Derm 1991;24:1002).

Equipment: LN2 (–196°C) is the standard freezing agent because it is readily available and not inflammable; however, it must be stored in a large Dewar flask, costing about $1000; replenishing because of evaporation and normal use costs about $50/mo; LN2 may be applied w a cotton applicator or GI swab, or sprayed w insulated cryosurgical canisters costing about $500; if using a small Thermos to hold LN2, provide a vent hole in cap to relieve pressure from evaporating gas.

Directions: The large cotton end of a GI swab holds sufficient LN2 to complete most freezings w 1 application; touch tip, twisted and shaped to a point slightly smaller than lesion, just to lesion, not to normal surrounding skin; freeze until a freeze zone extends beyond lesion; this takes 10–30 sec; freezing is painful, but local anesthesia is not necessary or practical; deeper freezing and greater destruction can be accomplished w a second freezing performed immediately after thawing of the first; LN2 cryotherapy is usually too painful to be used in small children; see alternative therapy for warts in small children in HANDS, 14.1.a.

- Aftercare: area frozen will be painful that d; offer ASA; dressings or special care are not needed; a blister, sometimes hemorrhagic, often forms during the next few d; if uncomfortable, pt may drain by puncturing it w a clean pin or razor blade; re-examine site 3–5 wk later and re-rx if persistent; cure rate for each rx is 50%–80%.

Warnings: *Skin cancer*: determining completeness of destruction is difficult because no tissue margins were determined (J Am Acad Derm 1991;24:653); specialists may use a tissue temperature probe inserted below the cancer; *wart on finger*: avoid damaging the digital nerve, located on each side of finger under the end of crease of skin seen when finger is flexed (BMJ 1985;290:188).

RX.19. 5-FLUOROURACIL (5-FU)

Purpose: To destroy actinic keratoses, superficial BCEs, Bowen's disease, and occas, resistant verrucae; 5-FU interferes w DNA synthesis by inhibiting thymidylate synthetase activity; 5-FU appears to select and destroy early lesions while leaving normal skin intact.

Preparations: Cr and soln forms are available (Carac cr, 0.5%, 30 gm; Efudex cr 5%, 25 gm, and soln 2% and 5%, 10 mL, and Fluoroplex cr 1%, 30 gm, and soln 1%, 30 mL, Rx, $$); percentage used appears to make little difference in outcome; for face, use either cr or soln; for elsewhere, add tretinoin cr 0.05%–0.1% (generic, 20/45 gm, Rx) concomitantly to improve penetration.

Directions: Pt applies 5-FU bid w fingertip; protection of fingertip w plastic glove or cotton usually not necessary unless fingertip becomes irritated; avoid eyes and mucosae; expect irritation, redness, crusting within 1–2 wk; continue applications for additional 1–2 wk until superficial erosions appear; generally f/u q 2 wk to determine depth of penetration and need to continue rx; after rxn has reached its peak and 5-FU has been dc'd: prescribe class II–III TCS oint qid × 1 wk.

Warnings: Occas contact allergy w edema, blisters, itching, esp w 2nd or later course of rx; bx any lesion still present after course of 5-FU; actinic keratoses lesions tend to reappear at 2 yr.

Index

Page numbers followed by *f* refer to figures; those followed by *t* refer to tables.